Textbook of
ILIZAROV SURGICAL TECHNIQUES
Bone Correction and Lengthening

Textbook of
ILIZAROV SURGICAL TECHNIQUES
Bone Correction and Lengthening

VLADIMIR GOLYAKHOVSKY MD, PhD, DSc
Attending Physician
New York University Hospital for Joint Diseases Orthopaedic Institute
Clinical Associate Professor of Orthopaedic Surgery
New York University School of Medicine
New York, NY 10003
Formerly Professor and Chairman of Orthopaedics and Traumatology
Moscow Institute of Medicine and Dentistry
Moscow, Russia

VICTOR H FRANKEL MD, PhD
President Emeritus
New York University Hospital for Joint Diseases Orthopaedic Institute
Professor of Orthopaedic Surgery
New York University School of Medicine
New York, NY

Illustrations and Photos by VLADIMIR GOLYAKHOVSKY

JAYPEE

JAYPEE BROTHERS MEDICAL PUBLISHERS
The Health Sciences Publisher
New Delhi | London

Jaypee Brothers Medical Publishers (P) Ltd

Headquarters
EMCA House
23/23B Ansari Road, Daryaganj
New Delhi 110 002, India
Landline: +91-11-23272143, +91-11-23272703
+91-11-23282021, +91-11-23245672
E-mail: jaypee@jaypeebrothers.com

Corporate Office
4838/24, Ansari Road, Daryaganj
New Delhi 110 002, India
Phone: +91-11-43574357
Fax: +91-11-43574314
E-mail: jaypee@jaypeebrothers.com

Overseas Office
J.P. Medical Ltd.
83, Victoria Street, London
SW1H 0HW (UK)
Phone: +44-20 3170 8910
E-mail: info@jpmedpub.com

EU GPSR Authorised Representative
Logos Europe, 9 rue Nicolas Poussin
17000, La Rochelle, France
Phone: +33 (0) 6 67 93 73 78
E-mail: contact@logoseurope.eu

Website: www.jaypeebrothers.com
Website: www.jaypeedigital.com

Textbook of Ilizarov Surgical Techniques: Bone Correction and Lengthening

First Edition: 2010

Reprint: **2026**

ISBN: 978-81-8448-933-0

Printed in India

To the memory of
Professor Gavriil Abramovich Ilizarov

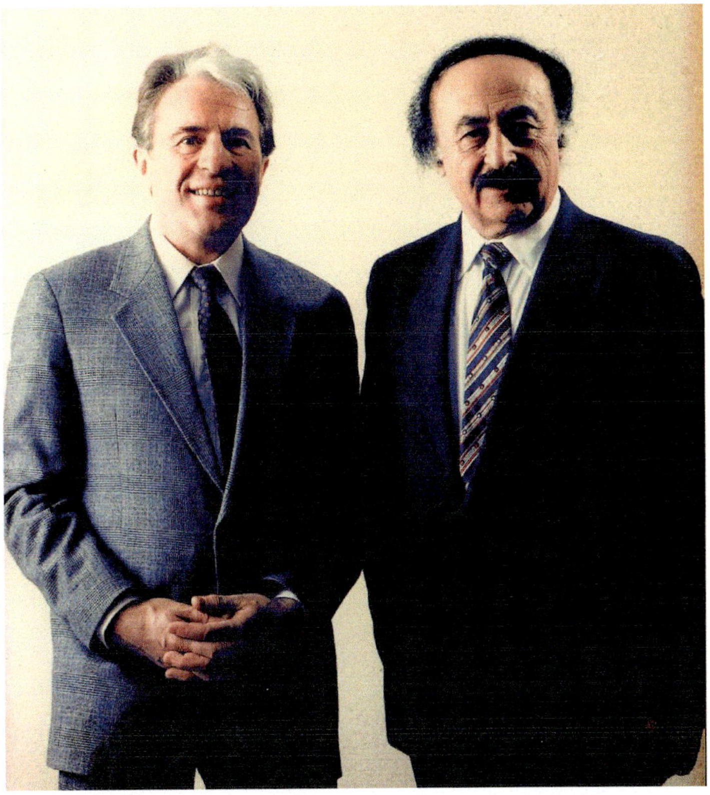

Portrait of Dr Ilizarov (Right) with the author
Dr Vladimir Golyakhovsky, 1988, New York

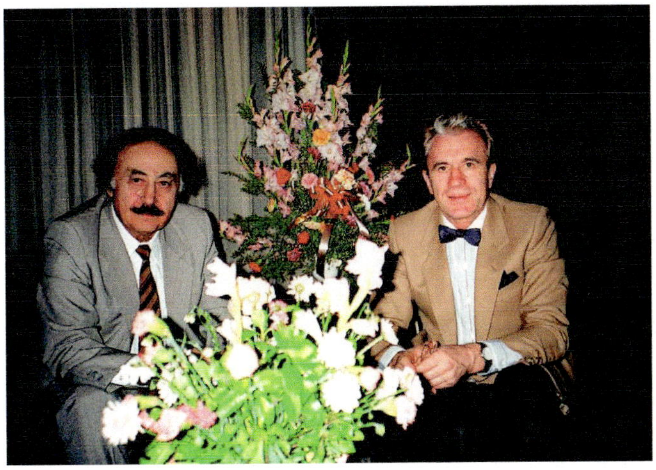

Sant Yago, Chily

Preface

Seventeen years passed since publication, in1993, the "Operative Manual of Ilizarov Techniques", a richly illustrated first American book about the Ilizarov techniques and methods. Utilizing the techniques developed by him, a circular external fixator, a Russian Doctor Gavriil Ilizarov, in 1950-1960s introduced principally new techniques for treatment bone fractures and deformities. With this innovation, he opened a new chapter in the subject of the whole orthopedic surgery—the minimally invasive methods of bone deformities correction. For many years, his name and work were not known in the Western countries because the communist Soviet Russia was isolated behind the so-called "Iron Curtain". With the fall of communism, in 1990s, the great interest and enthusiasm developed toward the Ilizarov work among European and American orthopedic communities. The "Operative Manual" was written at that time with the purpose to instruct the surgeons how to assemble and apply the configurations of a circular fixator for the bone correction and lengthening. In several years there were new editions of this book translated and published in Brazil and Russia. In this way the "Operative Manual" has served thousands of orthopedic surgeons as a guide to master Ilizarov's methods.

In the past 17 years the professional market of the books and articles on the subject of the Ilizarov methods had a plenitude of new ideas, and the "Operative Manual" was almost forgotten. In 2009, the Indian publisher company "Jaypee Brothers Medical Publishers", based in New Delhi, came across the "Operative Manual", which was not available any more. The Indian publisher discovered it and considered a classic book and offered to one of the authors (Vladimir Golyakhovsky) to have a new edition with revision of the recent advances happened during last several years. Indeed, there are new modifications of the Ilizarov fixator and the Ilizarov techniques developed in Italy, Germany, the US, and other countries. The author gladly agreed to have a new Indian edition, and to include the recent developments, together with the new illustrations, in the book. Authors also offered to the Publisher to write new chapters:

- Gavriil Abramovich Ilizarov—The Man, The Creator, The Teacher
- Biomechanics of the Ilizarov external fixator
- Ilizarov frame assemblage
- Biomechanics of the Ilizarov method
- Biomechanic considerations for the fracture treatment
- Basics of the method of distraction osteogenesis
- Basics of the method of compression osteogenesis
- Criteria of bone healing and fixator removal.

These chapters, composed together, have a purpose to serve as an introduction for the description of the Ilizarov techniques and methods. Some of these materials were scattered in the chapters of "Operative manual" but the author considers expedient for the reader to get to know these particular subjects before learning how to assemble and use the fixator.

The last chapter of the book "The New Modifications of the Ilizarov Technique" reflects the development of new innovations which were developed since circulation of the original Ilizarov's ideas in orthopedic community around the world. The apparent simplicity and clarity of the Ilizarov technique provoked many orthopedic surgeons to offer their own modifications, as it always happened to the great inventions. Some of the new modifications are based on advanced technology of new materials for fixator parts, there are introductions of aluminum rings, and carbon rings, and titanium rods. Some modifications consist of small technical innovations. All these modifications are governed by the principles discovered and technique developed by Dr Ilizarov.

The most essential innovation of the Ilizarov treatment is an addition of the computer programming to the calculation of bone deformity correction. The computer assisting control helps doctors and the patients to produce precalculated bone reduction, correction, compression and lengthening. Several special software programs including Internet-based programs are available in the US, Germany and other countries. But, as Professor Ilizarov was fond of saying: "To perform the treatment properly and successfully, one must know the method as well as the apparatus."

Dr Gavriil Ilizarov was in India, in 1983, with lectures and demonstrations. One of the authors (Vladimir Golyakhovsky) also was in India, in 1994, and gave lectures and performed surgeries at the hospitals in Mumbai and New Delhi. He was impressed by the great interest developed by the Indian orthopedic surgeons toward the Ilizarov's methods. He also traveled the country and became a fan of India and Indian people. We present the new edition of the book with a hope that this will make contribution to the practice of Ilizarov techniques.

Vladimir Golyakhovsky
Victor H Frankel

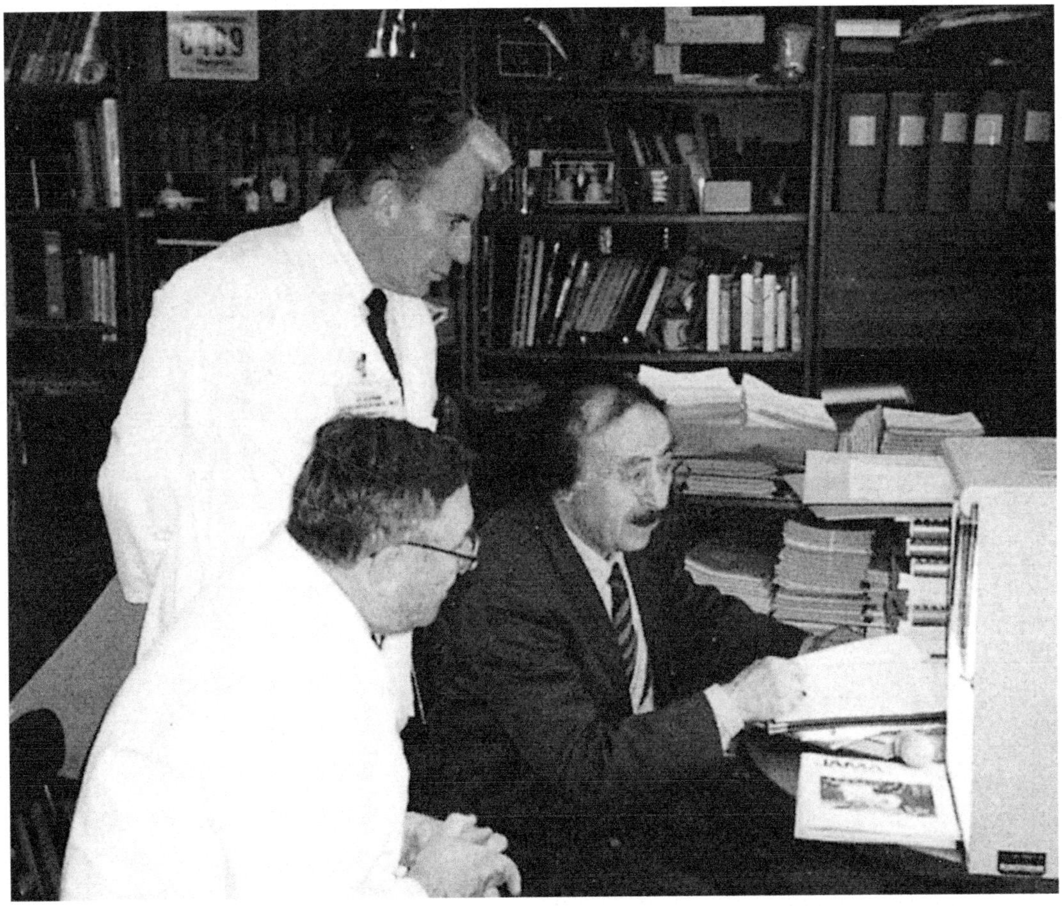

The authors, with Professor Ilizarov, at the Hospital for Joint Diseases in New York City, December 1991

Acknowledgments

The authors wish to thank Dr Svetlana Ilizarov (a daughter of Professor Ilizarov) for a help with the recommendation in writing the chapters of her father biography and of *New Modifications of the Ilizarov Technique.* Svetlana worked for several years in the beginning of her professional life as a doctor and researcher at the Kurgan Medical Center and Institute, in Russia, under the guidance of her father and is very much familiar with the main subject of this book. She is now working in New York City and is familiar with some of the new modifications of the Ilizarov technique. We also offer our gratitude to Mrs Irina Golyakhovsky, the wife of Dr Vladimir Golyakhovsky, who word-processed the introductory chapters with the patience and dedication. And we want to express our thanks to Shri Jitendar P Vij (Chairman and Managing Director) of Jaypee Brothers Medical Publishers (P) Ltd., for his high appraisal of the original book of "Operative Manual of Ilizarov Techniques", for offering us a new publication of the book, and his kind attention and support during our work of preparation of the manuscript.

Contents

Gavriil Abramovich Ilizarov—The Man, The Creator, The Teacher

The progress of science almost always is created by two types of geniuses: the first type brings about the conception of a new idea, this is the genius-discoverer; and the second type develops the existing idea, this is the genius of completion. Only in a very rare occasion the same scientist can become both the originator and developer of an idea. This rare type of genius creates a revolution in science.

Two names those of John Charnley (1911-1982) and Gavriil Ilizarov (1921-1992) are especially prominent in the history of Orthopedics of the 20th century. The success of Charnley's innovation of low friction arthroplasty revolutionized replacement of total joint in all of the major joints. The success of Ilizarov's circular fixator with multiplanar transfixation revolutionized the fracture, bone deformities, nonunion and other bone pathology treatment, leading to use of tissue generation for the lengthening and correction of all tubular bones.

Dr Charnley belongs to the second type of geniuses—he developed and completed the existed idea of joint replacement. Professor Ilizarov belongs to the rare type of geniuses who brought about the concept of a new idea and completed it by himself, developing the new chapter in orthopedic science. He was the first one to introduce a new type of the circular external fixator, in 1950s, and the first one to develop the Tension Stress concept for the direction and control over the tissue growth, and on the way he developed a new doctrine of tissue generation under the influence of bone distraction. The most surprising fact of his achievements is that he accomplished them under very poor and primitive conditions in a small and remote Siberian corner of Russia. In his creative work he encountered many people who did not believe the evidence of their own eyes. He had a very interesting life story full of numerous obstacles and heroic achievements.

Gavriil Abramovich Ilizarov was born in the small town of Beloveghsk in the Western Part of Whit Russia ("Gavriil" is the Russian interpretation of the biblical name Gabriel, "Abramovich" is the Russian patronymic name after Abraham). His father belonged to the little known Jewish community called Tats, "the Mountain Jewish" of the Caucasus Mountains. The family was extremely poor and to survive they moved to the father's native place the Caucasian village of Kussary, in the southern Republic of Russia Dagestan, Young Gavriil, the oldest of six children, had to help his mother to take care of his siblings, and he could not attend the school until he was eleven. Very early, however, he displayed great intellectual curiosity toward natural phenomena and science. The hard life of his boyhood gave him strong character, a desire to explore the possible, and an ability of great persistence. All these qualities would help him in the future. Moving forward through the ordeals, he took the school course just in five years, and then the three-year Rabfack course (Russian equality of the American College) in two years.

In 1939, he was accepted to the Simpheropol Medical School in Russian region of Crimea. In two years, in 1941, the War between fascist's Germany and communist's Russia erupted, and his Medical School was evacuated to the small town of Kzyl-Orda in the Soviet Middle East (Kazakhstan). The conditions of life and education there were extremely poor; most of the teaching staff went to the war, there was no clinical training at all. Nevertheless, the doctors were in great need in the country, and young Dr Ilizarov graduated from the school in 1944. Without any practical training, he was sent to work in the village of Dolgovka in the Kurgan district of Western Siberia. One has to imagine all difficulties at that war time in Russia. The working conditions for a doctor there were very primitive; he lacked much necessary medicine and essential equipment. During the five years of his sole practice there, Dr Ilizarov had no alternative but to overcome all the difficulties, and to become a self-trained internist, surgeon, obstetrician, pediatrician, and so on. There he developed some skill in conservative treatment of fractures.

In 1950, he was promoted to the position of a staff physician in the Hospital for the War Invalids in the small Siberian city of Kurgan, over 2000 km east of Moscow. At that time, there were thousands of wounded World War II veterans with bone nonunion, deformities and osteomyelitis. The small provincial Hospital had the shortage of vital equipment for such patients; the treatment was usually performed either by plaster casts application or by skeletal traction, and the results were unsatisfactory. Dr Ilizarov was determined to overcome that routine ways and to break through stagnation of the old conservative principles of treatment. The necessity is the mother of his first invention, and necessity combined with extraordinary talent helped him to make something from nothing: in 1951, he developed the ring and device for stable transosseus fixation. The Ilizarov's ring was first in the World with two K-wires in crossing directions.[1]

He himself told us the story how once he woke up during the night inspired by this idea. He had to immediately check up the idea. The only piece of wood to imitate the bone within easy reach was the handle of a spade. He used it as the model of a bone, introduced the two wires crosswise and fixed them to the improvised ring. This made the position of ring very stable. The idea behind was to use two rings connected to the bone above and below the fracture or nonunion, and then to connect to each other by the metal rods alongside the bone. In this way he developed a frame for a circular external fixator capable to bring about compression, distraction and correction of the bone fragments.

Dr Ilizarov did not have any training in engineering and did not have anybody to help him perfecting the model of a two-ring frame. Adding the dozens of new parts to the original construction, he overcame many difficulties by himself. Initially, for the purpose of support and stable position of the rings, he combined circular frame with the Böhler splint for skeletal traction (a popular 20th century tool for fracture treatment), then gradually he perfected the frame utilizing it for multiple purposes. Despite all his efforts, he did not get any respect and help from the bureaucratic organizations and manufacturing companies. All the frame parts were made by his grateful patients at the small local factory for repairing bus parts, and smuggled out a part at a time. Ironically, the officials in the Ministry of Health ignored the very existence of Dr Ilizarov, they called his innovations "a locksmith's approach to the surgery".

With enormous efforts, he was able to achieve good results from the treatment and, in 1958, he brought his fixator to Moscow, the capital of Russia, to present his invention to the attention of the leading orthopedists. He was allowed to demonstrate his fixator in action just in one experimental surgery at the Botkin General Hospital. At that time, the fixator still was the circular frame supported by the Böhler splint. The application of frame was combined with simultaneous regimen of skeletal traction, and to assist him was assigned a young resident, Dr Vladimir Golyakhovsky. Surgery was a success and provoked the impression of astonishment and great interest. But none of the leading professors paid much attention to the ideas of the unknown provincial physician from a remote Siberian town. He left Moscow very disappointed.

Fortunately, Ilizarov had a great amount of energy and determination. He continued perfecting the fixator and the technique of different methods of treatment, expanding the indications for fixator use. Over the years, his fame had spread and people throughout Russia learned of his existence only from the "grapevine", swapped stories about the miracles he performed in treating the hopeless invalids. His reputation for successful treatment slowly spread, and the patients from over the country traveled to the city of Kurgan, seeking relief from their misery. They started to call him "The Magician from Kurgan".

[1]The ring fixators were not widely known at that time although Dr Bittner, an American, introduced similar ring in 1934. But his invention had no farther practical development and is virtually unknown by the clinicians even now. In no way could Dr Ilizarov know about it in Russian Siberia.

Most of his brilliant findings came to him empirically. A particular anecdotal case illustrates this well: one of his patients, the World War II invalid, had a very short stump of the leg below the knee, and he suffered from inability to wear prosthesis. This man has begged Dr Ilizarov to do something for him just because he considered be a surgeon-magician. But the bone was too weak and even this "magician" did not know how to help him. At that time, he did not yet develop his well-balanced concept of the distraction osteogenensis. Yielding to that insisting patient, he reluctantly introduced through a short stamp of tibia two K-wires connected to the rings for gradual distraction. He made a careful cut through the bone, preserving medullar blood supply. His idea was to create a gap for filling it with a bone transplant. In three months, he ordered X-ray to calculate the size of a transplant for implantation. To his great astonishment, the traction gap was replaced by the newly formed bone. Dr Ilizarov realized that the new bone was grown in result of a slow gradual traction. Any doctor could be surprised by such observation and then forget it. But Ilizarov immediately recognized the great potentials of this observation: the distraction can produce osteogenesis.

He continued clinical experiments of the use of a careful bone cut with slow gradual traction, and almost always there was a new bone formation. This single empirical observation brought about the discovery of tension-stress phenomena and development of a new technique, the corticotomy or compactotomy. At that time, he put together a tiny experimental laboratory in which he performed solo research. Through his experimental work, he was the first to show that distraction rather than compression causes the healing of non-unions and pseudoarthrosis. This was the beginning of a new concept of conservation and exploitation of the bone's natural unlimited plasticity. In result, he introduced the concept of tension-stress effect of gradual tissue distraction.

Early in the 1960s, Dr Ilizarov reported the first successful lengthening of up to 25 cm of the shortened lower extremities. Nobody in the world could achieve such results. Undeterred, he continued to pester the professors and bureaucrats of various institutions in the attempt to gain recognition for his fixator and technique he had developed. The essence of his research and clinical findings—that the distraction but not compression is a mode of treatment—was disparaged as representing a contradiction of the fundamental principles of orthopedics. Dr Ilizarov seems to be upsetting those concerned with maintaining conventional levels of orderliness and humbleness. The envy also played an important part in this wrong attitude. As a result, his accomplishments were never reproduced in any of the major medical centers.

For 20 years, Dr Ilizarov continued to work in the same tiny hospital in Kurgan, Siberia, without support and understanding from the bureaucrats of science. He was not a communist party member in the society dominated by the communist doctrine. In 1965, at last his perseverance bore fruit: a decision was made by Moscow orthopedic bosses to send someone to Kurgan to see what that insistent Dr Ilizarov was doing and check his results. The trip to Kurgan fell on Dr Vladimir Golyakhovsky, the senior attending at the Central Institute of Traumatology and Othopaedics, and also not a communist. At that time, the Moscow orthopedic community had known practically nothing of the Ilizarov improvements in his methods. Nevertheless, the Golyakhovsky's bosses gave him this parting briefing: "Don't trust the Ilizarov stories one bit: he's a crook. Go to the Hospital and personally examine every patient, writing down notes of each case. Back to Moscow you'll present an annihilating report. It's high time that the con artist was exposed".

At the arrival to Kurgan, Golyakhovsky was astonished to discover that the city looked as Mecca for the crippled invalids, everywhere there were limping people with the crutches who came to seek healing by Ilizarov. The line of waiting Ilizarov surgery was more than 1000 patients. For two cold winter months, Golyakhovsky worked side-by-side with Ilizarov at rather primitive operating room, learning the techniques from that outstanding surgeon. He found that the fixator and the methods were perfected very much comparing to what he had seen 7 years before in Moscow. The conditions at the old small hospital were extremely difficult even by the Russian backward medicine: the dark rooms were crowded with a dozen or more cramped patients with the Ilizarov frames on their legs or arms, it was almost impossible to walk between the beds, the air was stuffy and stinking. But the results of the treatment were as incredible as the Ilizarov's surgical brilliance. He could gradually stretch the bone as much as twenty-five cm. Golyakhovsky was full of admiration for "Magician from Kurgan", and eventually they established a warm friendship. He wrote back to his Moscow bosses that Ilizarov methods are the new progressive development. There he made his first sketches of the techniques which made the framework of the illustration for this book, and he brought the sketches back to Moscow. He also brought with him an Ilizarov present—the two sets of his fixator to start to use them in Moscow. Dr Golyakhovsky delivered a report which was exactly opposite to the one expected from him. Presenting his impressions and findings, he tried to persuade his superiors that the Kurgan surgeon deserved all the support possible for development of his ideas and for spreading his methods. He described them as the original Russian discovery deserved to be widespread abroad, and he even predicted that Dr Ilizarov deserves the world fame. But all was in vain, for his "tactical mistake" Golyakhovsky was punished by a demotion and prohibited to do the Ilizarov surgery.

In 1967, the No. 1 athlete of the world, an Olympic champion, high-jumper, Valery Brumel sustained a compound leg fracture subsequently plagued with persistent nonunion and osteomyelitis. Millions of his fans followed his condition with great attention. Moscow professors recommended amputation of the leg. Dr Golyakhovsky referred Mr Brumel to Dr Ilizarov, and the Ilizarov's procedure saved his leg and his ability to jump came back again. The recovery of this prominent patient brought an excellent publicity to Ilizarov and this helped him to overcome the resistance of bureaucrats. After 20 years of persistent efforts, he was fully recognized in his country Russia, became a member of the Academy of Science and a member of Russian Parliament. He was granted permission and given sufficient state funds to build the new Institute of Experimental and Clinical Orthopedic Surgery in the city of Kurgan. There he established the largest medical center for the treatment of bone pathology by his own methods: 800 beds, huge rehabilitation clinic and large research department with dozens of laboratories. In Moscow, Dr Golyakhovsky was finally given permission to start using Ilizarov fixator for surgeries and the methods became popular all over Russia. Later on, Golyakhovsky visited his old friend Ilizarov now the Director of the Kurgan Institute and a professor. They published together several scientific papers. Dr Golyakhovsky became a professor in Moscow and soon after, in 1978, he immigrated to the United States. There he had to overcome all the immigrant's difficulties, and to start from the scratch a new surgical career. In New York City, he unsuccessfully tried to excite the curiosity of American doctors telling them of the Ilizarov techniques. But even though Ilizarov's work became highly recognized in Russia, the rest of the world knew very little about him and neither the method nor the Ilizarov name were known to the American orthopedic surgeons until the 1980s.

Meanwhile, in 1980, internationally-known Italian author and explorer, Mr Carlo Mauri, from the city Lecco, the member of the famous Kon-Tiki and Ra expeditions, went to Kurgan seeking Prof Ilizarov's help. Mr Mauri had a severe persistent nonunion and osteomyelitis of the leg. All prominent European orthopedic surgeons tried to help him but without success, and he was recommended to have an amputation. Ilizarov performed on him one of his trademark procedures of distraction for development of local osteogenesis, the bone healed and the leg was saved. Mr Mauri called Ilizarov "the Michelangelo of Orthopaedics". Impressed by the miracle of his recovery, the team of Italian orthopedic surgeons from the city of Lecco went to Kurgan to learn the technique. They invited Ilizarov to conduct a symposium in Italy, and they secured a license to manufacture his fixator. This catapulted Ilizarov to international fame, he was invited to visit many countries including India, in 1983. In 1985, Dr Victor Frankel, the President of the New York Hospital for Joint Diseases, has seen the Ilizarov procedure in Spain and Italy and developed a great interest in this pioneering technique. He brought the fixator to New York and performed the first Ilizarov surgery in America, in December 1986. At the same time, another American surgeon, Dr Stuart Green, of California, was also bringing the Ilizarov technique to America. In 1987, Drs Frankel and Green went to Kurgan and invited Professor Ilizarov to New York. At the same time, Dr Dror Paley, from Canada, also went to Kurgan, he learned the technique there and performed the first Ilizarov surgery in Canada, in 1987.

The first international Symposium of the Ilizarov technique was organized in New York, in October 1987, by the Hospital for Joint Diseases together with the Smith and Nephew Richards Medical Company. The symposium was a real triumph of Prof Ilizarov. More than 300 American orthopedic surgeons came to listen to his lectures and to start training in the techniques. The Smith and Nephew company started to produce the Ilizarov apparatus in America. At the Symposium, the first meeting in ten years between the two old friends professors Ilizarov and Golyakhovsky occurred.

Golyakhovsky was given by Dr Frankel a position at the Hospital, and they started to work together. The result of their joint work was the first American Manual of the Ilizarov technique based on 300 first surgeries, which is also the basis of this book.

Professor Ilizarov has published more than 600 scientific papers and the monographic creation "Transosseous Osteosynthesis", and he received almost 300 patents from many countries. He became a well-known scientist and surgeon around the world and was invited to lecture to dozens of countries. Dr Golyakhovsky's early prediction proved finally to be right.

Thousands of orthopedic surgeons around the world use now the Ilizarov methods and Ilizarov fixator performing the Ilizarov procedures. Even the title of procedure "Ilizarov" became itself the common noun. In many countries the ASAMI (Association for Study of the Application of the Method of Ilizarov) chapters have been organized.

On July 24, 1992, Professor Gavriil Abramovich Ilizarov suddenly passed away from heart failure, at the age of 71. The world lost the remarkable Man, the Creator, and the Teacher.

Vladimir Golyakhovsky

Professor Gavriil A. Ilizarov
Receiving
Inspiration for His External Fixator

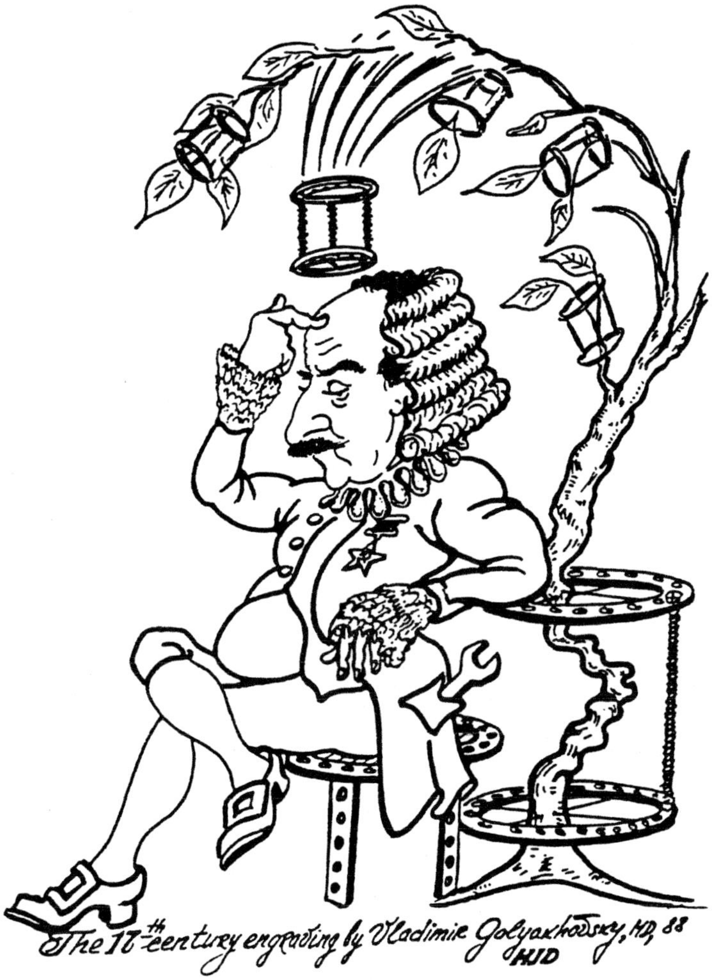
The 17th century engraving by Vladimir Golyakhovsky, MD, 88
MD

Caricature by Dr Vladimir Golyakhovsky presenting Dr Ilizarov in a pose and costume of Sir Isaac Newton at the historical moment of his Inspiration for Discovery from the falling apple. Dr Ilizarov liked this drawing very much because there were real similarities in both discoveries

PART ONE

Introductory Chapters

Chapter 1

Biomechanics of the Ilizarov External Fixator

The Ilizarov multiplanar circular external fixator is a remarkable versatile device; it possesses some of the most optimal biomechanical characteristics for the correction, distraction and compression of the bone. Unlike the uni- and biplanar large-pin fixators it can be used to treat virtually any type of limb deformities. When the bone is loaded, the fixator maintains higher axial elasticity and stiffness to bending, in comparison to other conventional fixators.

Various pieces of this device permit assemblage of many different frames combinations, and adjustment or reassembly during the long course of the treatment.

When connected to the bone, the resultant frame of fixator replicates the cylindrical shape of the tubular cortical bone shell, with greater diameter. This design allows the fixator frame to accommodate high axial, torsion and compression loading.

With the fixator in place, the mechanical action of compression or distraction can be performed in many different directions; in any of the positions fixator maintains proper bone fragment stability, important for achievement of tissue growth and regeneration.

There are several biomechanical factors related to the increase of the apparatus stiffness assisting to the necessary stability of fixation. These are the extrinsic factors as distinguished from intrinsic factors of the local tissues pathological changes. The extrinsic factors must be considered in advance before application of the apparatus. For intelligent use of the Ilizarov fixator the general recommendations are as follows:

1. Success of treatment depends on the frame proper composition. The main part of any type of frame is the ring with a flat surface and multiple holes. The number of the rings is most important factor for the frame stability – increased number brings about more stable construction. Simple two rings frame is recommended for the upper extremity. The optimal number of rings for lower extremity is four. The rings have to be allocated by two to each bony segment above and below fracture/nonunion. This design allows the frame to accommodate very high axial torsion, compression, shear, and combined torsion-compression loading. Biomechanical principles have shown that, for the strength and stiffness of frame, the distance between two neighboring rings must be not greater than that of the diameter of the ring.
2. The positioning, orientation, and number of rings are critical factors for deformity correction. In some cases two half-rings can be connected to form the full ring. Greater stability of the frame can also be achieved through introduction of additional half-rings connected to the full ring. Two half rings connected parallel to each other can be introduced into frame as a "puller" or "pusher" device for correction of an angular deformity.

3. It is preferable that the rings of the frame are of the same size. The important criteria for the consideration of the rings size is a maximal diameter of the limb segment. Because the breadth of extremity varies at different levels, the space between the skin and the ring also will vary. As a rule K-wire span must be at least 3 cm to prevent possible ring pressure in case of the soft tissue swelling.
4. Rings orientation must be aligned strictly perpendicular to bony fragments in a configuration with their inclination or angulation, with the corresponding holes of all rings along the same straight line, making rings connection with the threaded rods easy. In case of angular deformity the ring orientation establishes their positioning in relation to the long axis of each bone segment.
5. The central rings must be in a close position to the fracture/nonunion site. The closer the ring is placed to the tip of free bone fragment end, the more stable this fragment is during all necessary bone movements – compression, distraction or correction. The feeble bone structure and soft tissues condition have to be taken into consideration. In case of osteoporotic changes the central rings have to be located farther from nonunion site.
6. In many cases the two connected half-rings can be used instead of a full ring. They have the advantage of being easily reinstalled during the long course of treatment. The half-rings are mostly used for the upper and lower arm frames, and for the foot component of a leg frame. As the foot component the half-ring must be elongated by adding two connecting plates to each of its ends.
7. If the ring is situated close to the joint it can prevent or severely restrict the joint motion. In such cases it is useful to incorporate into frame a five-eighths ring or a half-ring with curved end plates. Both of these ring modifications are not so strong as full ring but their three-point connection to the adjacent ring permits it to bear any necessary loading stresses.
8. For use in the proximal part of the femur frame there is a special arch in two versions: 90- and 120-degree with slots. Assemblage of these components is facilitated by the introduction of two or three half-pins of 4 or 5 mm in diameter instead of wires.
9. Ring (and arches) connections play a crucial part in the assembly of any type of the frame, they determine rational distribution of frame strength, balance arrangement of different structural loading and stability of the frame attachment to the bone fragments. They serve also as ring direction guides. Main type of ring connector is the threaded rods of different lengths but with the same pitch (i.e. the distance between two threads) which equals 1 mm. This signifies that one full turn of the nut corresponds to a change also equal to 1 mm. At least four rods must be used to connect two neighboring rings, affixed at equal distance both vertically and horizontally on the rings. Biomechanically, four threaded rods provide much greater protection against bending.

   The slotted cannulated rod has special functions in connecting rings. This rod may serve as a connector and at the same time may be used as pulling device.
10. The graduated telescopic rods of four different lengths are the hollow aluminum cylindrical tubes with partially threaded shaft. They are significantly stiffer than threaded rods. One end of telescopic rod is fastened to a ring with a bolt, and a partially threaded shaft protruding from the cylinder attached to the next ring by the partially threaded rod. The smooth surface of the partially threaded rod provides greater stiffness to accommodate the stress of the tightened bolt connected to the ring.
11. The graduated telescopic rod is much like the telescopic rod. It is a cylinder with one end coupled to a ring via a tightened bolt. It has a square head that is adjustable by hand, permitting easier and simpler adjustment by a quarter of mm for compression and distraction. It locks after each turn, has visual references on the square sides, and clicks audibly after every turn.
12. Fastening of the frame is achieved with the nuts and bolts. Dr. Ilizarov consciously excluded anything sharp from his fixator system, in particular, the

screws and screwdriver, to prevent any serious injury to the surrounding tissue.

There are three types of hexagonal 10-mm nuts: a full or 6-mm thick nut, a three-quarter, or 5 mm thick nut, and a half, or 3 mm thick nut. One thread's pitch of all three nuts equals 1 mm; thus the full nut has six threads, the three-quarter nut has five threads, and the half nut has three threads. Depending on the number of threads, different nuts serve different purposes in the frame assembly. Inasmuch as one thread's pitch equals 1 mm, one full turn will produce 1 mm of movement on the rod, which recommended to average amount of distraction-compression in the lengthening method for 1 day. Thus the turn of the nut is used as a driving force in the technique.

To facilitate a one-fourth turn, Richards Medical Company introduced a special quadragonal nut with 15 threads; its head marked with dots from 1 to 4, signifying increments of the full turn.

13. Using bolts is the best and simplest way to tighten the parts of the frame. There are three types of connecting bolts with the standard hexagonal head. They differ from each other in leg length: 10-mm length, 16-mm length, and 30-mm length. The pitch of the thread in all three types is equal 1 mm. The 10-mm and 16-mm bolts are mostly used for connecting the post and plates. The 30-mm bolt is used to connect three or more parts.

    There are two types of bolts specially designed to fasten K-wires to the flat surface of the ring: the cannulated wire-fixation bolt and the slotted wire-fixation bolt.
14. Introduction of Kirschner wires (K-wires) for the bone fixation is a key technique for the apparatus application. It determines both the positioning and stability of rings. Drilling the smooth K-wires of small diameter (1.5 mm and 1.8 mm) creates small hole in the soft tissue, compact bone and bone marrow. Introduced multidirectional and transfixed to the rings under tension, K-wires bring firm stability of the bone fragments. The entrance and exit points of the K-wire must be located at least 1.5 to 2.0 cm from the major blood vessels and nerves. Each wire drilled through the bone must be introduced correctly at the first attempt. The rule is, *one wire, one hole.*
15. Multidirectional bone transfixation, called "transosseous osteosynthesis" by Dr. Ilizarov, is done by the K-wires, it brings maximum stability to the rings and to the bone fragments. This stability can also be reinforced by the offset K-wires connected to the ring by the supports, posts, and half-hinges. The number and configuration of the offset wires provide not only better ring stability but increases the stiffness of the whole frame.
16. For the proper K-wires introduction the ring must be equally centered to the bone axis. This helps to achieve a wide angulation between two K-wires. The wide spread between the two crossings K-wires brings about more even distribution of the loading forces on the bone cortex along the plane of the ring. This spread has to be as much as possible close to 90/90 degrees.
17. Introduction of the stopper wires with an olive shaped stoppers (a wire with a rounded bulge that becomes seated against the compact bone), adds to the bone and the frame stability. Use of the stopper wires is recommended for the fragment's deviation correction, technique of bone pulling, and inter-fragmentary compression, and at the sites of osteoporotic bone.
18. For correction of hand deformities there are specially designed miniparts of fixator, one-fourth of size of the original parts. With the transfixation of the metacarpal bones the special light frame allows to achieve lengthening and correction of the fingers. The same miniparts can be used for the toes deformity treatment.
19. Introduction of the hinges between two neighboring rings bring desirable gradual correction of angular deformities. A two-axis hinge consists of a single unit that permits rotation around two orthogonal axes. Used in combination with distraction-compression devices, the hinges help gradually to correct deformities, with simultaneous transformation of the bone and soft tissues. Subsequently, the hinges are used as pivotal (rotation) point components for

necessary straightening. The position, orientation, and number of hinges are critical factors for deformity correction. The advantages of using hinges are: they constrain motion in a specific plane or planes; they provide a specific fulcrum for calculation and control of correction of the bone fragments angulation or displacement; they provide biologic adaptation of tissues to new desired positioning.

Several important parameters must be considered in hinge positioning:

a. Two rings to which hinges are attached must be strictly perpendicularly to bone fragments; they either start perpendicularly to end angulated, or vice versa.
b. Two hinges located at the opposite sides of deformity usually required for stability.
c. Two hinges rotation axis must be situated on the same horizontal level of the deformity apex.
d. It is critically important that hinges of the same plane are oriented along the same plane as the deformity.
e. Movement of the axis of the hinges rotation to concave or convex sides of deformity produces corresponding compression or distraction of the fragments.
f. The positioning of the hinges can be used to achieve different types of deformity correction, such as opening wedge, distraction, compression, translation, and derotation.

20. In some cases there are the big posttraumatic or postsurgical skin scars, the introduction of the hinges between two rings can help for skin stretching by the local tissue sprain. This helps for development of neovascularization of soft tissue and brings about the softening of a scarred area – an important additional effect of treatment during correction of the bone deformity.

Most of the parts of fixator have been developed by Dr. Ilizarov during his work in very harsh and poor conditions at the Siberian city of Kurgan, in 1950-60s. Some of them may look today like the old fashion design (for example, the simple threaded rod). But they did work well for the treatment of thousands patients. Starting in 1990s, the new modern design of many of the same parts have been developed (for example the gradual telescopic rod instead of the threaded rod), and new lighter material is used for their production. Esthetically these modern parts look more attractive and up to date but they carry out essentially the same function as the old ones.

2 Chapter

Ilizarov Frame Assemblage

For the lower extremity, a four-ring fixator frame is most commonly used. In some cases, however, it may be necessary to apply up to six rings. For the upper extremity, a two of the three-ring frame is used. In each frame choice of a ring level determines distribution of the forces applied to the ring. Choice of the ring inclination determines the direction of the forces applied to each ring.

In constructing any type of Ilizarov frame, the main considerations are:

- The stability of the frame fixation to the bone;
- The prevention of gross bone fragments motion;
- The ability to manipulate and to perform necessary fragment movements such as straightening, bending, distraction, compression, rotation, of a combination of these movements.

There are two methods of frame construction:

1. The first and most recommended method is to assemble the main parts, the rings and connected rods in advance with consideration of all existing deformities.

   The motionless, main supporting ring supports the primary frame stabilization forces and bears the weight of the entire construction. This is stationary ring and always is located at the proximal base of the frame.

   The stabilizing ring determines the force of stabilization and balance of the frame and always is located most distally. Both of these rings must be positioned with consideration of correct inclination and perpendicular to the corresponding parts of a bone (if there is a deformity). To stabilize the frame an extremely strong force must be applied when tightening the wires to the rings, sometimes as much as 300 kg.

   The rings between the supporting and stabilizing are called pushing-pulling rings and they determine the directions of the forces of distraction-compression. They must be placed close to the fracture/nonunion site, or to site of the planed osteotomy.
2. The prepared frame is placed sterilized as a whole over the limb in the beginning of surgery. After necessary correction of the distances between rings, the frame has to be transfixed to the bone with the K-wires. The proximal supporting ring must be transfixed the first, then follows the distal stabilizing ring. After that the intermediate rings also have to be transfixed.

   The frame must be able to bear the patient's weight, to sustain distraction-compression forces, and support the patient's physical activity during many months of treatment, and the rule no. 1 is the fixation must be absolutely firm.
3. During bone lengthening, muscle tension can cause a deviation in the distracted bone fragment. This must be taken into account when setting the inclination of the proximal main supporting ring to ensure preservation of deformity development. To prevent this, 5 to 7 degrees of recurvature and varus positioning of the

main supporting ring will bring correct direction of distraction.

The main advantages of frame preassembly are that it saves time during the surgical procedure and gives the surgeon the latitude to try some component variations. The disadvantage is that it may require adjustments, because it is impossible to foresee all necessary modifications, especially in complicated cases.

4. The second method of the frame assemblage is to construct it during surgery piece-by-piece over the limb. To do this the K-wires first have to be introduced into the bone, starting at the site of the proximally situated main supporting ring. The sterilized ring has to get connected to the wires, and they are properly tensioned. Next step is the wires introduction for the neighboring pushing ring, and connection of this ring to the wires and tensioning them. The same has to be done to all rings situated distally.

The chief advantage of this method is that it affords a surgeon great experience in practical frame construction details and may help avoid some corrections during the procedure. The primary disadvantage is that piece-by-piece frame assembly requires a great deal of time and the help of many trained assistants to hold the limb and to direct the wires introduction.

This is a slow and more cumbersome method of frame assemblage.

3 Chapter

Biomechanics of the Ilizarov Method

In the preface to his monographic creation "Transosseous Osteosynthesis" (Springer Verlag, 1992, 800 pages) professor Ilizarov wrote: "Our research in medicine, biology and engineering has led to the evolution of more than 800 unique, highly effective methods of treatment that extend beyond the realm of traumatology and orthopaedics". Most of methods have been shown in that book. All of them are more or less based upon discovered by Ilizarov important biologic law of the tissue genesis and growth. He coined for this law a term "Tension-Stress Effect" and formulated it thus: "*slow, steady traction of tissues caused them to become metabolically activated, resulting in an increase in the proliferative and biosynthetic function*".

When used in conjunction with the Ilizarov fixator, attached to the bone fragments, the tension-stress effect permits the development and formation of new tissues. Gradual traction applied on living tissues creates stresses that stimulate the regeneration and growth of tissues structures. If subjected to slow, steady traction, the tissues become metabolically activated. This is a phenomenon characterized by the stimulation of both proliferative and biosynthetic cellular functions. Regenerative processes depend upon the adequacy of the local blood supply. Local neovascularization is a principal force responsible for all tissues neogenesis. An increase in local and regional vascularity helps to provide an adequate and sufficient blood supply.

Ilizarov was the first to observe that under influence of forces of particular rate and frequency the motion of distraction produces effect of neogenesis and growth of virtually all the local tissues involved: bone, muscles, tendons, fascia, vessel's walls, nerve's intercalary growth of existing trunks and growth of new nerve fibers, and the skin.

Observing the progress of treatment of thousands of his patients Ilizarov discovered that the early bone formation occurs by the inframembranous ossification, and is located parallel to the applied force. This observation served as a basis for the second important biologic law: *the shape forming processes acting upon bone tissue are dependent upon the magnitude of the applied load and the adequacy of blood supply.* The early bone formation occurs by the inframembranous ossification, and is located parallel to the applied force.

For development of the bone collagen columns deposited along lines of the mechanical stress of the slow gradual motion, the first and most important condition is preservation of local blood circulation. Normally, two-thirds of the cortical blood supply comes from the nutrient artery located in the bone marrow. The periosteal arterioles provide one-third of the blood supply. In the case of any bone distraction, with partial or complete bone marrow interruption, the periosteal arterioles begin to increase and extend their function as the main source of the cortex blood supply. Therefore, in order to optimize the anatomic and physiologic condition for new bone formation, the preservation of both endosteal and periosteal blood supply is of great importance.

The biomechanics of Ilizarov method have a main fundamental distinction from the other types of external fixators. It consists of careful approach and particular attention to preservation and stimulation of local and regional blood circulation. This is the essence of the Ilizarov procedures of the frame application and subsequent manipulations of the bone fragments. The Ilizarov procedure is essentially a bloodless surgery, majority of the cases allow to achieve good result without wide skin opening. The correctly performed introduction of the wires can be done with only of a drop of blood lost. The open reduction or correction osteotomy, is indicated relatively rare. In most of the cases the fragments correction can be achieved by the close technique. Thus, in majority cases the blood loss during procedure can't exceed 100 cc.

The technique of corticotomy (or compactectomy) is the only part of procedure requiring skin incision and complete bone cut. This is a circumferential transection of the cortex of tubular bone (femur, tibia, humeral bone) for the purpose of distraction and correction, and can possible produce a hemorrhage. This elegant and intricate surgical technique was developed by Dr. Ilizarov in 1960s as opposed to a wide-open osteotomy cut through the vasculature. The Ilizarov corticotomy consist of cutting a compact wall of a bone with simultaneous preservation of the periosteum and bone marrow. This technique allows to save the periosteum and the bone marrow in order to preserve local and regional blood circulation. It is strongly recommended to perform the corticotomy after the fixator frame is assembled properly and transfixed securely to the bone in order to keep the osteotomized fragments in steady position. Cortical bone is remodeled, after it is cut, by bone cells deposited on the periosteal, endosteal, and haversian canal surfaces. With gradual dilatory lengthening through the bone cut, billions of new cells develop. Depending on the goal of treatment, the corticotomy can be performed at one level (monofocal) or two levels (bifocal) on the same bone. In general, the monofocal corticotomy is indicated for: (1) lengthening of the bone up to 5 cm; (2) bone fragment transportation up to 5 to 7 cm; (3) stimulation of local and regional blood circulation in the limb for generation of osteogenesis without significant bone lengthening (e.g. in pseudoarthrosis or nonunion); and (4) gradual correction of bone deformity.

For preservation of the limb function the Ilizarov method include early mobilization of the patient. Beside the activation of regional blood circulation, the axial loading on the limb fixed with the frame stimulates micromotion of tensioned K-wires. It may seem puzzling that the thin 1.5 mm, or 1.8 mm K-wires can withhold the enormous stress of axial loading over a course of several months of treatment and also can bear the forces of distraction-compression without breaking or cutting bone tissue. The unique wire-ring combinations in the Ilizarov fixator produces a much lower axial stiffness and axial loading force, which distributes the load to all parts of the frame, than do the uniplanar and biplane fixators that use much heavier pins of 4.5 mm. At the same time the K-wires show higher axial stiffness against loading from bending forces.

The wires combined with the rings allow the optimal biomechanical characteristics for the bone fragment stabilization. In addition to serve as a structurally supportive network, the wires translate distraction-compression forces and execute bone fragment alignment along with all the other necessary fragment position corrections. The wire is the part of the fixator that determines how the treatment proceeds, and the final result.

For the cortical bone drilling there are wires with bayonet point tips, and for the cancellous bone drilling there are wires with the trocar point up. Each wire must be introduced slowly by the low-power drill with a speed of no more than 30 to 40 rpm. This permits moving aside such movable soft tissue structures as blood vessels and nerves, thereby avoiding serious complications. Each wire must be introduced correctly at the first attempt. Multiple holes resulting from incorrect drilling destroy compact bone through mechanical damage and through burning. Multiple drilling through bone marrow significantly destroys it and blood circulation, causing hematoma formation, delaying its ability for new cell development, and may even contribute to infection. Beside of this, with multiple wire holes the subsequent loading from the distraction-compression movement at the same cortex location will farther hasten bone destruction and resultant wire fixation weakening.

The half pins measuring 4.0 and 5.0 mm in diameter were not the parts of the set of Ilizarov fixator, and have been introduced by the Italian surgeons for use in special frame for proximal femur fixation. They are two types: 4-mm half-pin with bayonet-pointed end, and with interrupted threaded section, and 5-mm half-pin with bayonet-pointed end and with continuous threaded end. With use of both types they have to be introduced so that both threaded portions are immersed in the bone cortex.

The use of the half pins contradicts the Ilizarov doctrine of the importance of stiffness and elasticity achieved through small-diameter tensioned wires. But occasionally they may be used for the reinforcement of the fixation of nonmovable supporting ring or arch, where they do not interfere significantly with the tissue regeneration resources.

The indications for use of half pins arise when the application of a ring is impractical and has to be replaced by the arch, and also when necessary additional support is required, after wire fixation already has been applied.

The tensioned wires are remarkably resistant and in addition they have enough elasticity so as to allow a proper biological stimulus to bone healing. The restricted elasticity of the tensioned K-wires allows for cyclic micromotions at the site of fracture or osteotomy (corticotomy). This was shown to activate the piezoelectric phenomena in the cells of bone marrow, in compact bone, and in the newly developed regenerate. This has long been considered to be stimulatory to bone healing. If the tissues are stimulated by the elastic micromotion, the nerve impulses are activated, and help control the passage of electrically charged ions through the cells activating their ion channels. Because of tensioning effect of the wires, the bone is continuously loaded unlike a plate or any other type of internal fixation. This limited-elasticity type has a particular advantage: it generates more rapid callus formation and maturation. Dr. Ilizarov considered this mechanism to be an analog to the mechanism of the fetal growth plate activity. The exact mechanism of existing micromotion-cellular development is not completely known.

As a part of biomechanics of the Ilizarov method, the obligatory rule is that wire fixation to the rind must be properly tensioned. The quality of bone healing and/or bone regenerate development depends on the strength of wire tensioning. Increased K-wire tensioning brings about a suitable balance in the stability and flexibility of the frame. The exact strength of tensioning depends on the frame construction, local bone condition (osteoporosis vs. normal bone) and functional wire loading (stabilization vs. distraction-compression). Only tensioned wire can sustain the required loading forces and perform the task of stable frame support over the long course of treatment. The range of the wire tensioning strength depends on the frame construction, local bone condition, weight of the patient, and on the functional wire loading. The range of wire tensioning strength is 50 to 130 kg:

- Wire on half-ring: 50 to 70 kg
- Offset wire: 50 to 80 kg
- Two wires on a ring in a child: 100 to 110 kg
- Two wires on a ring in an adult patient: 120 to 130 kg.

The strength of tensioned wires is not the constant during treatment, but can decrease or increase depending on the movement of frame parts due to distraction-compression. The clinical signs of a decrease in tension strength are pain and skin irritation at the wires site. The radiographic signs of tension strength increase appear as concave wires bending with compression, and convex wire bending with distraction of the bone fragment.

Retensioning of the slack wire is performed by application of two wrenches to the head of a fixation bolt and nut and a slow turn both of them a quarter-turn or half-turn. If it is a need for significant wire retensioning, it is performed with reapplication of a wire tensioner.

In the bone fragment distraction there is always a possibility of fragment deviation. For axial stabilization and prevention of deviation of the fragment is recommended to use a guidewire introduced into the bone canal, proximal end of the guidewire must be above and its distal end below the fragment level. One of its ends (usually proximal) is buried in the bone canal, and the opposite end attached to a nonmovable ring of the frame.

During drilling the guidewire can become arched (or curved) and with harder drilling can destroy the internal organization of the bone marrow. That is why as soon as the wire tip penetrates the trabecular part of the bone the drilling must be stopped, and farther wire introduction has to be performed with gentle hammering.

In the technique of internal bone transport the two K-wires with stoppers can be used for pulling or traction of bone fragment. Only wires with stoppers can be used for pulling. Balancing the traction forces requires two symmetrically placed wires. If one pulling wire is used, the guidewire must be used to prevent fragment deviation. The stoppers must be situated distal to the level of the bone osteotomy (corticotomy) at the proximal half of bone fragment. Introduction of the pulling wires must be performed before the corticotomy, to prevent excessive bone fragment shifting and bone marrow damage.

The beauty of Ilizarov method is that they are universal for almost all types of bone deformity treatment. The basic of the method can be presented thus:

- Anatomical reduction and stabilization of bone fragments
- Correction of different types of displacement
- Correction of angular deformity
- Bone fragments compression
- Bone fragments distraction
- Combined bone fragments compression-distraction (for correction)
- Internal bone transport within a frame (replacing bone grafting)
- External bone transport with the movable part of a frame
- Correction of joint deformities
- Limb lengthening or correction of growth retardation
- Correction of congenital or traumatic pseudoarthroses of long bone
- Elimination of joint's contracture.
- Epiphyseal distraction for lengthening
- Correction of achondroplastic dwarfism by lengthening of limbs
- Compression arthrodesis of the knee
- Knee arthrodesis with compression-distraction for simultaneous leg lengthening
- Rotation of bone fragment inside a frame
- Filling bone defects (monolocal and multilocal)
- Widening of long bone diaphysis for strengthening or cosmetic correction
- Correction of resistant and relapsed club feet.
- Correction of the foot equines (with associated deformities)
- Eliminating of foot supination deformity
- Calcaneal correction and lengthening
- Correction and lengthening of the metacarpal bones
- Correction and lengthening of metatarsal bones
- Lengthening of short fingers
- Lengthening of short toes
- Lengthening of tibia short stump
- Lengthening of femur short stump
- Hand skin stretch for syndactyly correction.

Inside of each of these groups there are multiple variations for the treatment of individual types of deformities.

4 Chapter
Biomechanic Considerations for the Fracture Treatment

Dr. Ilizarov's initial intention was to use the circular fixator for fracture treatment. In its early version the frame was connected to a massive Böhler's splint to start the procedure by the simultaneous regimen of skeletal traction. The traction aids in reducing deformities and correcting shortness of the limb. Later on Ilizarov completely dismissed traction and performed fracture treatment by direct application of fixator.

Frame for fracture treatment cannot be assembled in advance because the varieties of fracture lanes and fragment displacement are too diverse and cannot be anticipated. In acute trauma cases is recommended so-called progressive-concentric construction of the frame. It is done piece-by-piece over the fractured limb. The sites of K-wire introduction are chosen in accordance with the type and level of fracture. In case of open fracture the main indicator is the site and size of wound. It is always important to start wires introduction and ring fixation proximally to fracture location. As soon as the proximal ring is placed and stabilized, the next stop is wires introduction and ring fixation distally to fracture. To make the frame stable, the intermediate rings must be assembled of two half-rings because it is impossible to introduce the full rings between the proximal and the distal ring.

In case of very unstable fracture and the muscles retraction a skeletal traction can be recommended as a temporary measure during a procedure. After frame application the traction has to be removed because it may prevent the necessary manipulation for the fragments correction.

In essence, the circular fixator application can be considered as an alternative to cast application and to skeletal traction. The frame of Ilizarov fixator actually replicates the cylindrical shape of tubular cortical bone shell. This makes the fixator very suitable for all manipulations necessary for the reduction and fixation of bone fragment. Indications for the Ilizarov fracture treatment are as follows:

1. Complex open and closed fracture of long bones
2. Intraarticular fracture
3. Comminuted fracture
4. Compound fracture
5. Grade C-3 fracture.

The main difference of biomechanics in fracture treatment with the correction procedures consists of the speed of the fragments manipulation. In some cases of fresh fracture reduction and stabilization of the fragments can be achieved straightaway. In other cases with the significant fragments displacement it can be achieved only gradually. For this the crossing wire (or wires) has to be introduced "off center" of the ring. The subsequent correction has to be done via this wire tensioning. Compression and distraction can be done during first two to three days, if necessary.

The advantages of using the Ilizarov fixator in fracture cases are:

1. Possibility of simultaneous anatomical reduction

2. Stable fixation by multiplanar direction with the K-wires
3. Introduction of olive stop wires for correction of deformities
4. Early functional treatment, including joint range of motion and weight bearing
5. Possibility of correction of the secondary displacement by the frame adjustment
6. Reinforcement of the frame with secondary displacement
7. Easy approach to the wound in case of compound fractures.

5 Chapter

Basics of the Method of Distraction Osteogenesis

Despite the generally accepted view of compressive forces as the only stimulus for bone neogenesis, Dr. Ilizarov demonstrated that stimulation of certain tissue growth and regeneration can be achieved by gradual distraction. At first it was just an empirical observation on the effect of bone stretching. He discovered that gradual distraction applied on living tissues creates stresses that stimulate the regeneration and growth of tissues structures. With the series of clinical observation he established that with rigid bone fragment fixation, proper speed and frequency of distraction it is possible to stimulate the latent resources of tissue necessary for their potential neogenesis, bypassing the compression stage. Distraction forces can create tissue stress capable of stimulating local metabolic activity with cell transformation. This eventually leads to the development of bony regenerate. Farther on, in 1960s, he introduced and developed the method of distraction as a well-balanced teaching, so called distraction osteogenesis.

Lengthening and deformities correction by the method of distraction osteogenesis are based upon the low of tension-stress, which is the effect of a gradual forced motion applied to the bone fragments by the circular external fixator. Tension-stress effect permits the development and formation of new tissues and treatment of many complex injuries and diseases of the locomotor system.

Method of distraction is used primarily for bone lengthening, for the correction of bone deformities, for bone segment transport (replacing the bone grafting). The regenerative processes depend upon the two main factors: the adequacy of the local blood supply and the stimulating effect of microvibration of the tensioned K-wires. Quality and quantity of newly formed bone depends upon several factors:

- The regidity of bone fragment fixation
- The degree of damage of the bone marrow, the periosteal, soft tissues and the nutrient blood vessels at the level of the osteotomy
- The speed of a distraction (rate)
- The rhythm (frequency) of a distraction
- The distribution of forces on the bone circumference.

It took Ilizarov years of clinical observations to work out the proper speed and rhythm of distraction. One of the problems was that after discharge from the hospital the patient had to do lengthening by himself, and must have an exact doctor's instruction. The early observations have shown that the rate of distraction of 0.5 mm per day often drives to premature consolidation of the lengthened bone, and that of 2.0 mm per day often results in delay of a new bone tissue formation. Ilizarov established the optimum distraction rate as 1.0 mm per day divided by four times - with a rate of 0.25 mm performed every six hours. With correctly chosen speed and rate, the growth of bone is visible on X-ray film in 2-3 weeks as a relatively dense cloud of connective tissue, eventually after 10 to 12 weeks this tissue would look like a newly formed bone.

The X-ray examination is not the only way to follow the bone formation at the site of distraction. It can be also shown as a formation of a dense tissue with the ultrasound examination.

The speed and rhythm of distraction are adjustable. With periodic control they have to be changed up to 1.5 mm/day, by the six 0.25 mm/turn, especially for the kids and young healthy patients. In some cases they have to be reduced to 0.5 mm/day by the two 0.25 mm/turn, mostly for the patients with osteoporosis. The motor forces in both situations must be distributed evenly on the moving bone fragment circumference. The optimum distribution of distraction forces is point of application with 90-degree between them.

There are two ways to perform distraction. The first is by applying two #10 wrenches simultaneously to the nuts attached to the fixator's ring, and to loosen and to tighten the nuts by a quarter of turn. The second and the most reliable method of distraction is achieved by using the graduated telescopic rod, which has a rotating head with a ratcher mechanism. One-quarter of the turn corresponds to 0.25 mm of distraction.

Dr. Ilizarov also discovered that the corticotomy of the same fragment near the nonunion site and simultaneous distraction both the nonunion and corticotomy sites increase the potential to stimulate tissue resources to healing at the nonunion. It was proved that in such cases distraction at the corticotomy site leads to increased local neovascularization. This, in turn, brings additional stimulus to the mechanical effect of tissue tension stress. In many cases of nonunion distraction becomes a powerful tool for treatment.

In certain cases of severe deformities with limb shortness and bone loss it is necessary to use distraction at one level combined with compression at another level. Depending on the predominant deformity, this may be primarily a case of distraction with compression as an additional treatment element. With significant bone loss this combined technique is called the segmental bone transport technique.

6 Chapter
Basics of the Method of Compression Osteogenesis

Compression of the bone fragments is the most traditional way of the fracture and nonunion treatment. With discovery of the method of bone osteogenesis stimulation, Dr. Ilizarov broadened the indications for compression and started to use it as a method of the bone deformities correction, bone segment transport, arthrodesis (fusion), and reversing distraction in case of hypoplastic bone regenerate development.

In most situations compression is produced in the same manner as distraction, but in the opposite direction. The same techniques used to produce distraction also are applicable to compression but in reverse direction: slow rhythmic movement of the one bone fragment toward the other. As with distraction, the same parameters of operation effect compression: speed, rhythm, distribution of forces on the bone circumference, rigidity of the bone fragment fixation, and the degree of damage of the bone marrow, periosteal, soft tissues and nutrient blood vessels at the level of fracture or nonunion. The task of compression is to stimulate a new bone tissue development but in much lesser quantity. Depending on a type of nonunion this has to be done with different speed: in hypoplastic type of nonunion a quarter of mm of compression twice a day for 4 to 6 days, then to stop for 4 to 6 days, and after this to continue compression again for 3 to 4 days. The chief indication for reduction of the compression speed and rhythm is severe pain at the site of compression, which can be a reflection of neurovascular deficiency.

In many cases of hypertrophic and normotrophic nonunion, the alternating compression with subsequent distraction maneuver is used two or three times to stimulate bone neogenesis. In cases of hypoplastic nonunion to stimulate an inert bone neogenesis it is recommended to reverse compression for a slow distraction for 3 to 4 days, then to stop, and after that to continue compression again for 5 to 6 days. This can be repeated for two-three times. This is so called compression-distraction method.

With primarily indications for compression, such as in hypertrophic nonunion with bone shortness, distraction can be used as an additional alternative method for a next stage of treatment element to stimulate bone neogenesis. This can produce lengthening of the bone at the site of nonunion healing.

Chapter 7

Criteria of Bone Healing and Fixator Removal

As it was originally intended, the distraction-compression techniques must be produced by the properly instructed and trained patient, or by the parents of a sick child, under periodical control of a doctor. The physician can coordinate the rate and rhythm of distraction at the particular stage. In 1980s Dr. Ilizarov developed a electromechanical autodistractor, programed to produce a 1 mm revolution per day. The battery for the motor were provided on the patient's belt. The device was a nonstop motor connected to the telescopic rod. Four autodistractors were attached to four telescopic rods. The device worked well but at time there were no micro-batteries and no computer programming. The autodistractor made the fixator frame heavier and more expensive, and did not become popular. With all new technical advances the simple turning of the rods by hand is the most acceptable method up to now. The real question is – at what point it has to be stopped?

The defined columns of new bone usually appear radiographically in 6 to 8 weeks of distraction. If the regenerate maintains a constant diameter, normal development is taken place. Tomographic evaluation of regenerate quality is recommended at least ones before the end of the distraction-compression period. It is also possible to do evaluation of quality of regenerate sonographically. At the stage of a regenerate development the distraction-compression must be stopped but the frame has to stay in place at least twice as longer as was the distraction period. Criteria for removal of the Ilizarov frame is the clear radiographic appearance of the regenerate calcification with its recanalization.

The tension of all K-wires must be released before they are cut. When the wire is cut while still under tension, severe pain, microinjury and even stress fracture in the regenerate may be provoked. After the wires are cut near the rings and the half-pins are screwed out, the rings must be separated by removing the connecting rods and taken out one by one. Clinical and radiographic evaluation of healing must be done with anteroposterior and lateral images. Careful checking with both hands determines strong or weak healing.

After many months of having a relatively heavy fixator the muscles of a patient's limb are weak, and the application of a plaster cast or splint for two to three weeks is recommended to protect new regenerate. In certain cases, with the regenerate of questionable strength, the two wires above and below the regenerate must be left in and incorporated into the cast walls.

PART TWO

Assembly of the Circular Fixator

8 Chapter

Rings and Arches

Several types of external fixation devices are in use today. These fixators differ (1) in the manner by which they are attached to the bones, either in one plane or by a multiplanar method, and (2) by frame shape and construction. The various types of pins and wires used also differ.

The Ilizarov device is a circular external fixator. Its principal component is a ring with a flat surface and with multiple holes. In a complete set of Ilizarov fixators there are 12 sizes of rings, which differ in diameter, corresponding to the different diameters of patient limbs. When the Ilizarov fixator rings are connected to the bone and to each other, the resultant frame actually replicates the cylindrical shape of the tubular cortical bone shell, but larger (Fig. 8.1). This design allows the fixator frame to accommodate very high axial, torsion, compression, shear, and combined torsion-compression loading (Fig. 8.2).

The Ilizarov ring serves three main purposes:

1. It supports transfixional K-wires and/or half pins, which can be fixed at the many hole sites on the 360-degree ring.
2. Two or more connected rings form a frame of the apparatus.
3. The rings bear supplementary parts of the frame necessary for dynamic bone treatment.

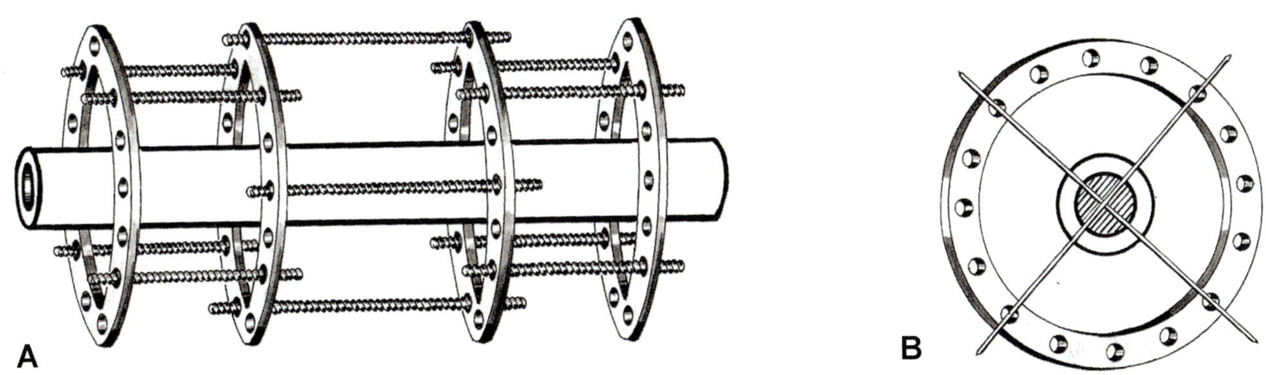

Figure 8.1: Schematic representation of a standard Ilizarov frame consisting of four rings connected to each other and transfixed to the tubular cortical bone. A, side view. B, cross section. Frame replicates the cylindrical shape of the bone shell, but larger

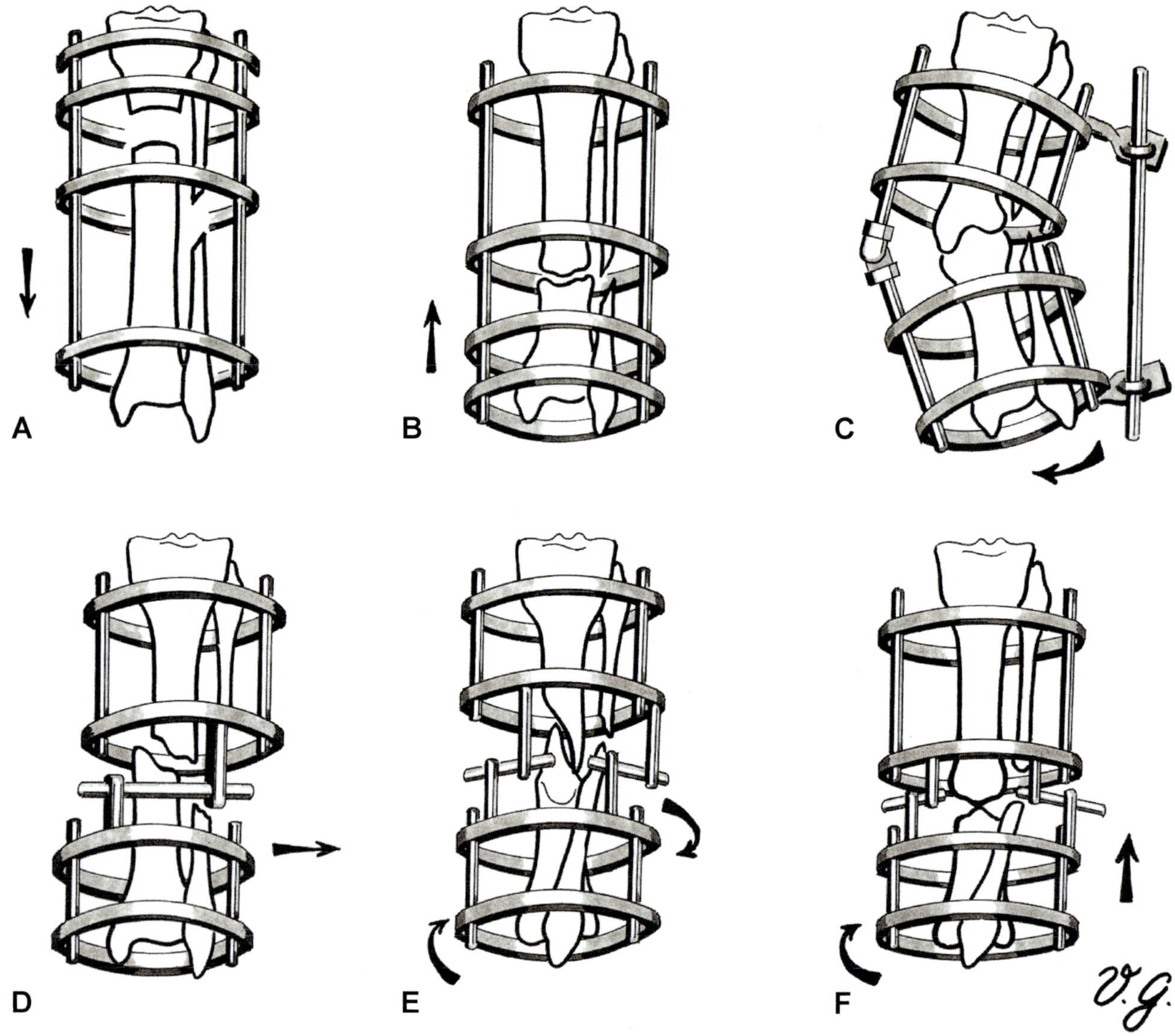

Figure 8.2: Schematic representation of the forces exerted on a four-ring Ilizarov frame in various loading modes for six different tibial-fibular deformities. *Arrows* indicate direction of forces. A, bone shortness. The frame is loaded in tension for bone and soft tissue lengthening. Distraction forces are applied through the frame to the site of osteotomy, resulting in significant tensile loading forces on the frames, which in turn increases tensile loading on the transfixion pins. B, bone nonunion. The frame is loaded in compression for bone fusion, which also increases tensile loading on the transfixion pins. This frame permits consecutive application of tensile loading for subsequent lengthening at the already fused site, so-called compression-distraction or "accordion" technique. C, bone with bending deformity. The frame is constructed with hinges to correct the bending deformity by applying forces opposite the direction of the deformity to achieve axial restoration. Olive wires are used to control or stabilize the bone position. The hinges on the middle rings are located on the convex side of the deformity, with force applied on the opposite side. This frame (and those in D, E, and F) allows consecutive application of compressive loading for bone fusion, and tensile loading for lengthening at the already straightened and fused site, the so-called straighten-compression-distraction technique. D, bone with shearing deformity. The frame is constructed to restore the normal axis of the bone by applying shearing forces to the site of displacement. E, bone with torsion deformity. The frame is constructed to rotate the distal fragment about an axis opposite the direction of the deformity by applying torsion forces to the site of displacement with a rotational mechanism (hinges and advancement screws) located between the middle rings. F, bone with combined deformities (e.g. compression-bending-torsion deformity). The frame is constructed to restore bone shape. It can be performed in a particular consecutive sequence (length-angulation-torsion) or in a combined process

To simplify frame assembly and disassembly, especially intraoperatively, the rings consist of two equal semicircular halves, connected by bolts and nuts (Fig. 8.3).

The perforated holes in the rings provide the basis for the Ilizarov system's flexibility; that is, multiple configurations are possible. The holes are situated on the same midline of the ring surfaces, equidistant from each other, and are of the same diameter. These factors make the rings easily connectable to each other and highly versatile in the construction of multiple types of frames.

The flat surface of the rings supports the heads of the bolts and nuts. The surface—bolt or nut interface ensures firm fixation of the wires, threaded rods, and bolts during the long course of treatment. Moreover, because all rings of the frame must be aligned perpendicular to the midline of the bone, the flat ring surface is paramount in achieving a secure wire inclination and plane orientation. The rings bear the stress of the tensioned wires (as much as 150 kg each) and provide rigid support for the entire frame.

The fixator components derive their strength and stability from their materials as well as from their design, being made of high-quality stainless steel alloys.

HALF-RING

The entire Ilizarov apparatus set contains half-rings in 12 sizes, each measured in its internal diameter in millimeters (i.e. 80, 100, 110, 120, 130, 140, 150, 160, 180, 200, 220, and 240 mm). Sizes 80 to 140 mm generally are used in pediatric patients, and sizes 150 to 240 mm in adult patients. Each half-ring, depending on its size, has 18 to 28 holes for the introduction of bolts or threaded rods. Each hole is 8 mm in diameter, and the distance between the holes is 4 mm (see Fig. 8.3B).

The diameter of the hole is slightly larger (2 mm) than the diameter of the rod and bolt, making introduction and alignment highly flexible. The difference of 2 mm between the diameter of the hole and the threaded rod has an important practical implication in assembly of the apparatus because, in this very complex procedure, it allows the surgeon greater flexibility in the angle of rod introduction.

Connecting Half-Rings

Figure 8.4 illustrates how two half-rings are joined to form a full ring. It is important that the surface is on an even plane when the half rings are joined. The connec-

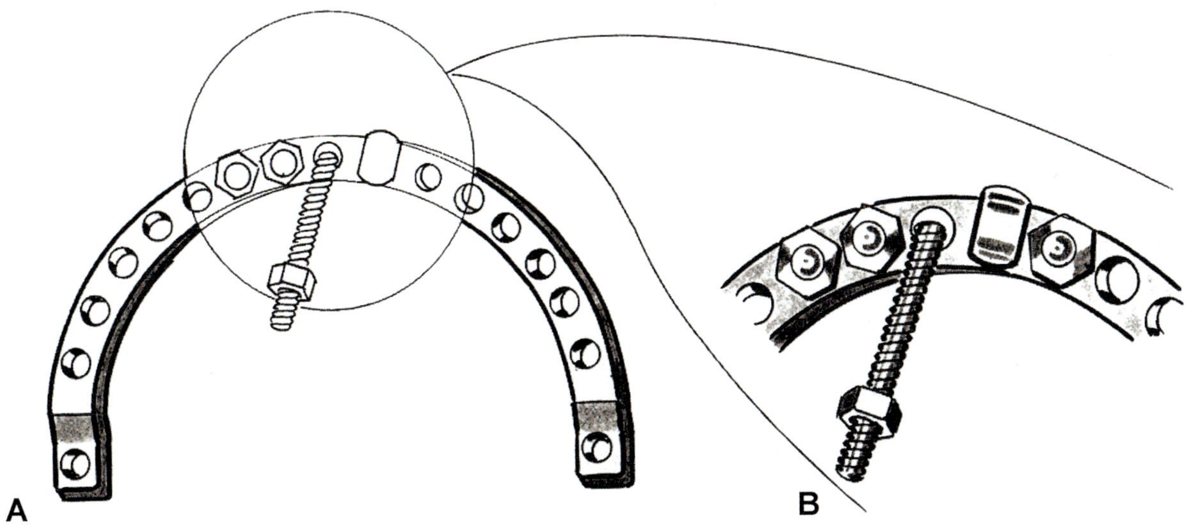

Figure 8.3: A, half-ring. Note two ledged areas on each end that serve to properly connect two half-rings. B, enlarged view of the half-ring shows a perforated hole and the flat surface, with a short connecting rod with nut. The diameter of the hole is 2 mm greater than that of the rod or bolt, allowing the surgeon flexibility of angulation and introduction of a bolt

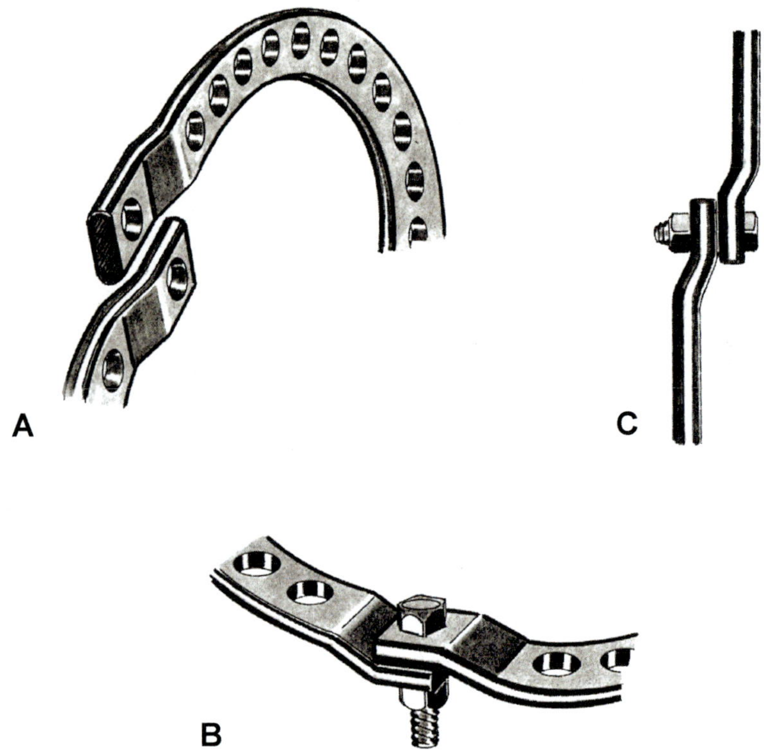

Figur 8.4: A, partial view of two half-rings in position to be connected. Note that the offset, ledged ends of the half-rings fit together on an even plane when correctly connected. B, partial view of the connected half-rings, connected correctly. C, partial view of two half-rings incorrectly connected, creating two discontinuous planes on each half-ring

tion of two half-rings to form a full ring is a crucial element in frame assemblage. After the half-rings are aligned, they are fixed with a bolt and nut (Fig. 8.4B). If they are connected incorrectly the surfaces will not be on an even plane (Fig. 8.4C). Two half-rings assembled on unequal planes cannot function properly because both will be at a different distance from the adjacent rings of the frame.

There also are full, one-piece circular rings of corresponding sizes in the complete fixator set, and other specially shaped half-rings.

Figures 8.5 and 8.6 show a full ring vs. half-ring construction. Each half-ring has one less hole on each side of the connection site than a full ring does. Thus at each connection site the ring has three holes less, and when assembled as a whole ring has six holes less than a full ring. This gives a full ring some advantages: It is slightly lighter because it does not require bolts and nuts to connect half-rings; and it has six more holes (Fig. 8.7A), which can be used for different purposes, such as the introduction of a connected plate, a threaded rod, or a hinge (Fig. 8.7B).

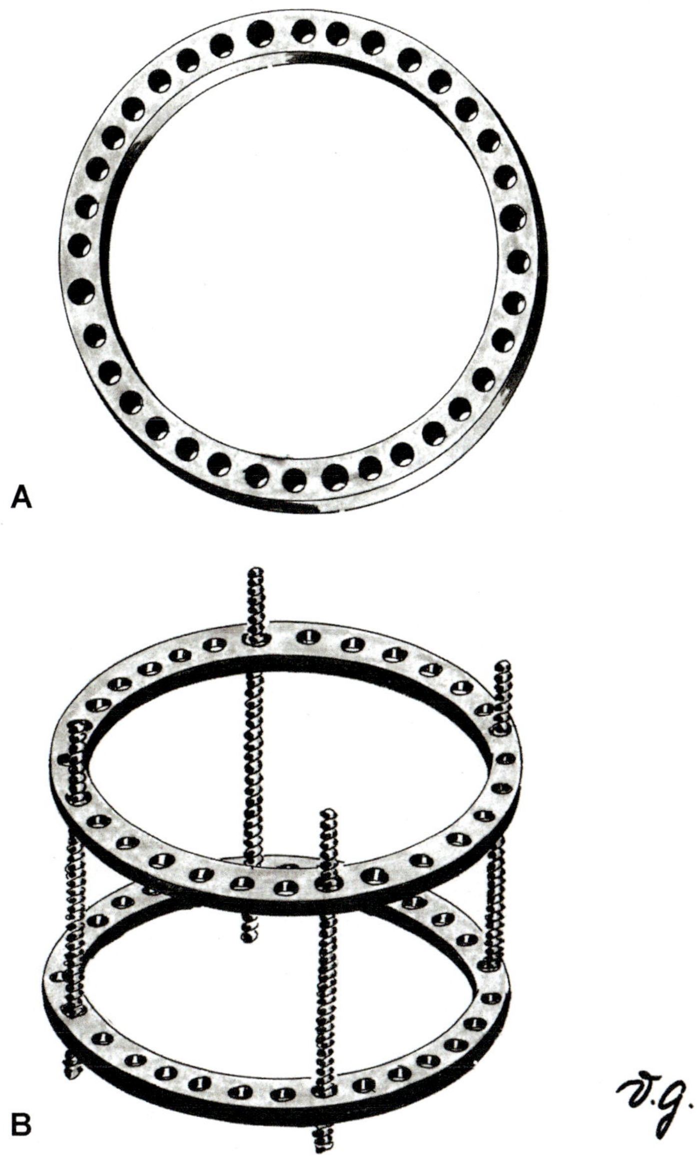

Figure 8.5: **A,** full ring. **B,** two full rings connected by four threaded rods, forming a component of the frame. Note that the threaded rods are equidistant and that the planes of both rings are strictly parallel

The full ring does have some disadvantages. For example, if the frame is assembled on the patient during surgery, the full ring must be positioned before introduction of the wires. Once the wires have been introduced, the full ring cannot be placed over them. Moreover, if for some reason there is tissue swelling and the full ring must be removed from the frame, it cannot be taken off over the other rings. A high-speed rotary

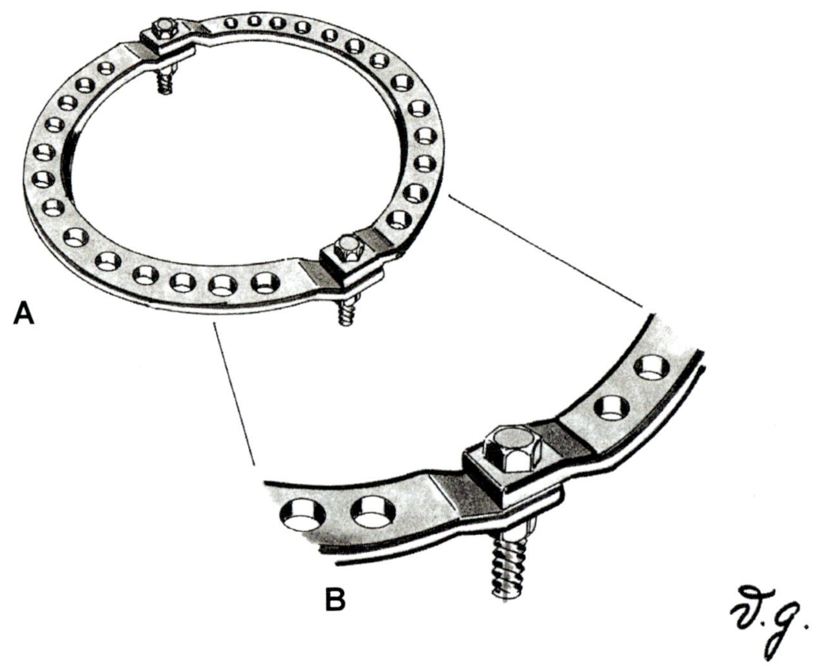

Figure 8.6: A, two connected half-rings. Note that at the sites of connection one hole is occupied by the bolt and nut and that for the purpose of frame strength there are no immediate holes on either side. B, enlarged view of the connection site of two half-rings

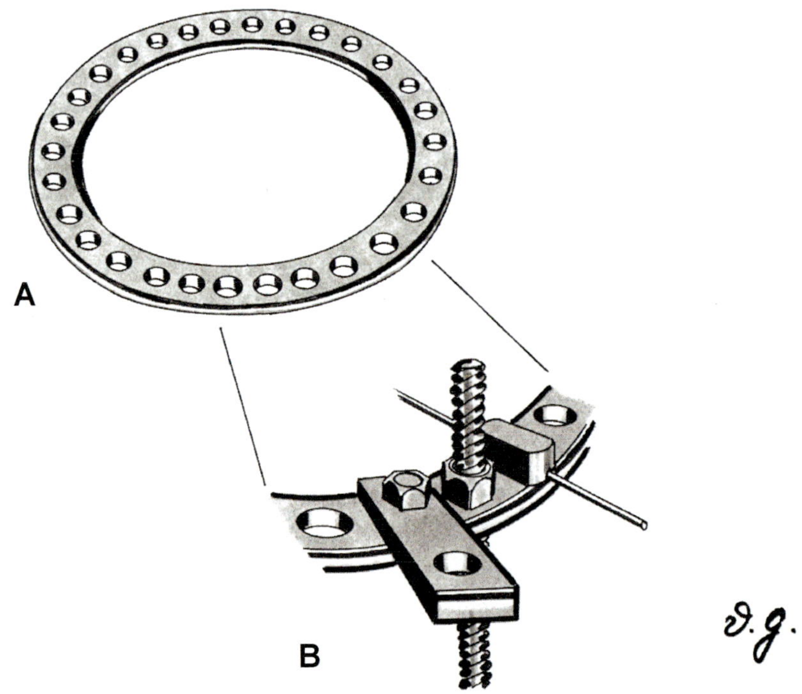

Figure 8.7: A, full ring. B, enlarged view of the full ring. Note that this segment corresponds in size to the enlargement in Figure 8-6B and that there are more holes to work with on the full ring than on the half ring

diamond saw (Anspach or Midas Rex) must be used to remove the full ring.

In some cases two half-rings can be connected, leaving a gap in the semicircle where the two ends do not meet. To construct this, a post and a support are fixed to the edged holes and are connected to each other with threaded rods (Fig. 8.8). This oval ring can be used to correct a displaced bone fragment or to lengthen a foot .

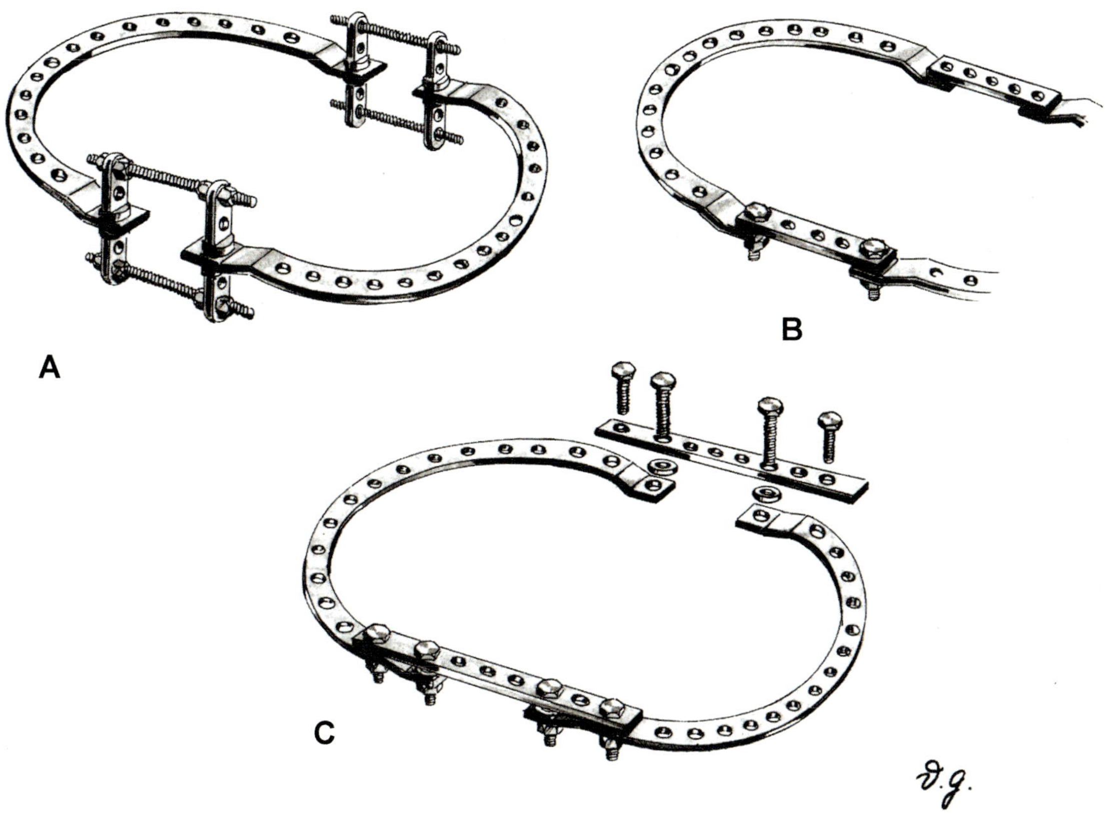

Figure 8.8: Three ways to connect two half-rings to form an oval ring, which can be used as a component of any frame, but usually as a foot component. A, two half-rings connected by four threaded rods. The post-support pair is fixed to each edged hole; then the rods are introduced on each side. The advantage of this configuration is that the distance between half-rings can be regulated simply by turning the nuts (shown on one side). B, two half-rings connected by two short connection plates (partial view). The plates are fixed to the ledged holes. C, to reinforce the oval ring, the two long connecting plates are used to connect the two half-rings. Note that washers must be used at the half-ring offset ends to securely tighten this connection

If only the small ring is needed at a particular level (e.g. in the forearm, hand, or a child's foot) the combination of three half-rings assembled in the shape of a clover is used (Fig. 8.9A). This cloverleaf increases the space between the ring and the limb (shown as a dotted triangle).

On rare occasions the combination of four half-rings can be used. This construct nets an even larger interior space (dotted lines in Fig. 8.9B), but makes the frame cumbersome.

Half-rings also are used for the foot component of a leg frame (Fig. 8.10). The half-ring at the calcaneal site usually must be elongated by adding two connecting plates to each of its legs. This permits more space for the obliquely introduced fixation wires. For stability and reinforcement, the second half-ring (usually the same

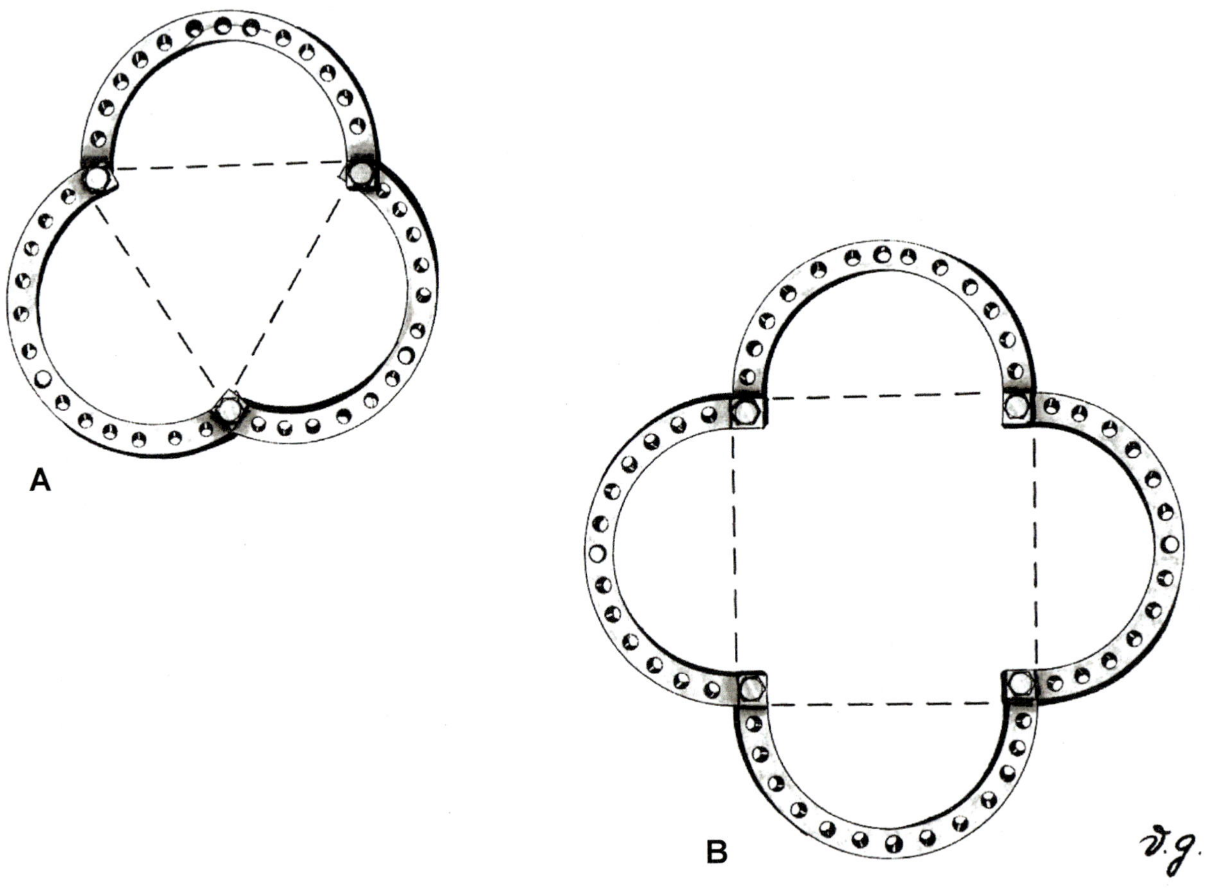

Figure 8.9: Clover-shaped rings are used to increase the space between the ring and the limb. A, three-leaf clover ring combines three half-rings. Increase of effective space is shown by *dotted triangle*. B, four-leaf clover ring combines four half-rings. Increase of effective space is shown by *dotted square*

size) is used at the forefoot section, and is connected to the plates with half-hinges (Fig. 8.10B). For forefoot stabilization, one half-ring can be attached to the leg frame (Fig. 8.11).

Two half-rings connected parallel to each other by the threaded rods can be used as a "puller" or "pusher" device inside the Ilizarov frame (Fig. 8.12). This device may be useful in correction of an angular deformity, as

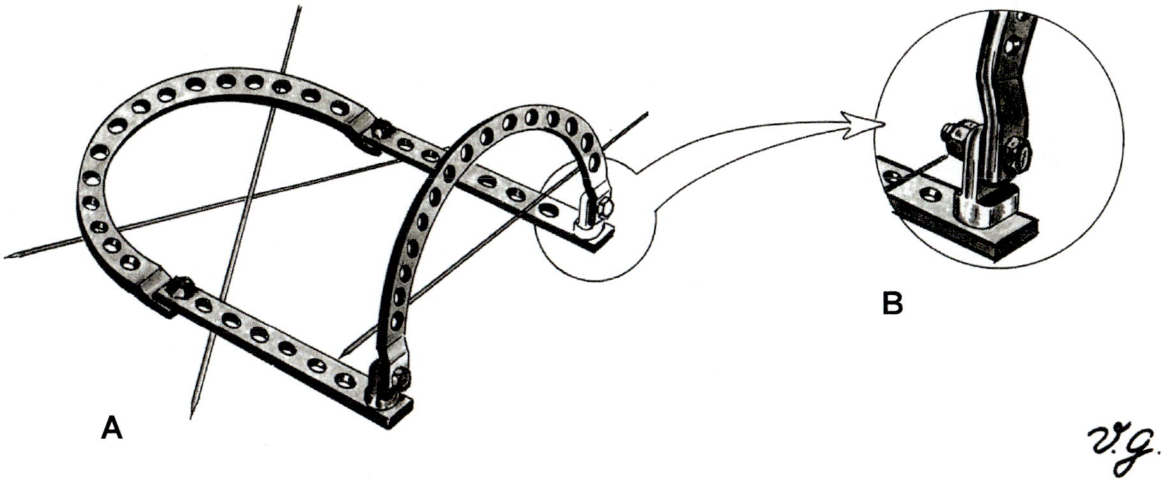

Figure 8.10: Use of two half-rings for the foot component of the leg frame. This component can be used for foot stabilization and for prevention of equinus deformity. A, foot component. The calcaneal half-ring is placed horizontal to a plane parallel to the plantar foot surface. By connection with two long plates, it supports a vertically placed forefoot half-ring. The advantages of this configuration are provision of effective space for the obliquely introduced K-wires and greater flexibility in using various planes for forefoot K-wires. B, enlarged view of foot component shows the connection between the horizontal plate and the vertically placed half-ring, accomplished with a half-hinge

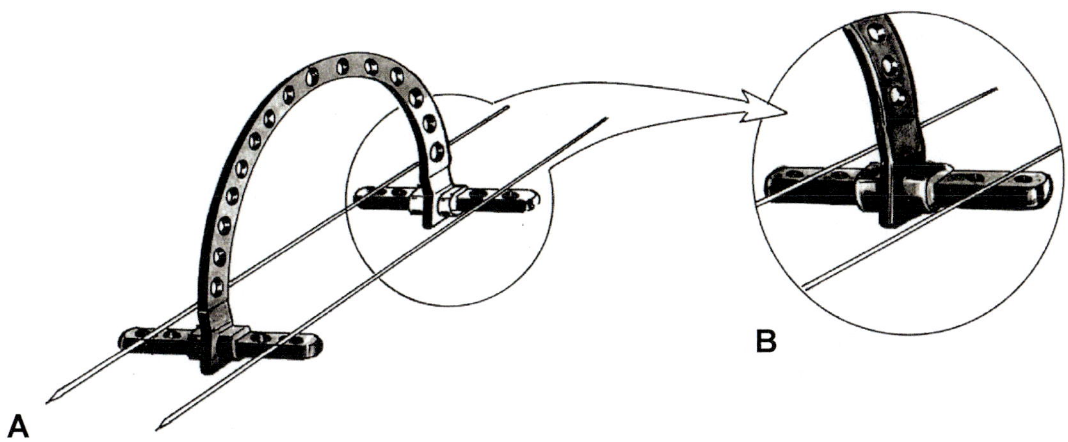

Figure 8.11: Half-ring can be used as a separate forefoot supporter. In this case the forefoot has to be transfixed by two parallel K-wires, for stability and to decrease pain. A, half-ring forefoot supporting component. A post-support pair is attached to each hole at the offset configuration at the end of each half-ring. The half-ring then is attached to the leg frame by two threaded rods placed at each side. B, enlarged view of same component consists of a post-support pair fixed to the offset end of the half-ring. This allows introduction and fixation of two parallel K-wires equidistant to one another

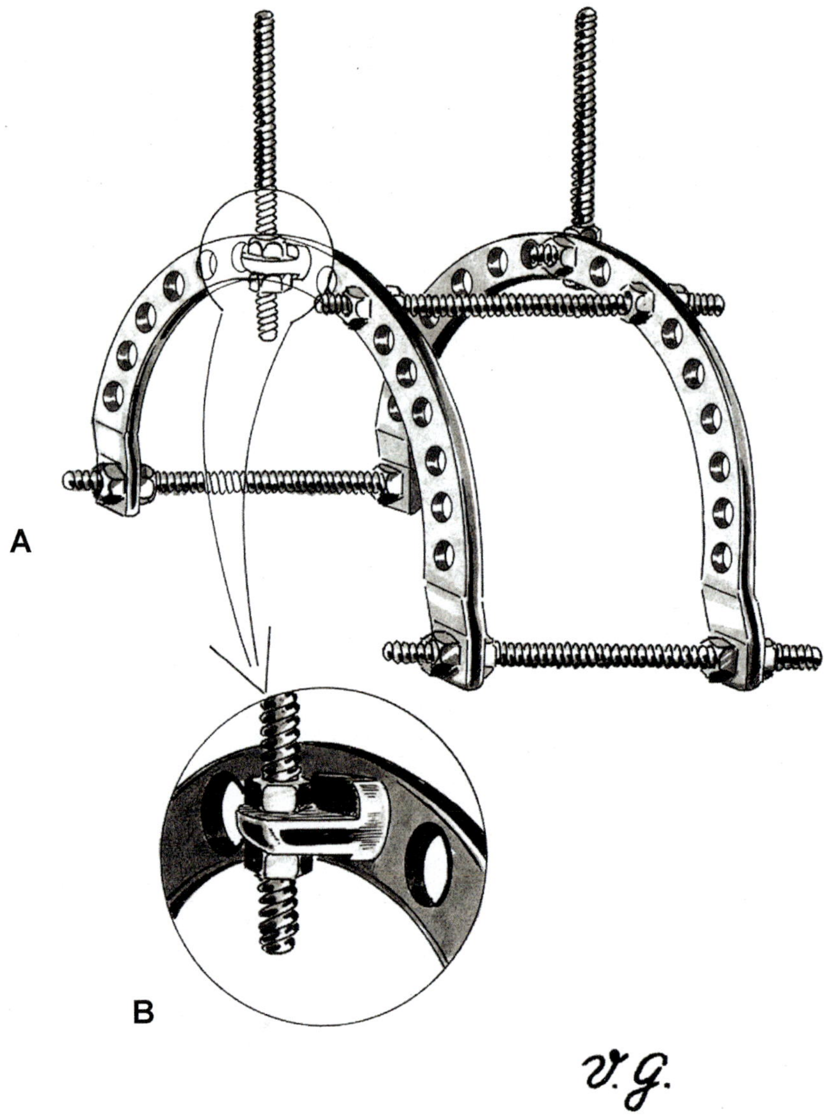

Figure 8.12: A, puller-pusher device. It consists of two parallel half-rings, each of which is attached to the motionless component (not shown) of a main frame by threaded rods. B, enlarged view of the half-ring connection to the motionless component of a frame. As shown, it consists of a half-hinge fixed to a half-ring and a threaded rod

in pseudoarthrosis or nonunion with angulation. Because this puller-pusher device is used to shift the bone fragments perpendicular to the longitudinal axis, it must be fastened to a fixed part of the frame. This is accomplished with a distraction-compression device (Fig. 8.13), consisting of two hinged supports connected by threaded rods. One connection site is on the half-ring, and the other on the long plate (Fig. 8.13).

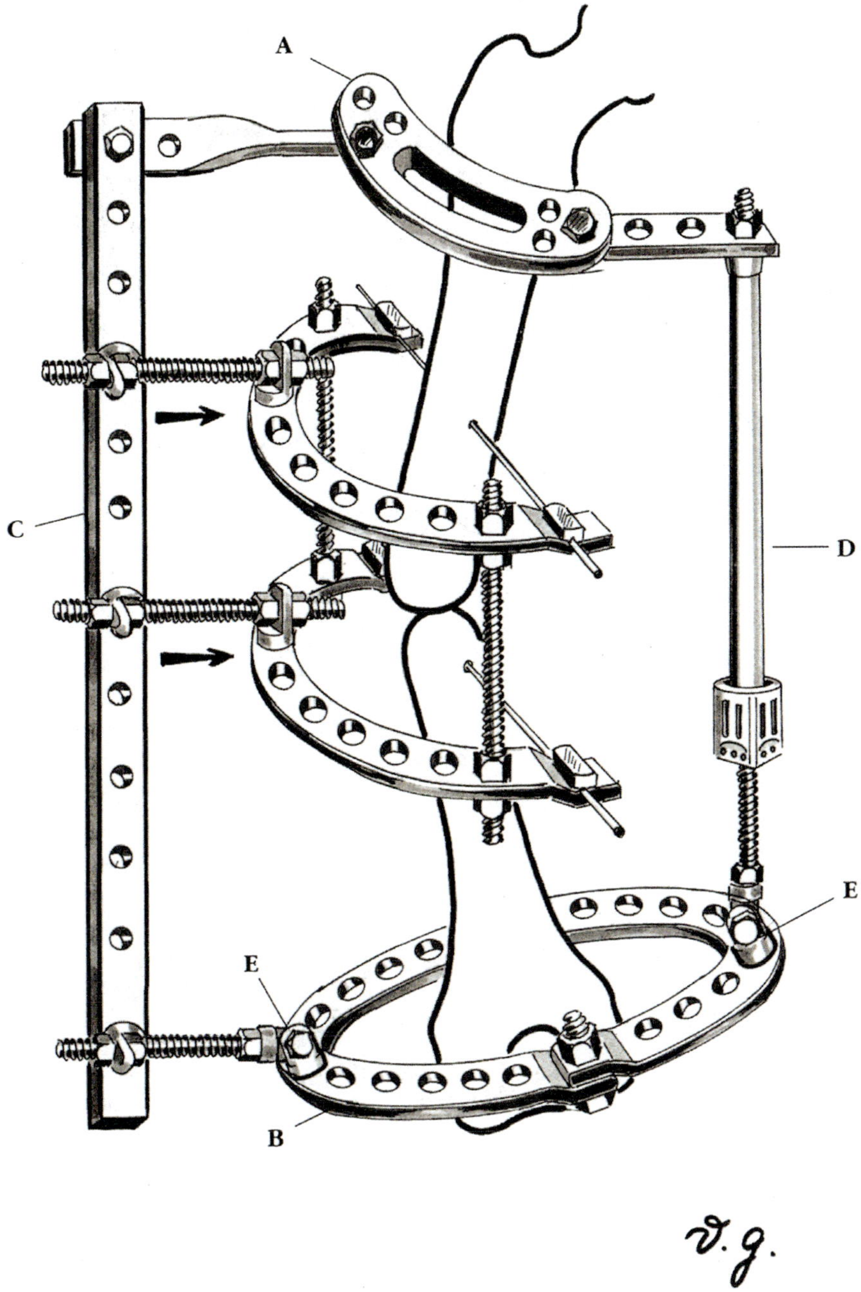

Figure 8.13: Schematic representation of an angulated femoral bone pseudoarthrosis with an applied Ilizarov frame. The frame consists of a proximal arc (A) and a distal ring (B) connected by a long plate (C) and graduated telescopic rod (D). For the purpose of angulation correction, the puller-pusher device (two half-rings) is included. *Arrows* show the direction of the applied forces. Note that the distal ring is connected to the frame with two hinges (E). Hinges are used so that the distal ring can move as the bone is straightened gradually

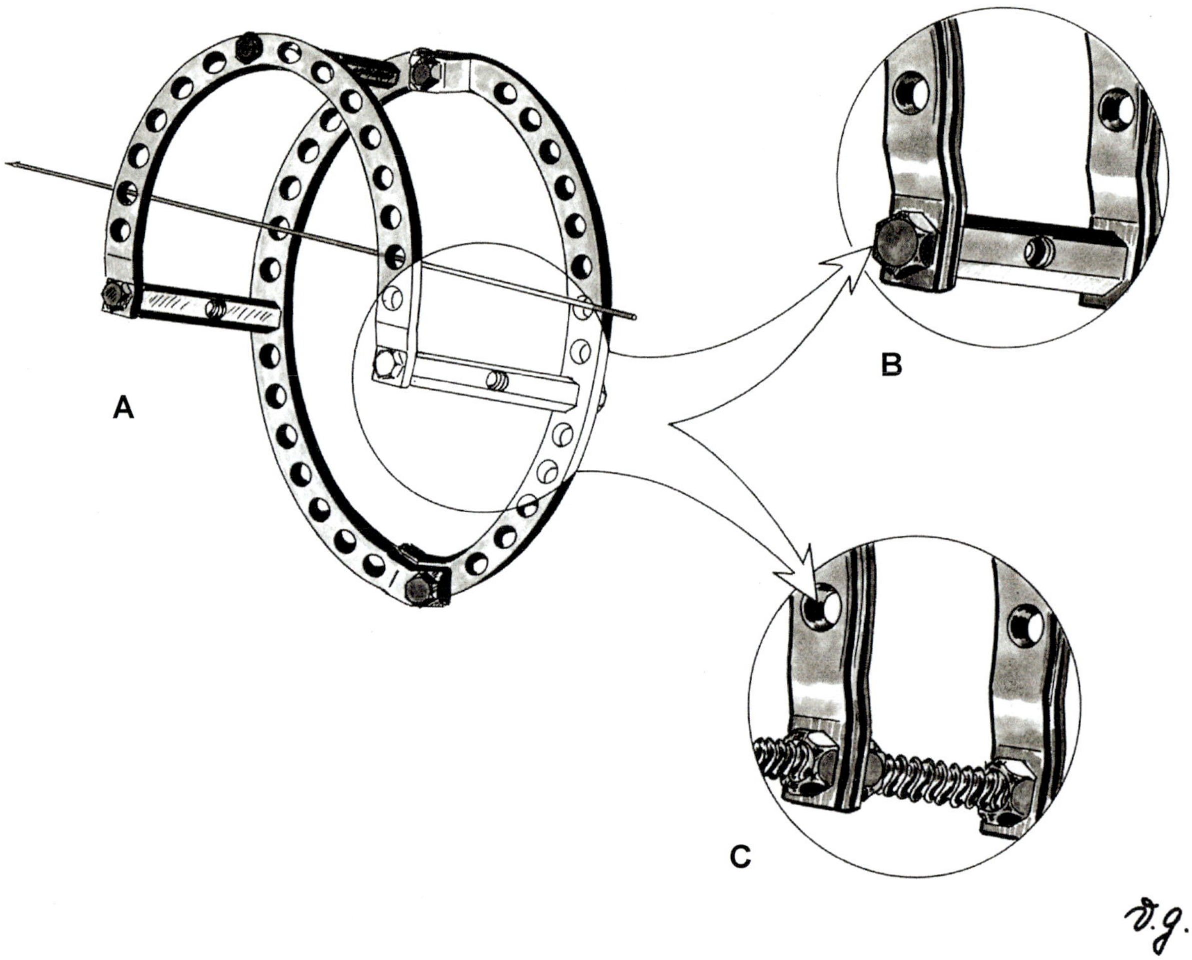

Figure 8.14: A, frame component for use near the knee joint, proximally or distally. It consists of a half-ring connected at three points to a full ring by threaded hexagonal sockets. Note transversely placed K-wire. B, enlarged view of component in A illustrates the method by which the hexagonal socket connects the ring and half-ring. C, enlarged view shows use of a threaded rod rather than a hexagonal socket, as a connector

Another use of half-rings is in combination with a full ring in the metaphyseal region (Fig. 8.14A). This construct permits free range of motion in the nearby joint, and at the same time reinforces the frame. For stability, the half-ring must be connected to the full ring at a minimum of three points. The connection usually is accomplished with threaded hexagonal sockets (Fig. 8.14B) or with short threaded rods (Fig. 8.14C). The half-ring is fixed to the bone with one wire because this configuration does not permit significant angulation between two wires. For stabilization, however, it is better to use two crossed wires, and thus a five-eighths ring.

FIVE-EIGHTHS RING

If the ring is situated close to the joint it can prevent or severely restrict motion. In such cases it is useful to use a five-eighths ring because this configuration eliminates the normal circumference, thus permitting less restricted joint motion (Fig. 8.15A). This situation arises primarily with knee and elbow joints, and is difficult to avoid because the wires must be introduced at the level of the tibial condyles (Fig. 8.15B) or the humeral epicondyles (Fig. 8.15C). Another advantage of the five-eighths ring is that there is more room for introduction of two cross wires. The five-eighths ring is not, however, strong enough by itself, especially for the load of the tensioned Kirschner wires; thus it must be used in combination with a full ring. The three-point connection to the full ring reinforces it and makes it almost as strong as the full ring.

Five-eighths rings are made in three sizes: 130, 150, and 160 mm in internal diameter. The 130-mm ring is used mostly near the elbow or in the pediatric knee, whereas the other two often are used for the adult knee.

On rare occasions the five-eighths ring also may be used in the middle of a regular frame configuration if there is a need for special care of soft tissues. It is easier to provide this care with part of the frame circumference opened. Indications for this usage include the existence of a myocutaneous flap, a large open wound with skin and soft tissue defect, or a large deep incision (as in compartment syndrome). In all such cases the five-eighths ring must be positioned with its open section over the area of special care, and must be connected at a minimum of three points to the adjacent rings in the frame (Fig. 8.16).

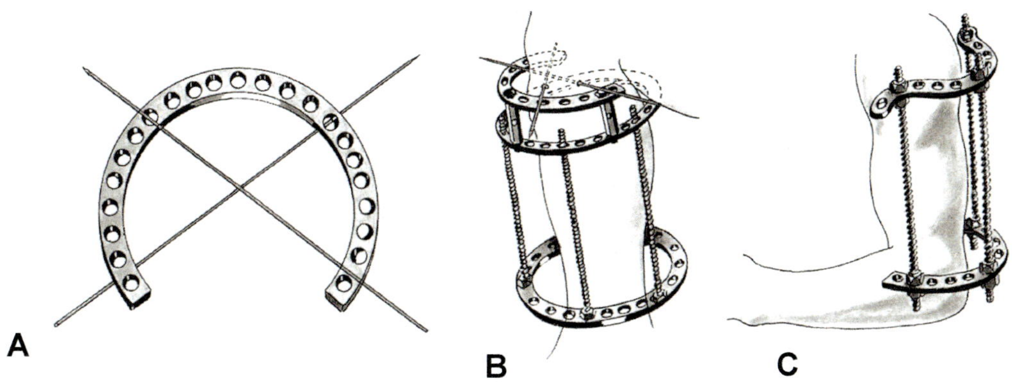

Figure 8.15: A, five-eighths ring with two crossed K-wires, used in areas where range of motion is essential, primarily in the knee and elbow. This ring gives the surgeon more working space for introduction of K-wires, as in the tibial condyles (B) and the humeral condyle (C)

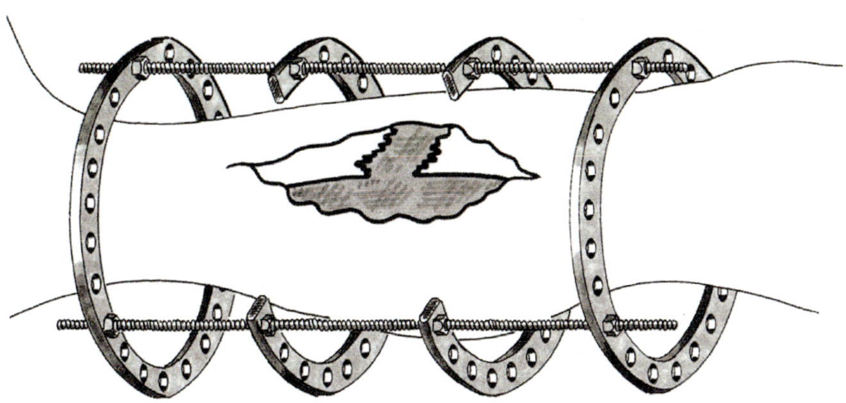

Figure 8.16: On rare occasions five-eighths rings also may be used as middle components of a stable full frame, particularly when the surgeon needs access to an open wound with bone and soft tissue defect. To use five-eighths rings in this configuration a high degree of frame stability must be assured. Thus the rings must be attached to the proximal and distal full rings at a minimum of three connection sites (with rods and bolts)

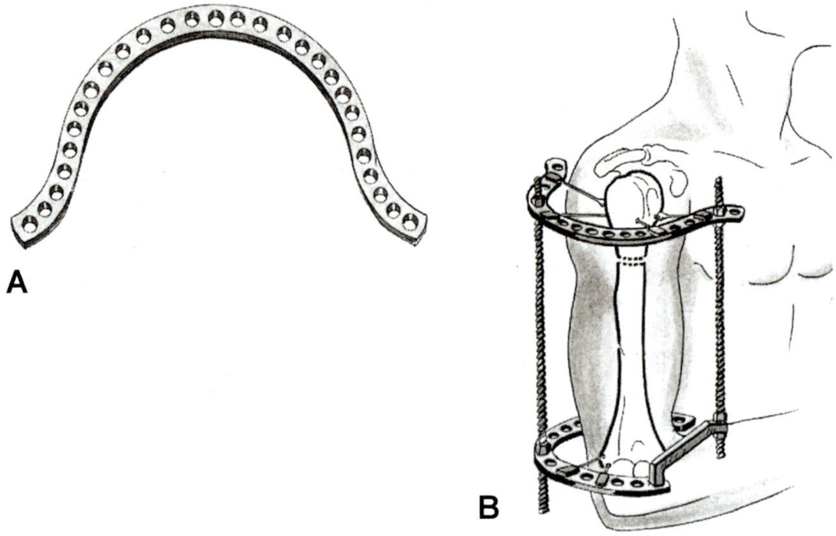

Figure 8.17: A, half-ring with curved ends. B, because of its shape, this half-ring is used exclusively in the deltoid area of the shoulder

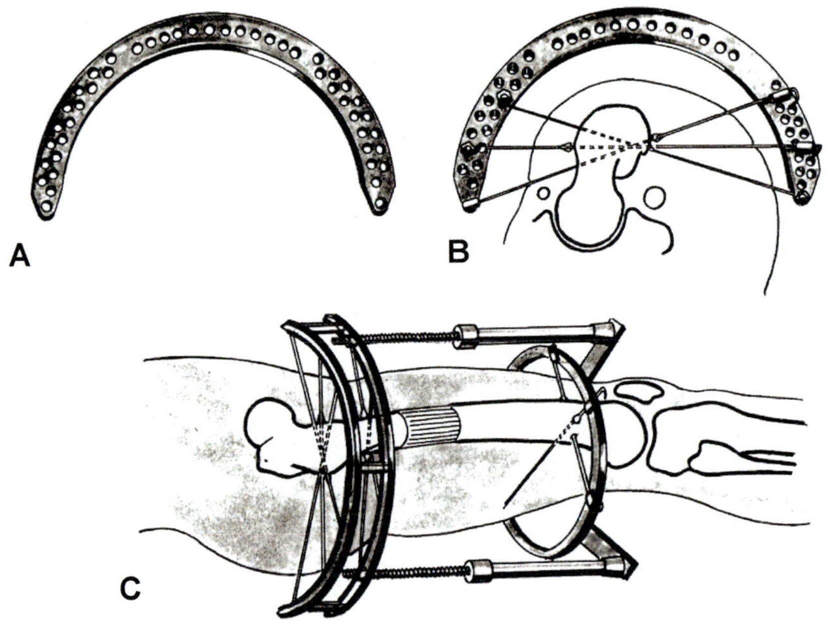

Figure 8.18: A, semicircular arch with wide walls and double row of multiple holes. These arches are much larger than five-eighths rings. B, the arch is used for femur fixation, with K-wires inserted at the level of the greater trochanter. C, K-wires are introduced in a fan-like pattern, and the sciatic nerve must be avoided carefully

HALF-RING WITH CURVED ENDS

The half- ring with curved ends extremities is essentially a modified five-eighths ring in which the ends curve outward (Fig. 8.17A). This configuration fits perfectly the deltoid area of a shoulder, and thus is used exclusively for the shoulder section of an upper extremity frame. The half-ring with curved ends is not

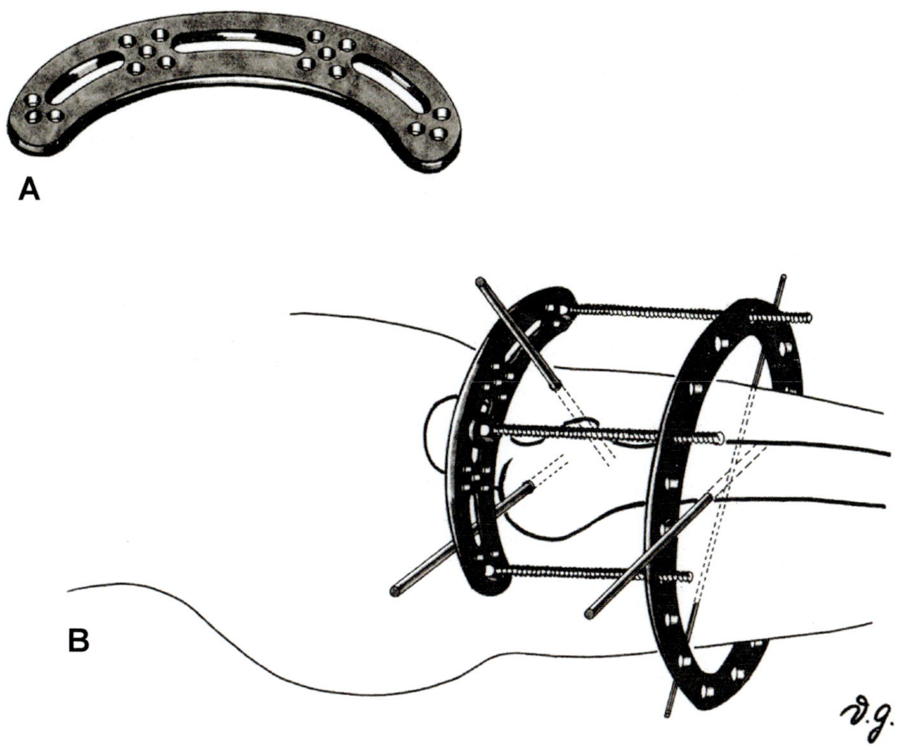

Figure 8.19: A, 90-degree femoral arch. B, schematic representation of a proximal part of the femoral frame component. The 90-degree arch and the full ring are connected by three threaded rods. Note that on the lateral side both the full ring and the arch are fixed to the bone by half-pins

so strong as a full ring, but its three-point connection to the adjacent ring permits it to bear any necessary loading stresses. Figure 8.17B shows an Ilizarov frame for the upper arm that uses the half-ring with curved ends in combination with a five-eighths ring.

ARCHES

In the original Ilizarov set there were large-diameter (290 to 300 mm) semicircular arches with wide walls and double rows of multiple holes (Fig. 8.18A). This arch was constructed for upper femur fixation, with five to six wires at the level of the lesser trochanter (Fig. 8.18B). The arch must fit the trochanteric area along with the adjacent buttocks soft tissue. The wire must be arranged fan-like, at approximately 30-degree angles. It is inevitable that some wires will be very close to the sciatic nerve (Fig. 8.18C).

Dr. Ilizarov and his assistants, as well as other orthopedists in the Soviet Union and other eastern European countries, have used these upper femoral arches for years. Despite their experience, there are some disadvantages to using such a large component with dangerously placed wires. Drs. Cattagni and Cattaneo, of the Lecco District General Hospital in Italy, in the 1980s introduced a new component for use in the proximal femur. An essential part of this component is a modified arch in two versions. Instead of a large semicircular construct with wide walls, they developed 90- and 120-degree arches with slots (Fig. 8.19). Assemblage of this new component is facilitated by the introduction of two or three half-pins instead of wires. The half-pins are drilled in two cortices of the anterior and lateral subtrochanteric regions, and do not come close to the sciatic nerve (Fig. 8.19B). A detailed description of this frame is provided in Chapter 11.

9 Chapter

Ring Connections

BOLTS AND NUTS

Rule number 1 in the assembly of any type of Ilizarov frame is that all parts must be fastened together firmly with bolts and nuts. No matter which part of the frame is being connected, it must be fastened immediately to another component. Immediate, firm tightening achieves the stability necessary for the frame assemblage. Fastening is achieved with the bolts and nuts. No screws or screwdrivers are used. From the beginning, Dr. Ilizarov consciously excluded anything sharp from the system, in particular, a screwdriver, to prevent any serious injury to the patient.

Use of bolts and nuts is the best and simplest way to tighten the parts of the frame together. Several types are used.

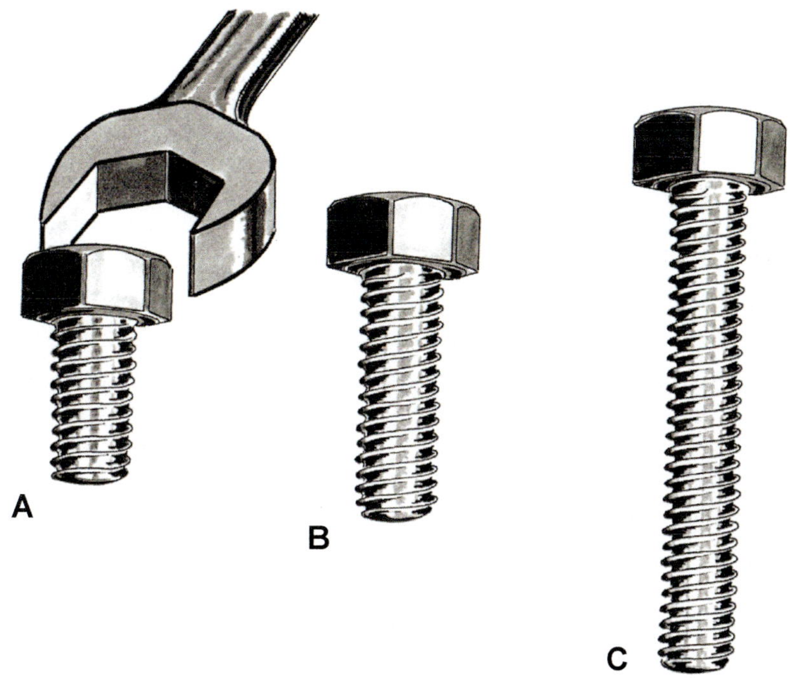

Figure 9.1: Three types of bolts with the standard hexagonal head. They differ from each other in leg length. A, 10-mm length bolt shown with the standard 10-mm wrench, which fits all types of bolts. B, 16-mm length bolt. C, 30-mm length bolt

Connecting Bolts

There are three types of connecting bolts in a set. Common features are the threaded leg, 6 mm in diameter, with a pitch equal to 1 mm between each thread, and a standard 10-mm hexagonal head, 4 mm thick. The bolts differ from each other in length, being 10, 16, and 30 mm (Fig. 9.1). Recently some companies in Europe and the United States have added a 25-mm bolt, but it is not included in a standard set. Each type of bolt has its own purpose.

The 10-mm connecting bolt is too short to connect all types of parts. It is used only for connecting the threaded sockets and bushing to the rings or connecting plates and for fastening the rods and half-pins through the apertures of the socket, bushing, and Ilizarov telescopic rod (Fig. 9.2).

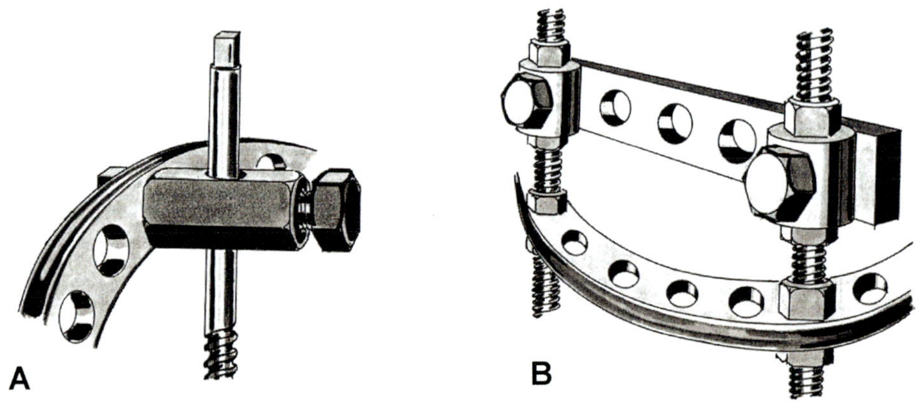

Figure 9.2: Two frame components consisting of parts connected by 10-mm bolts. A, frame component used for half-pin introduction. The 10-mm bolts are used to tighten the threaded hexagonal socket to the ring and to lock the half-pin into the socket aperture. B, frame component for ring segment reinforcement. The 10-mm bolts are used to tighten two bushings to the threaded rods. Two additional 10-mm bolts (behind the plate) are used to fasten the transverse connected plate

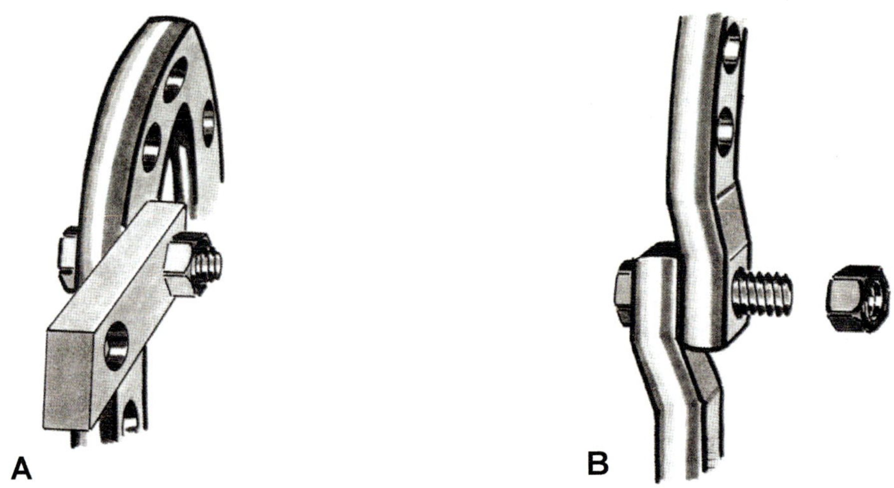

Figure 9.3: Parts of a frame connected with a 16-mm bolt. A, short connection plate connected to a ring with a 16-mm bolt. Note that the bolt length is particularly suited to connecting the ring, the plate, and the nut (16-mm total). B, offset ends of two half-rings are connected by the 16-mm bolt. The nut is shown separately

The 16-mm bolt is one of the most important parts of the set. It is used to connect all main parts. Because the thickness of most parts is equal (5 mm), this bolt is long enough to fasten two parts together and still allow enough space to tighten the nut (Fig. 9.3). The 16-mm bolt also can be used instead of the 10-mm bolt by screwing one 5-mm thick nut onto it.

Both the 10-mm and 16-mm bolts are used for connecting the female post to the rings and plates. The 16-mm bolt penetrates deeper into the threaded hole of this part, and can be used for two-, three-, or fourhole posts. The 10-mm bolt alone can be used for the female hinge because it has a short threaded hole.

The 30-mm bolt is used to connect three or more parts (Fig. 9.4). It is also useful in cases in which a gap must be left between two parts.

Nuts

The smallest component of the set is a 10-mm nut, which serves multiple purposes in the frame assembly. It is used to:

1. Tighten the connecting bolts
2. Stabilize the connecting rod
3. Tighten the wire fixation bolt
4. Act as driven force for the ring in a distraction-compression movement

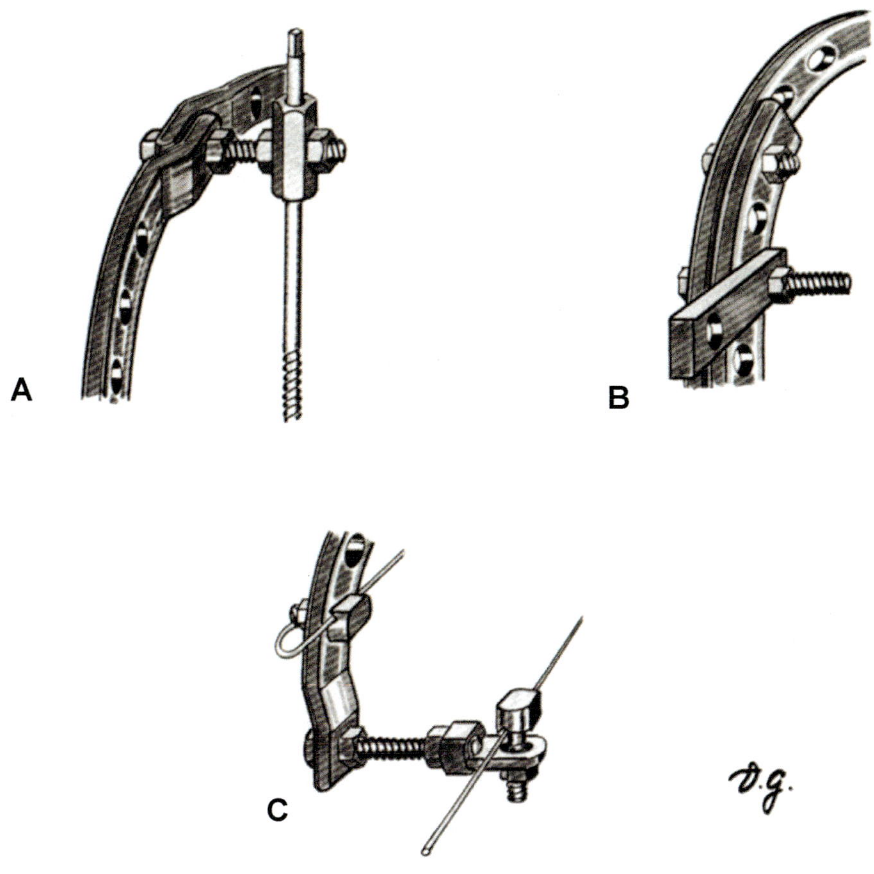

Figure 9.4: Three possible uses of the 30-mm bolt are represented on three sections of the ring. A, 30-mm bolt is used to connect two half-rings and to support a half-pin by attaching a threaded socket to its free end. B, one section of a ring is reinforced by attachment of a five-eighths ring with a 30-mm bolt and a short connecting plate. Note the 16-mm bolt, above the plate, which is only long enough to connect two parts. C, 30-mm bolt is used here to support an offset (drop) wire. A half-hinge supporting a fixation bolt is attached to the bolt to effect this function, and the fixation bolt purposely is open. Note the second K-wire attached to the ring with a wire-fixation bolt

5. Lock the socket and/or bushing onto a threaded rod
6. Affix the pulling wire of a distraction device
7. Achieve fixed positioning of a male support
8. Secure hinge clearance
9. Secure a gap on the threaded rod.

There are three types of hexagonal 10-mm nuts: a full, or 6-mm nut; a three-quarter, or 5-mm nut; and a half, or 3-mm nut (Fig. 9.5).

To stabilize the frame an extremely strong force, sometimes as much as 300 kg, must be applied when tightening all nuts. The frame must be able to bear the patient's weight, to sustain distraction-compression forces, and support the patient's physical activity during many months of treatment. Because of the intensity of this tightening, it is easy to damage or even break some of the fine threads of the nut and bolt. In fact, this is why a bolt and nut, once used, should never be reused for a second frame. Reused bolts and nuts may break and seriously weaken the entire frame.

The thickness of the three types of 10-mm nut corresponds to the number of threads of each. One thread's pitch equals 1 mm, thus the full nut has six threads, the three-quarter nut has five threads, and the half nut has three threads. Depending on the number of threads, different nuts serve different purposes in the frame assembly. Inasmuch as one thread's pitch equals 1 mm, one full turn will produce 1 mm of movement on the rod, which is the recommended average amount of

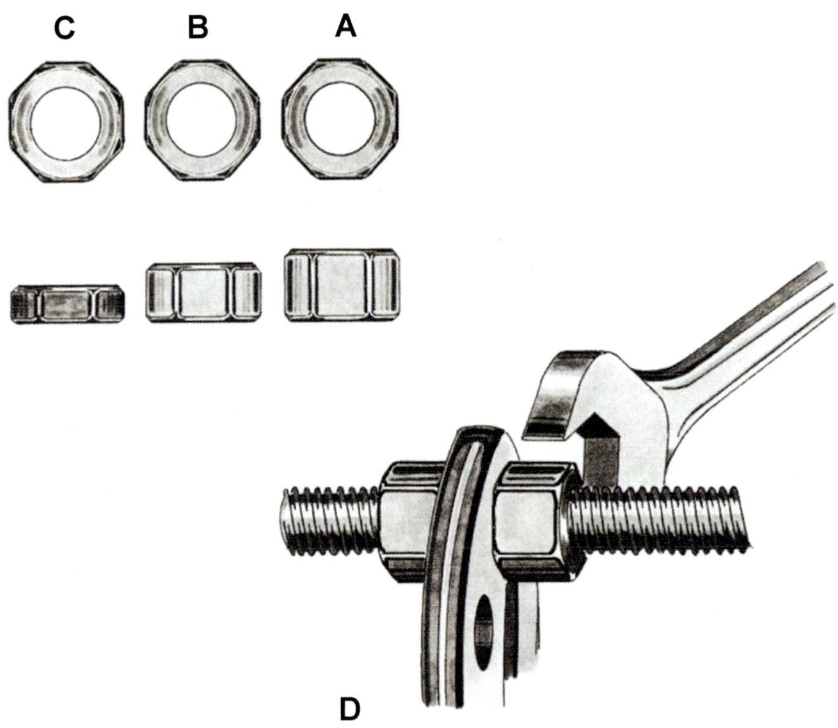

Figure 9.5: Three types of hexagonal nuts from the Ilizarov set. A, full, 6-mm nut. B, three-quarter, 5-mm nut. C, half, 3-mm nut. D, two 6-mm nuts typically are used to secure a long connecting rod to a ring

distraction-compression in the Ilizarov lengthening method for 1 day. Thus the turn of the nut is used as a driving force in the Ilizarov technique (Fig. 9.6). Usually, one-fourth turn four times a day is the recommended distraction-compression rate for 1 day.

A completely stable nut that can be fixed securely after each one-fourth turn is needed for this purpose. The full 6-mm nut perfectly matches this requirement. It has 6-mm threads and is secured on the threaded rod, even if damaged. This nut is used to connect a frame with multiple rods (Fig. 9.7A). Four 6-mm nuts are required

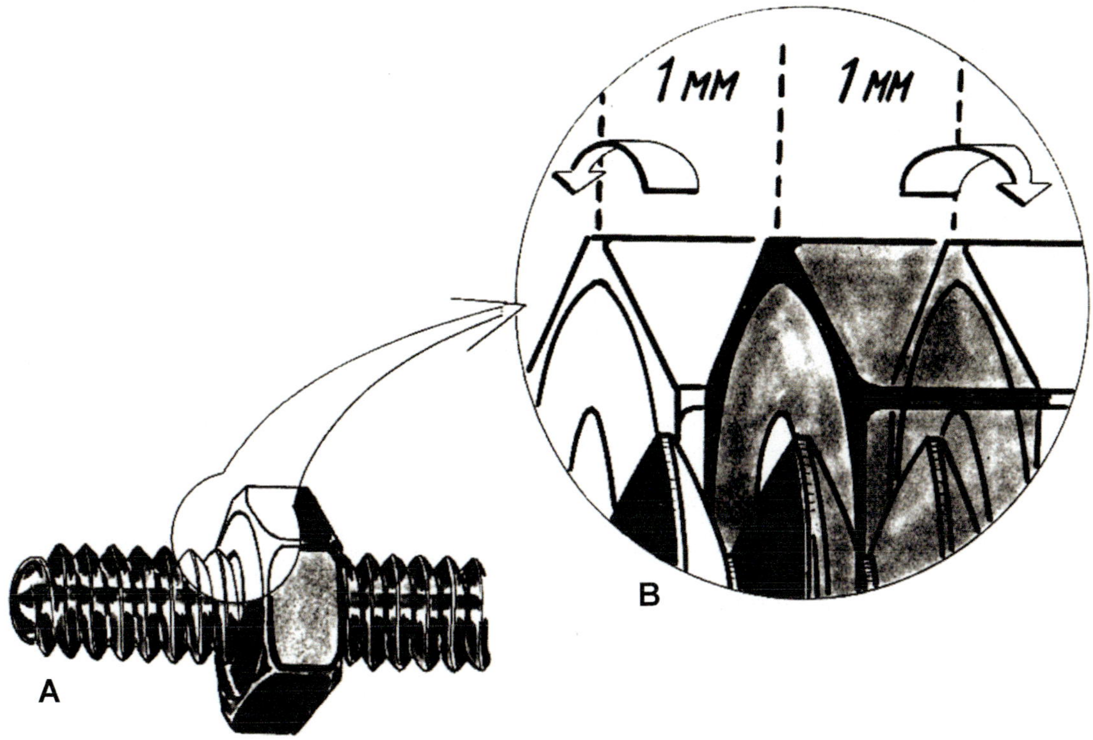

Figure 9.6: Position of a nut as it turns along a threaded rod. A, the nut is screwed onto the threaded rod. B, schematic of an enlarged section of the nut and rod. *Arrows* indicate the direction of the tightening nut; with each full turn it advances 1 mm

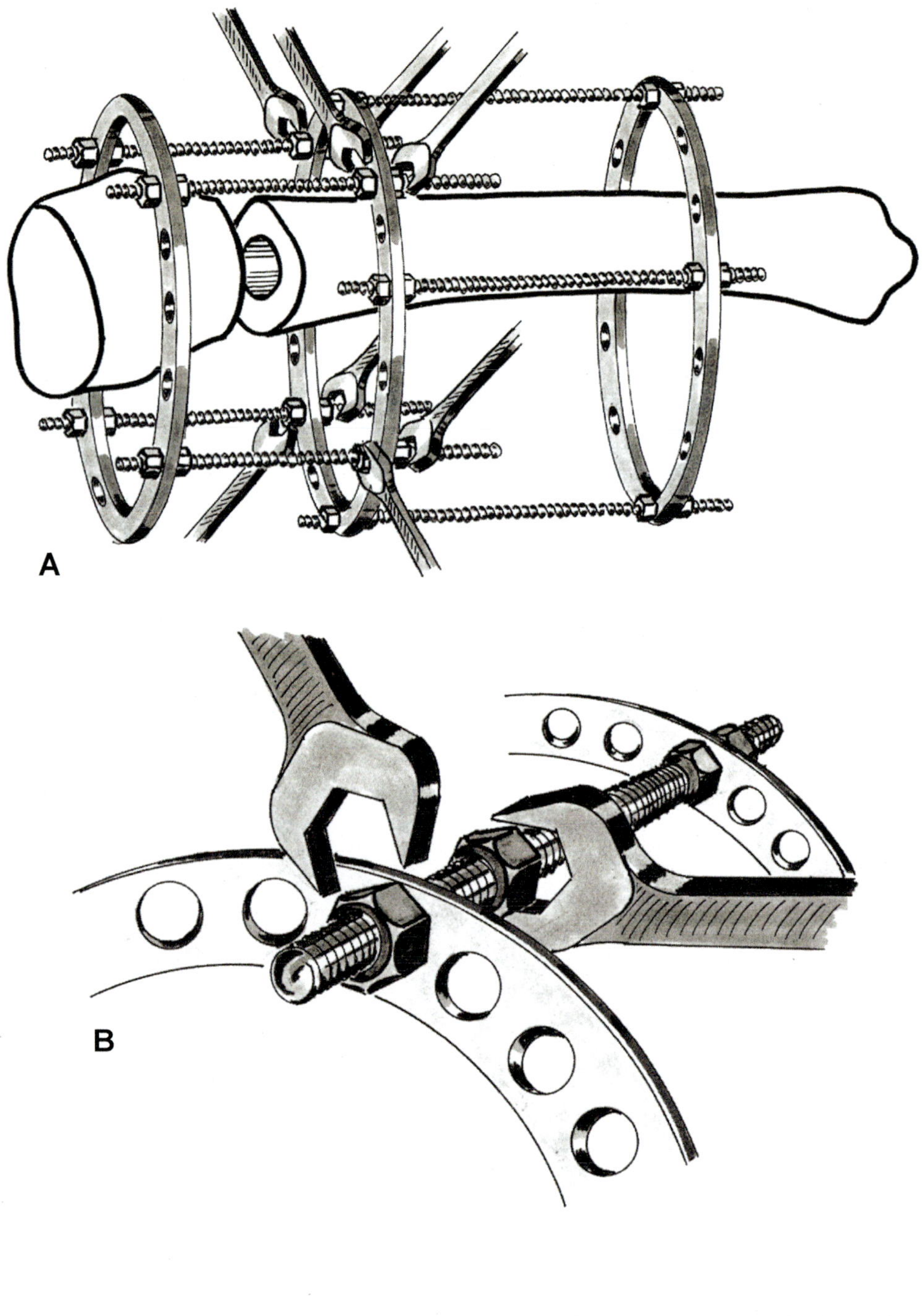

Figure 9.7: A, schematic of the osteotomized tibial bone with a three-ring frame. Four pairs of full (6 mm) nuts are attached to the middle ring. Distraction-compression forces are brought about by turning the nuts with four pairs of wrenches. *Note:* In reality, this technique of distraction-compression is performed with just one pair of wrenches, applied consecutively to each pair of nuts. B, enlarged section of ring, with two pairs of full-size nuts and two wrenches used for fixation and for compression-distraction

for fastening when the distraction-compression technique is used (Fig. 9.7B).

To facilitate a one-fourth turn, Richards Medical Company introduced a special quadragonal nut. It is 10-mm long, with a 10-mm quadragonal head marked with dots, from 1 to 4, signifying increments of a full turn. The quadragonal shape is convenient for distraction-compression movements and is very stable with 15 threads (Fig. 9.8).

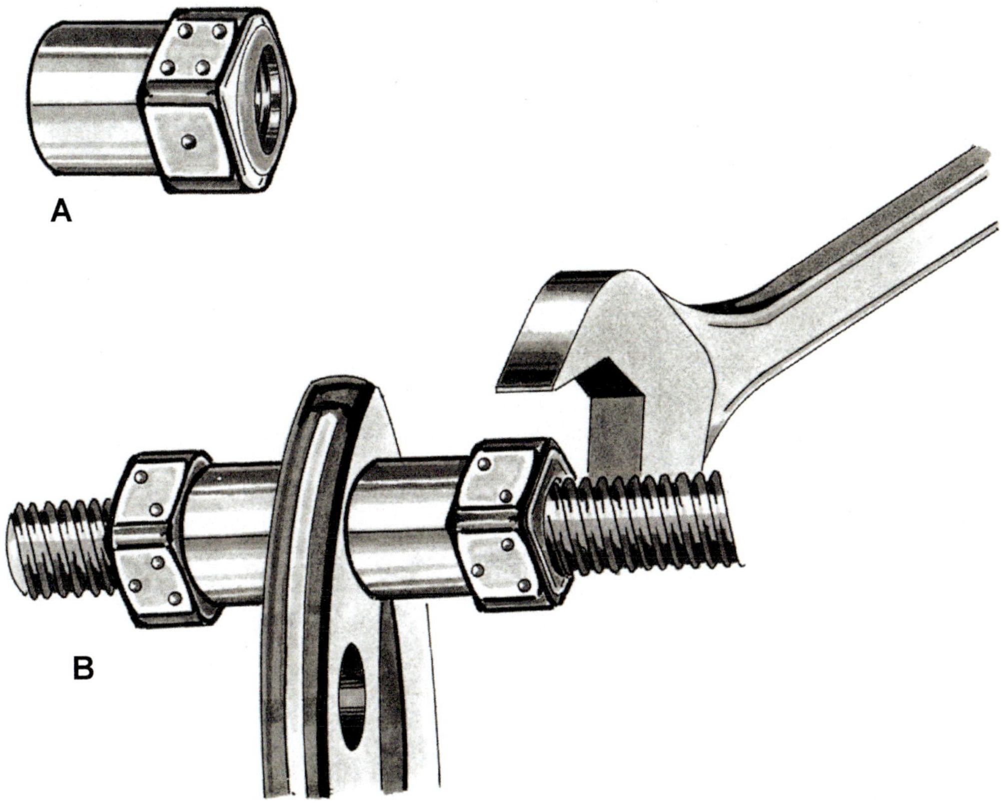

Figure 9.8: A, combined nut with quadragonal head for use in distraction-compression technique. B, section of a ring with two combined hexagonal nuts attached to the threaded rod. Two wrenches used for one-quarter (0.25 mm) turn

The three-quarter (5-mm) nut is the most widely used in all frame constructions. It is completely stable, and at the same time is narrow. The 5-mm nut is highly convenient for frame stabilization (Fig. 9.9A), for connecting two half-rings, and for bolt fixation and tightening (Fig. 9.9B). It cannot be considered strong enough by itself for use with distraction-compression devices.

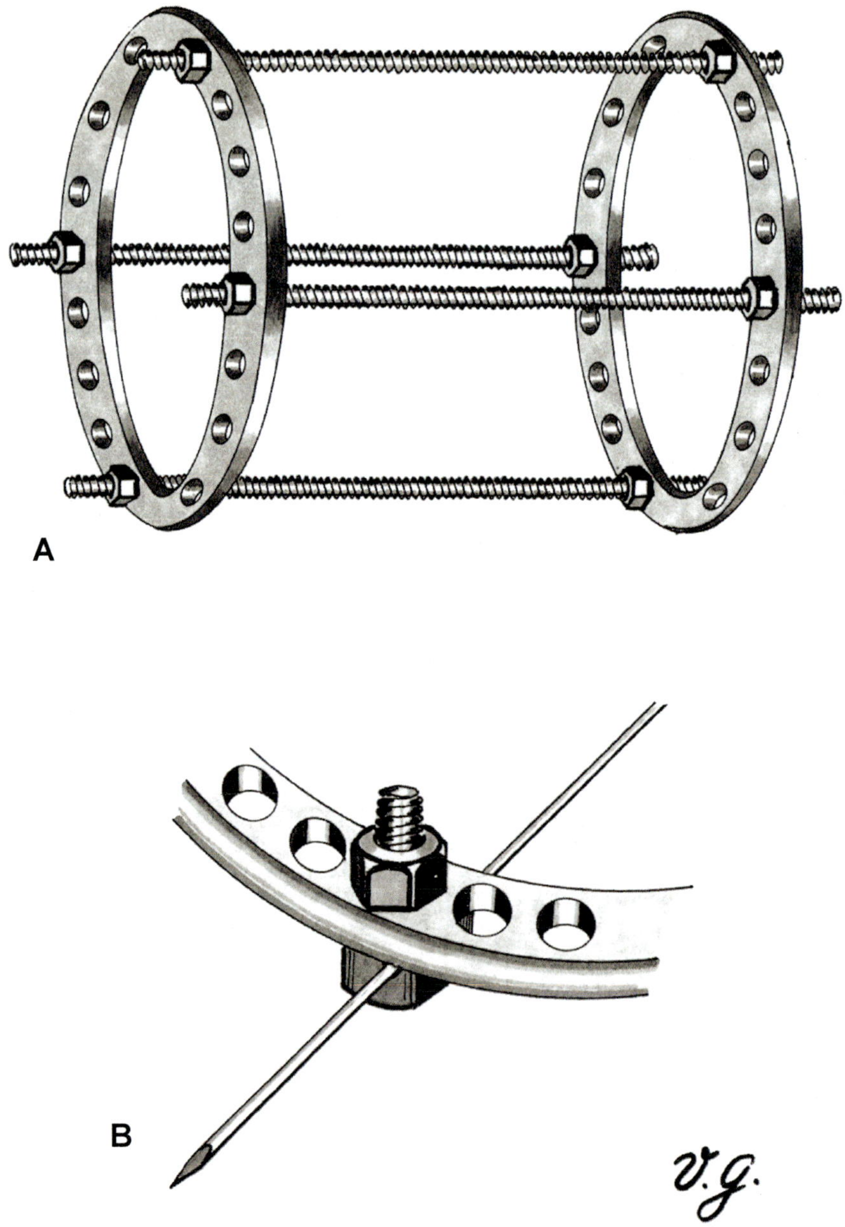

Figure 9.9: A, two-ring frame connected by four threaded rods, which are fixed to the rings with 5-mm nuts. B, wire fixation bolt fastened to the ring with a 5-mm nut

The 5-mm (three-quarter) and 6-mm nut combination is used in some frames, notably to construct the distraction-compression device. This pushing-pulling device consists of a threaded rod with one cannulated end to which a K-wire is attached. The K-wire then is bent and tightened between two 5-mm nuts, while on the opposite end of the rod two 6-mm nuts are fastened. These 6-mm nuts serve the purpose of distraction (or pulling the K-wire), which requires the strength to withstand forces equal to distraction-compression (Fig. 9.10). The 6-mm nut is stable enough for this purpose.

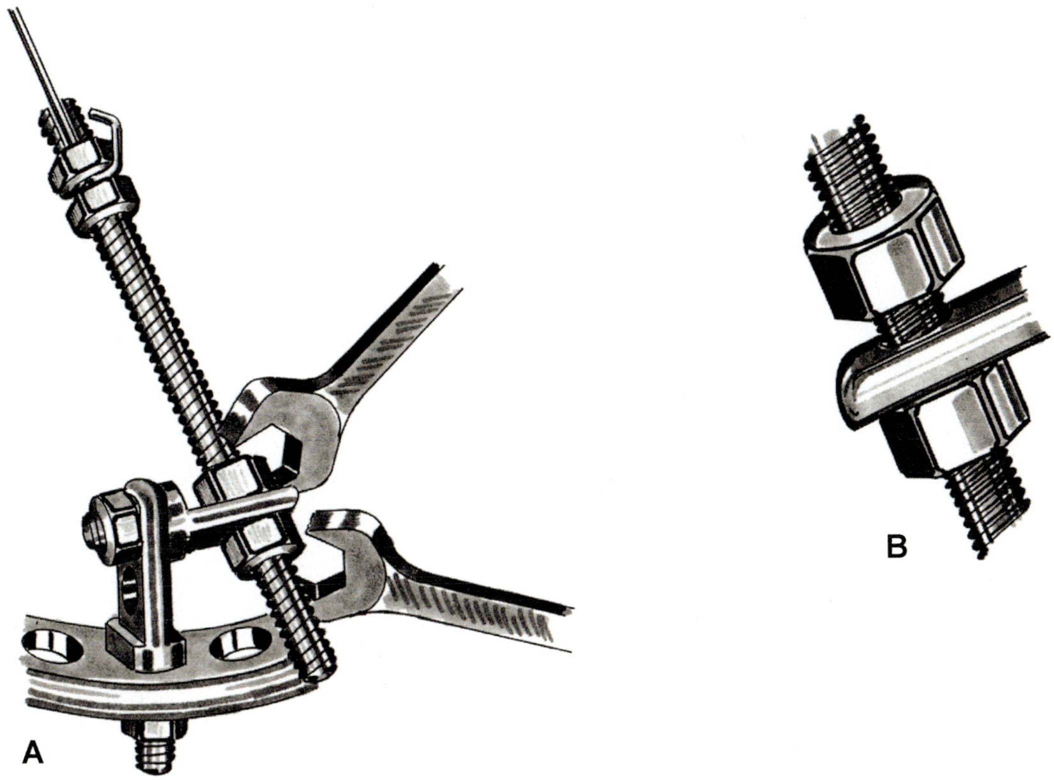

Figure 9.10: A, section of a ring showing an attached pushing-pulling device and two wrenches. Note that four of the nuts are all 5-mm (three-quarter) nuts, and that the two nuts near the wrenches are 6-mm (full) nuts. Only the full nuts may be used to produce movement of the slotted threaded rod, and thereby the pulling force of the tensioned wire. B, enlarged section shows two 6-mm nuts on the threaded rod. The upper nut is turned so that it is three threads from the supporting half-hinge. To produce downward movement of the rod, the lower nut must be turned upward three full revolutions

The 3-mm thick half nut has only three threads, and cannot produce a bond secure enough to fasten main components. It is used as a supplementary nut only, chiefly for hinge construction, to lock the 5-mm nut in a position to secure a gap between two connected half-hinges (Fig. 9.11).

A special type of stopper nut with a nylon insert also is used for hinge construction. The nylon stopper nut enables the surgeon to achieve lock-tight fastening in any desired position, producing a secure gap (Fig. 9.12). This stopper nut turns very stiffly, and cannot be used for any other purpose.

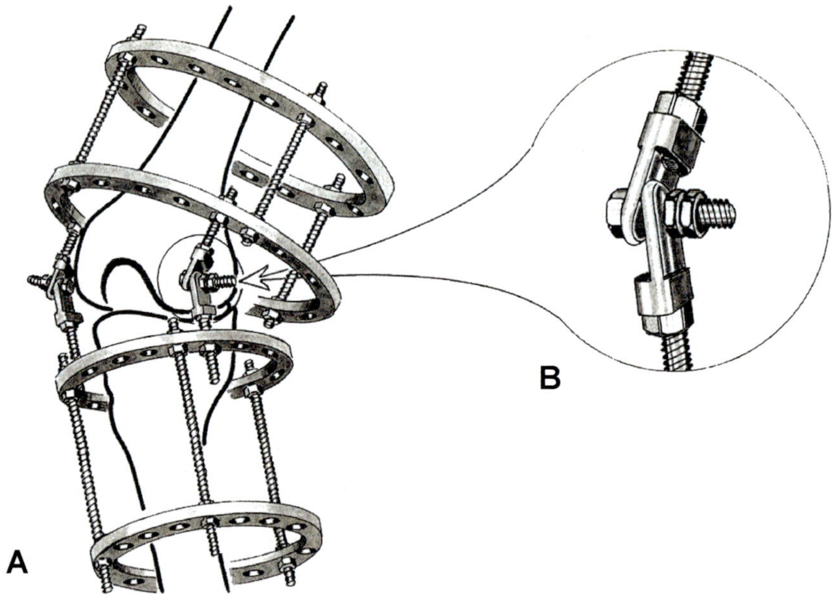

Figure 9.11: Use of hinges and 3-mm nuts. A, schematic of the knee joint in a position of flexion with two Ilizarov frames attached. One frame (shown partially) is attached to the femoral bone, the other to the tibia. The two frames are connected to each other by two hinges. Note that the hinges are placed at the level of the knee joint instant center. B, enlarged view of the hinge. Two half-hinges are shown connected by a 16-mm bolt, leaving a 2-mm gap between their flat surfaces. This gap is secured by two tightened 3-mm nuts. Each nut serves as a stopper to the other

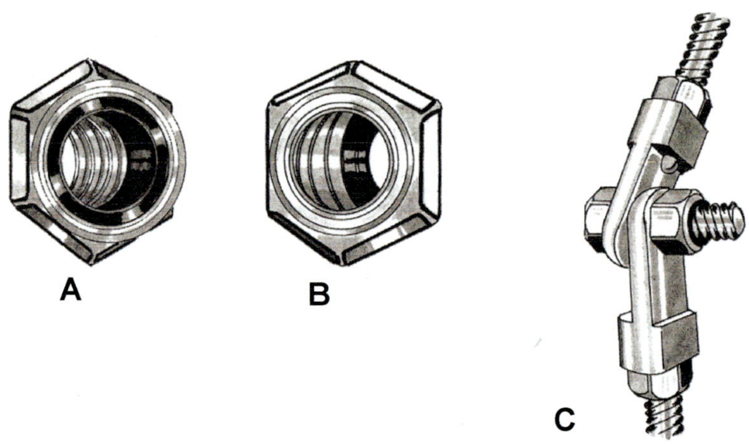

Figure 9.12: Nut with nylon insert and its usage with the hinge. A, frontal view of the nut. Note that only three threads are shown, and the smooth surface of the nylon insert occupies the rest of the aperture. This smooth area of elastic nylon serves as a stopper. B, reverse view of the same nut. There is no nylon stopper on this side, and thus the nut is placed on the threaded leg of a bolt with its back facing the bolt head. C, hinge, consisting of two half-hinges connected by a 16-mm bolt. The 2-mm gap between the surfaces of the half-hinge is secured with the nylon stopper nut

RODS AND PLATES

Ring connections play a crucial part in the assembly of any type of frame. They determine rational distribution of frame strength, balanced arrangement of different structural loading, and stability of the frame attachment to the bone fragments. The proper types and sizes of ring connectors and the way they are fastened predetermine the success of treatment.

The seven types of ring connectors in the Ilizarov set include threaded rods, partially threaded rods, telescopic rods, connection plates, graduated telescopic rods, threaded sockets, and oblique support connectors. The first five ring connectors are in the original set; the last Itwo were added by the Italian orthopedic group, The Association for the Study and Application of the Methods of Ilizarov (ASAMI). Each of the ring connectors has its purpose and must be used accordingly. Some ring connectors must be used in combination with others, for reinforcement of frame stability. Furthermore, some of the connectors are suitable for very different purposes. Knowledge of these many purposes and skillful use of the connectors are essential to facilitate frame assemblage.

Rods

The main type of connector in the Ilizarov system is the 6-mm in diameter stainless steel threaded rod. The threaded rods come in 10 lengths: 60, 80, 100, 120, 150, 200, 250, 300, 350, and 400 mm.

All rods share the same pitch (i.e. the distance between two threads), which equals 1 mm. This is important because it signifies that one full turn of the lock nut corresponds to a change (e.g. in distraction or compression) also equal to 1 mm (see Fig. 9.6). In fact, the threaded rods serve not only as the primary ring connectors but also as ring direction guides in the crucial distraction and compression motion.

The threaded rods have high strength characteristics for axial loading, but their ability to withstand bending decreases dramatically with increased length. Thus at least four rods must be used to connect two neighboring rings, affixed at equal distance both vertically and horizontally on the rings (Fig. 9.13). *To assure equality of distance when affixing connecting rods, a practical tip is to count the holes of the ring and divide by four.*

Biomechanically, four threaded rods provide much greater protection against bending than three rods do.

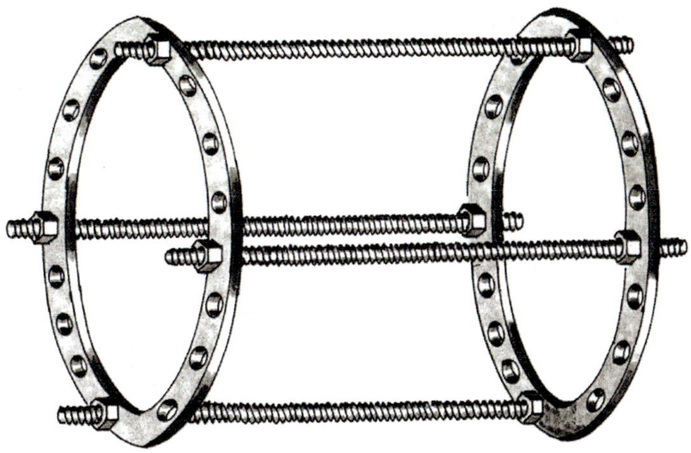

Figure 9.13: Threaded rod exhibit characteristics of high axial load stiffness, but their ability to withstand bending forces decreases significantly with length. Thus four threaded rods always must be used to connect two rings

Biomechanical principles also have shown that, for reasons of strength and stiffness, the distance between two neighboring rings must be not greater than that of the diameter of the ring.

Slotted Cannulated Rod

The slotted cannulated rod has special functions in connecting rings. This rod may serve as a connector and at the same time may be used as a pulling device (Fig. 9.14).

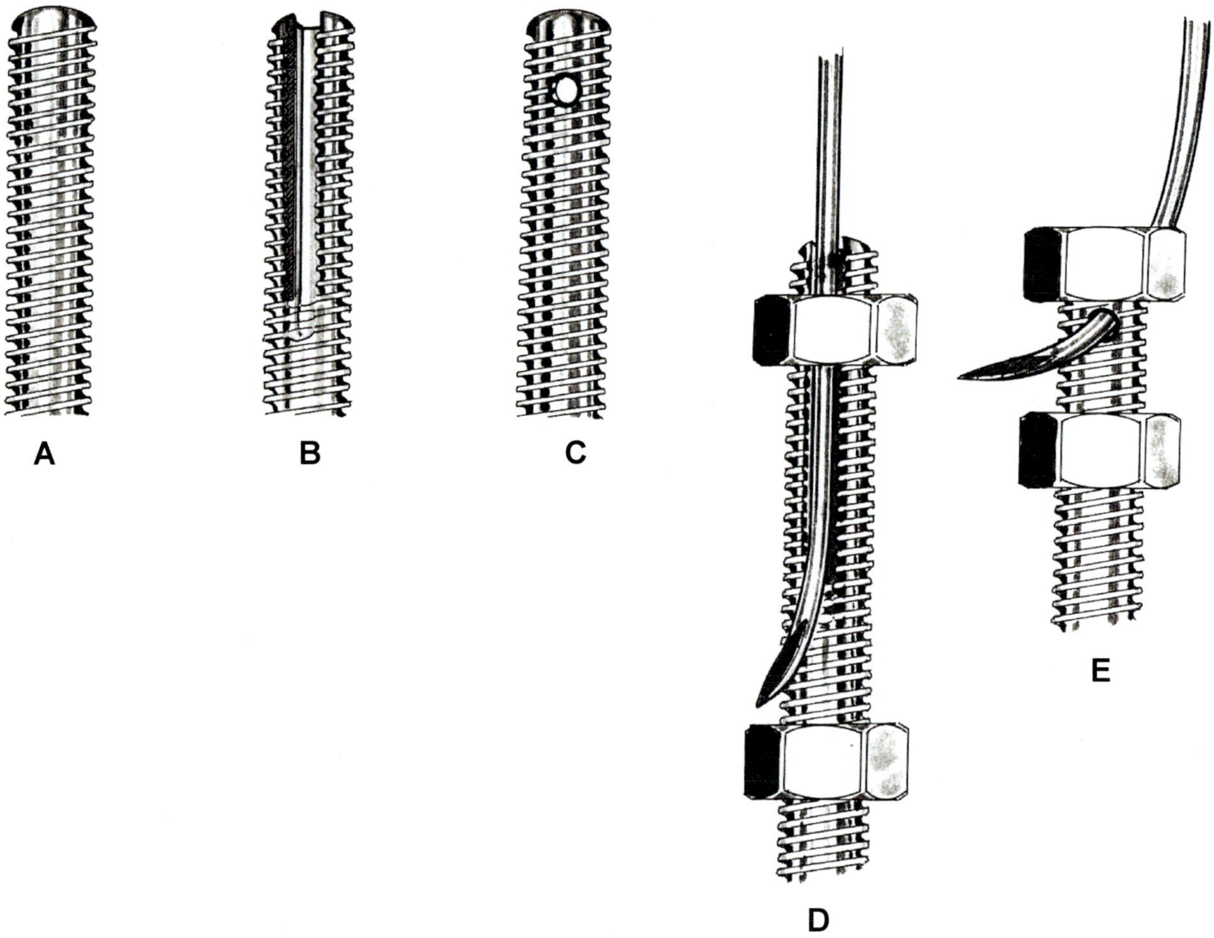

Figure 9.14: Partial views of three types of threaded rods. A, end of a standard threaded rod. B, end of a slotted threaded rod. 2 x 2-mm slot extends the length of 20 threads. C, end of a cannulated threaded rod. A 2-mm aperture is drilled out at the top. D, slotted threaded rod with an introduced K-wire. The K-wire must be bent 90 degrees and locked in by the two 5-mm nuts. E, cannulated threaded rod with an introduced K-wire. To tension and affix the K-wire, it must be bent 90 degrees and locked in by the nuts

Telescopic Rod with Partially Threaded Shaft

The telescopic rods are the mainstays of ring connection in the original Ilizarov set. Telescopic rods are used to connect arches and rings and are significantly stiffer than threaded rods. A telescopic rod with a partially threaded shaft is an aluminum alloy cylindrical tube with one end fastened to a ring with a bolt and a partially threaded shaft protruding from the cylinder attached to the next ring in the frame (Figs 9.15A and B). These telescopic rods are 100, 150, 200, or 250 mm long.

Partially Threaded Rod

Partially threaded rods are the same diameter (6 mm) as the fully threaded rods, but they have a smooth, unthreaded surface in the middle section of the rod (Fig. 9.15C). This smooth surface provides greater stiffness to accommodate the stress of the tightened bolt. The partially threaded rods are produced in the sizes of 130 mm, 170 mm, and 210 mm, and they easily fit in the telescopic casing.

It is possible to use the regular, fully threaded rods instead of the partially threaded rods for similar purposes, but tightening is more stable with the latter. Moreover, this tightening possibly may destroy the threads, and a rod with destroyed threads cannot be used again for any purpose.

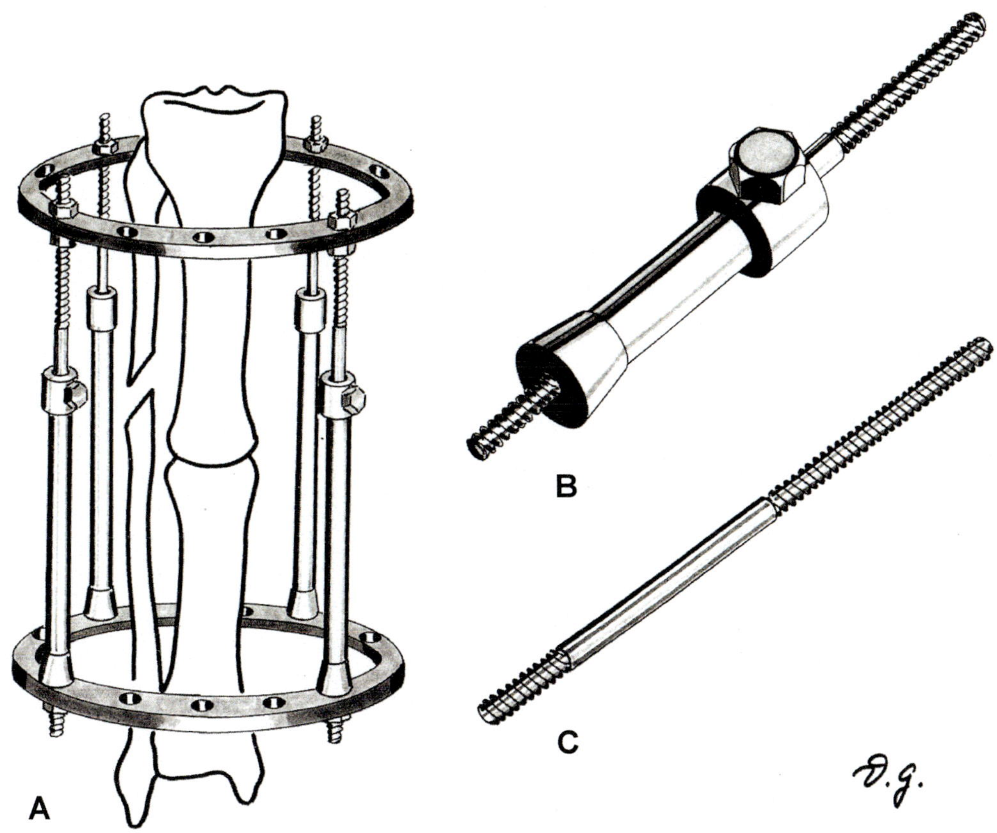

Figure 9.15: Use of the telescopic rod with partially threaded shaft. A, schematic of the tibia, with compression of nonunion, and the fibula partially resected, with a two-ring frame attached. The rings are connected to each other with four telescopic rods with threaded shafts. Compression is produced by turning the four pairs of nuts fixed to the upper ring. Note that the bolts are fastened to the smooth portion of the rods. B, short telescopic rod assembled with a partially threaded rod. C, partially threaded rod. Note that the smooth portion is in the middle of the rod, and one threaded area is shorter than the other, which enables the surgeon to use rods of the same length with telescopic cylinders of different lengths

Graduated Telescopic Rod

The graduated telescopic rod is an invention of ASAMI—Italy, and is included in the complete Ilizarov set. Much like the original telescopic rod, it is a cylinder with one end coupled to a ring via a tightened bolt. The graduated rod has two major features: the inside of the cylinder is fully threaded, and it has a square head that is adjustable by hand, permitting easier and simpler adjustment for both surgeon and patient (Fig. 9.16). This square device has an automatic locking system that is released by a small lever on its side (Fig. 9.16C).

This graduated telescopic rod system locks after the surgeon turns the device one-quarter turn, which corresponds to one-fourth of the desired distraction or compression (Fig. 9.16C). To turn the device beyond 0.25 mm the safety lever must be released. Moreover, each side of the square-headed device has numbered indented dots that signify the amount of turn in one-quarter increments, and the direction of turn. Turns that increase in number (1 to 4) are made in the direction of distraction; those that decrease (4 to 1) are in the compression mode. To determine the exact amount of movement in millimeters this graduated rod has a scale of numbers on the side of the cylinder and a hollow section that shows the rod within.

The graduated telescopic rod makes it easier for the surgeon to control the rate of distraction and compression. Several important, redundant safety features are built into

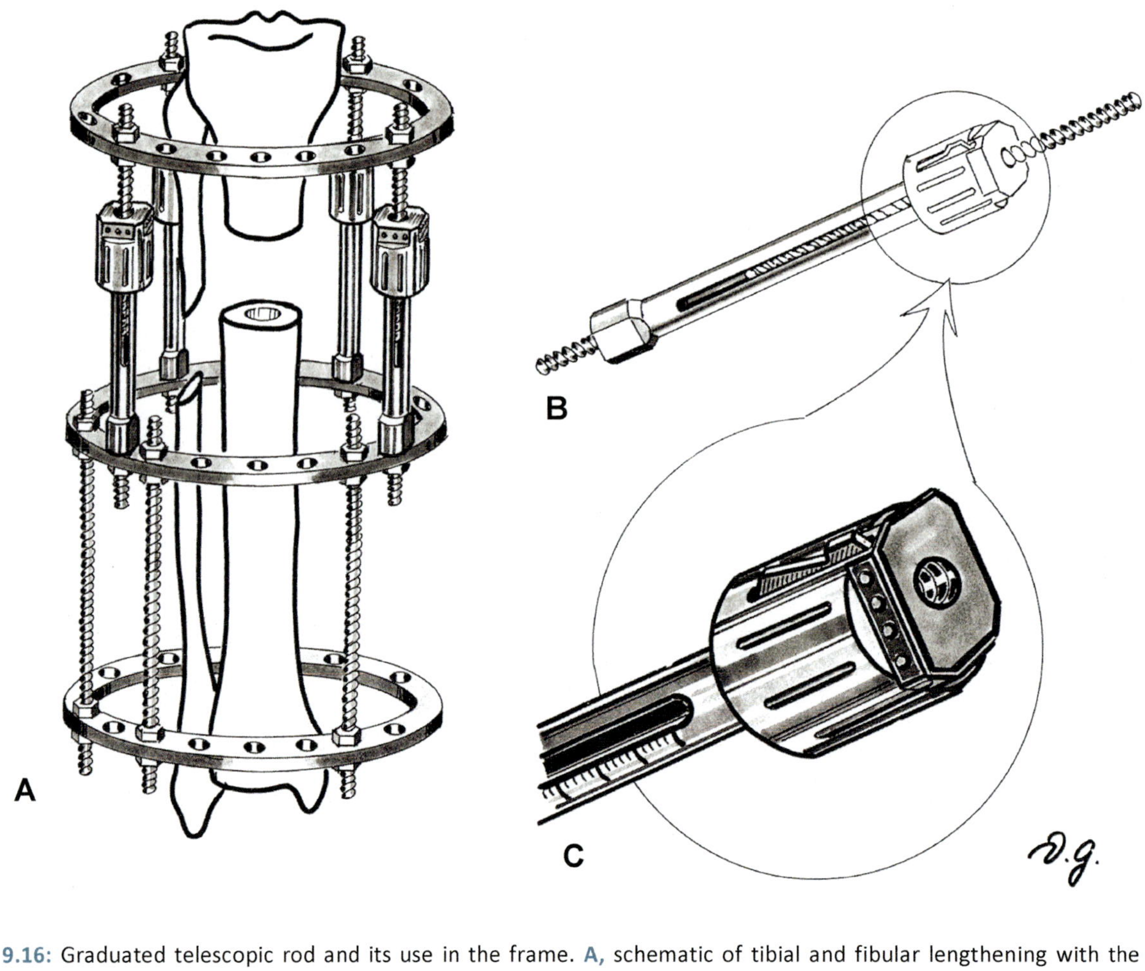

Figure 9.16: Graduated telescopic rod and its use in the frame. A, schematic of tibial and fibular lengthening with the distraction gap at the site of the proximal bone. A three-ring frame is shown. The proximal and middle rings are connected by four graduated telescopic rods that produce the distraction of the bone. Note that these rods are equidistant on the rings. The middle and distal rings also are connected by four equidistant threaded rods. B, general view of a graduated telescopic rod, with threaded rod inserted. C, enlarged view of the locking mechanism on the graduated telescopic rod

it; for example, it locks after one turn, has visual references on its square sides, and clicks audibly after every turn.

Connection Plates

Many clinical situations require the Ilizarov apparatus to be reinforced on either a temporary or permanent basis. In cases of multilevel bone fractures, multilevel osteotomies (corticotomy), and bone lengthening, such reinforcement with connection plates is routinely necessary. Connection plates also are used in the assemblage of the oval ring, for the foot component, for large frames, and for such correction of bone deformities as the simultaneous treatment of pseudoarthroses and angulatory deformity.

In some situations connection plates also are used to extend the main frame construction or to connect two or more components on different planes. There are five types of connection plates in the Ilizarov system:

1. Short connection plates
2. Long connection plates
3. Connection plate with threaded end
4. Twisted connection plate
5. Curved connection plate.

All plates are 5-mm thick, 14-mm wide, and have 7-mm diameter perforated holes. These same dimensions are shared by the rings.

Short Connection Plate

Short connection plates are available in nine sizes: 35 mm with two holes, 45 mm with three holes, 55 mm with four holes, 65 mm with five holes, 75 mm with six holes, 85 mm with seven holes, 95 mm with eight holes, 105 mm with nine holes, and 115 mm with ten holes

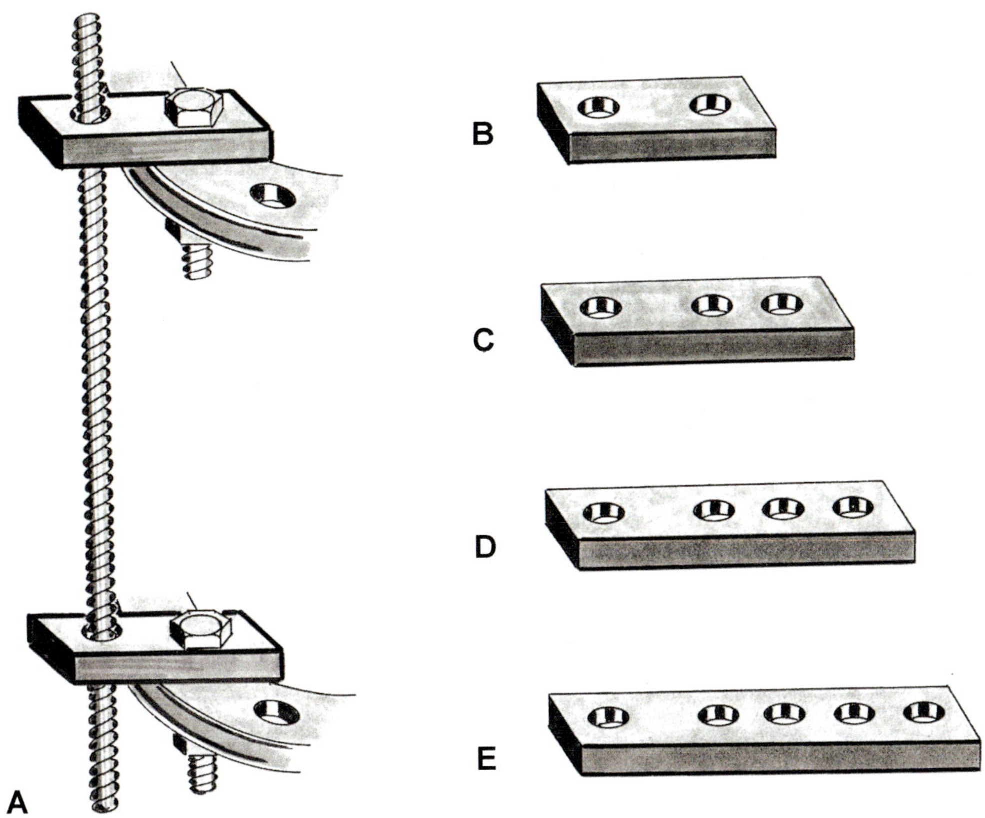

Figure 9.17: Short connection plates of different sizes. A, partial view of a two-ring frame connected by the threaded rod attached to a two-hole (short) connection plate, which serves as an extension of the rings. B, two-hole connection plate. C, three-hole connection plate. D, four-hole connection plate. E, five-hole connection plate

Plates with two and three holes are the most useful, and are applied often in frame construction (Fig. 9.17). In many situations connection plates serve as extensions of the main frame. The feature common to all plates is that the hole that is affixed to a ring always is separated from the next hole on the plate by a distance equal to one hole diameter.

Long Connection Plate

The average Ilizarov frame length for use in an adult is approximately 30 to 35 cm for the lower extremity and 20 to 25 cm for the upper extremity. In children, the frame length is 15 to 25 cm for the lower extremity and 12 to 18 cm for the upper extremity. These large frames sometimes must be reinforced by stiff supporting components, that is, the long connection plates in the Ilizarov set (Fig. 9.18). In some cases there is need for extended support to adjust the middle ring when the patient is further into the treatment program. Long connection plates are available in three sizes: 155 mm

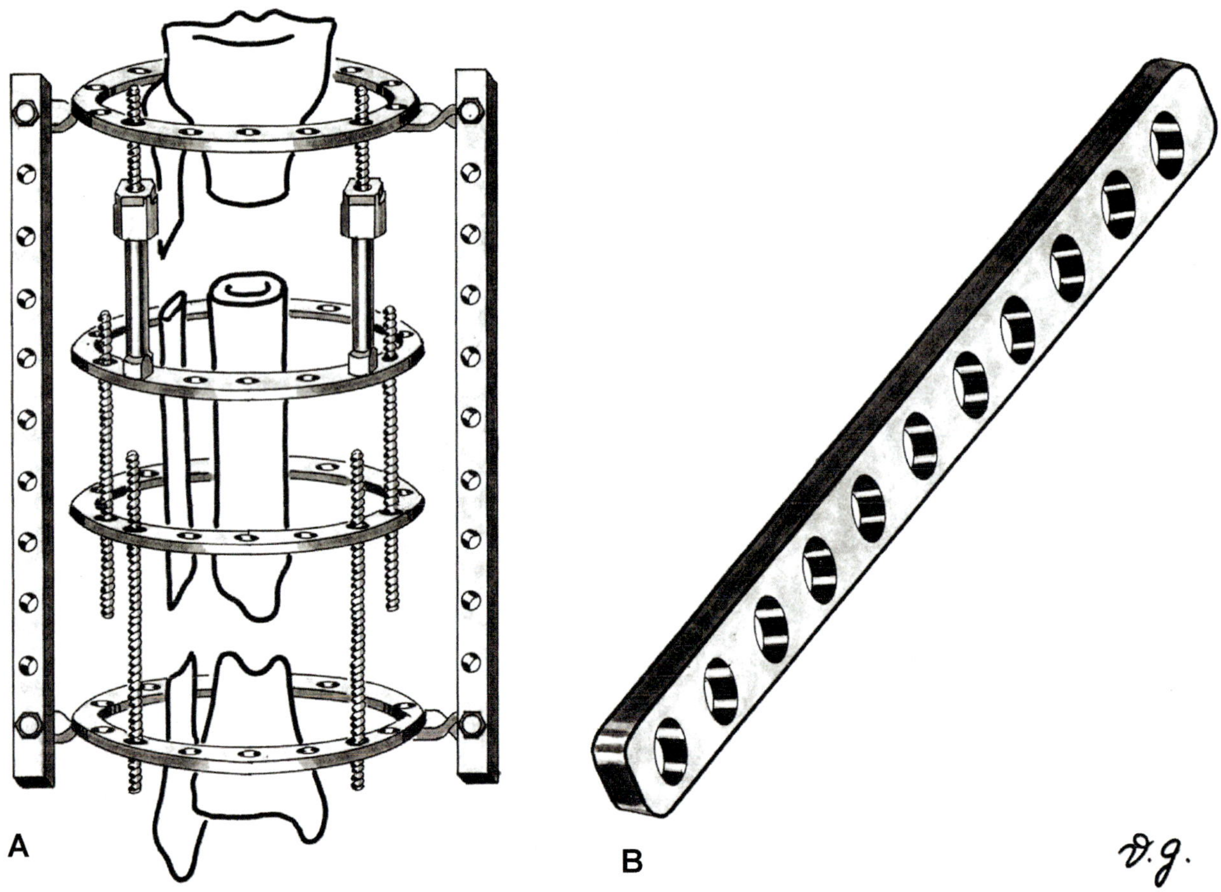

Figure 9.18: A, long plates are used to reinforce large frames during bone fragment transport and as extensions of the frame. B, long connection plate. Long connection plates are available in three lengths: 155, 235, and 335 mm

with eight holes, 235 mm with twelve holes, and 335 mm with seventeen holes. The shorter the plate the greater the distance between the holes (12 mm and 5 mm; Fig. 9.19).

Twisted Plate

Because the long connection plates are placed in line with the frame axis, their surfaces are at 90 degrees to each other. A special twisted plate is used as a connection from a horizontal to a vertical plane in the frame assembly. Twisted plates are available in three sizes:

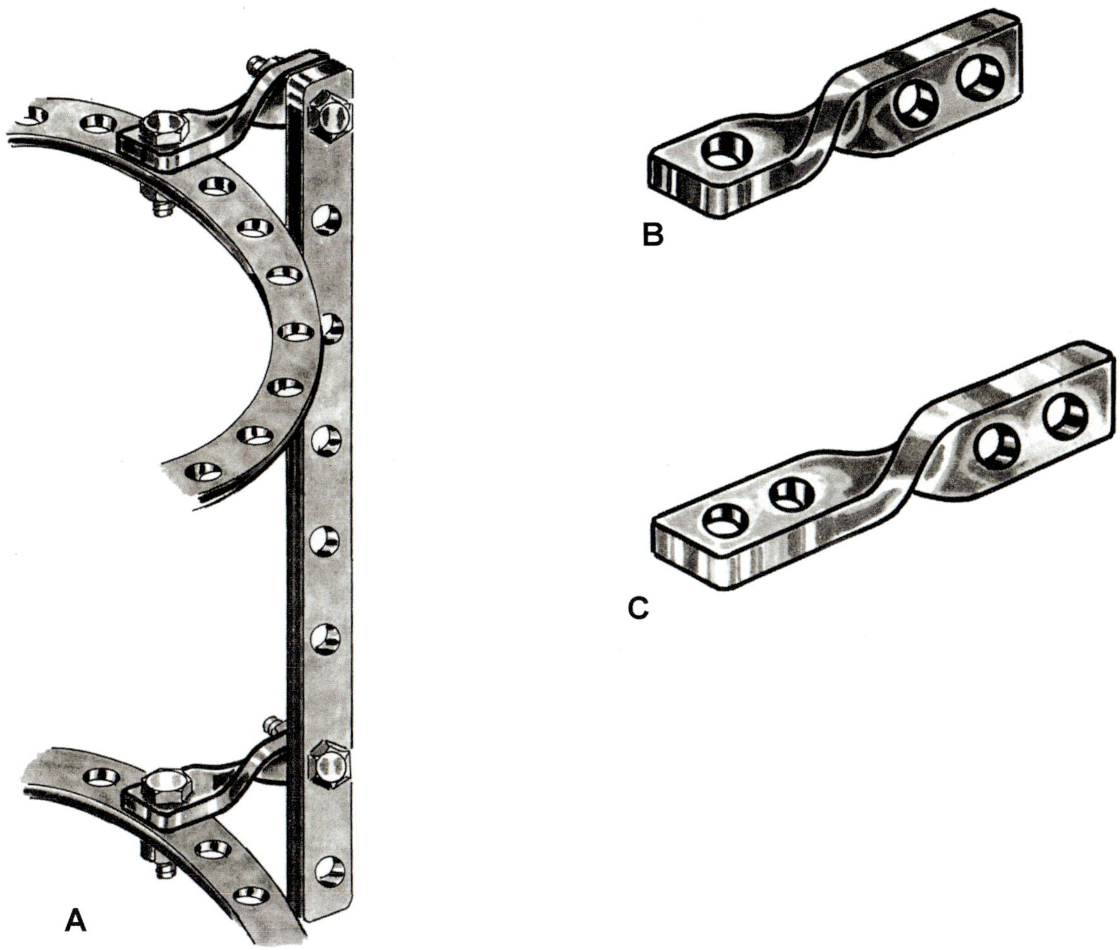

Figure 9.19: Twisted plates of different sizes. A, section of the frame consisting of two rings connected outward by the long connection plate is represented. Two-hole twisted plates supporting this connection are shown. Note that the long plate surface is situated in a 90-degree plane to the ring wall surfaces. Twisted plates are adjusted perfectly to this because their twist is equal to 90 degrees. B, three-hole twisted plate. C, four-hole twisted plate

45 mm with two standard holes, 65 mm with three standard holes, and 85 mm with four standard holes. These twisted plates also can be used to extend the frame outward (Fig. 9.19).

Connection Plate with Threaded End

Both short and long connection plates may be fixed to the frame with a variety of additional parts. Moreover, in some frame assemblies it is necessary to connect the plates at their butt ends with an appliance. A connection plate with a threaded end is provided for this purpose (Fig. 9.20).

There are four types of plates with threaded ends. Their common characteristic is a standard threaded rod protruding from one butt end. This threaded rod is part of the plate, which is made from one piece of metal. These plates are available in four sizes: 135 mm with five holes, 175 mm with seven holes, 215 mm

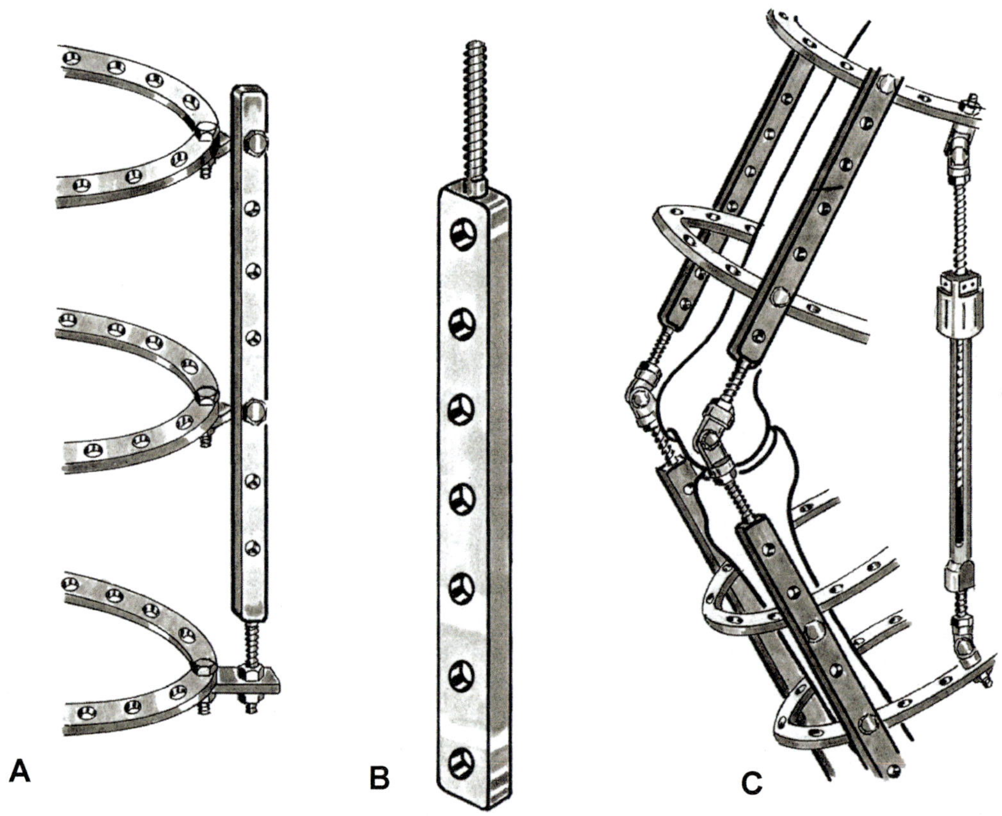

Figure 9.20: Connection plate with threaded rod. A, section of the frame showing three rings connected outward by the connection plate with threaded rod. Note that upper and middle ring connections are supported by two twisted plates, and the lower ring support consists of a short plate connected to the threaded end of the long plate. B, seven-hole connection plate with threaded rod. C, schematic of knee flexion contracture (partial view). A four-ring frame is applied, connected by two pairs of plates with threaded ends and a graduated telescopic rod. The threaded ends of these plates are connected with hinges. Use of plates with threaded ends for hinge support in the distraction frame makes this frame very stable

with nine holes, and 255 mm with 11 standard 7-mm holes.

The connection plate with threaded end can be used as a long supporting plate and also for construction of additional components.

Curved Plate

As an independent part of a frame, the half-ring has one disadvantage: It allows very little room for K-wire angulation. This can be corrected by adding a three-hole curved plate to the half-ring (Fig. 9.21A). Connected by a bolt and nut to a half-ring, the curved plate becomes a continuation of the curve. A curved plate increases the circumference of a half-ring (Fig. 9.21B) and connects frame areas where a straight connection plate will not fit. The curved plate is raised in the center so that it can be attached easily to the right and left half-ring ends. This curved plate is particularly useful for foot and forearm frames, but also can serve as a component of any type of frame.

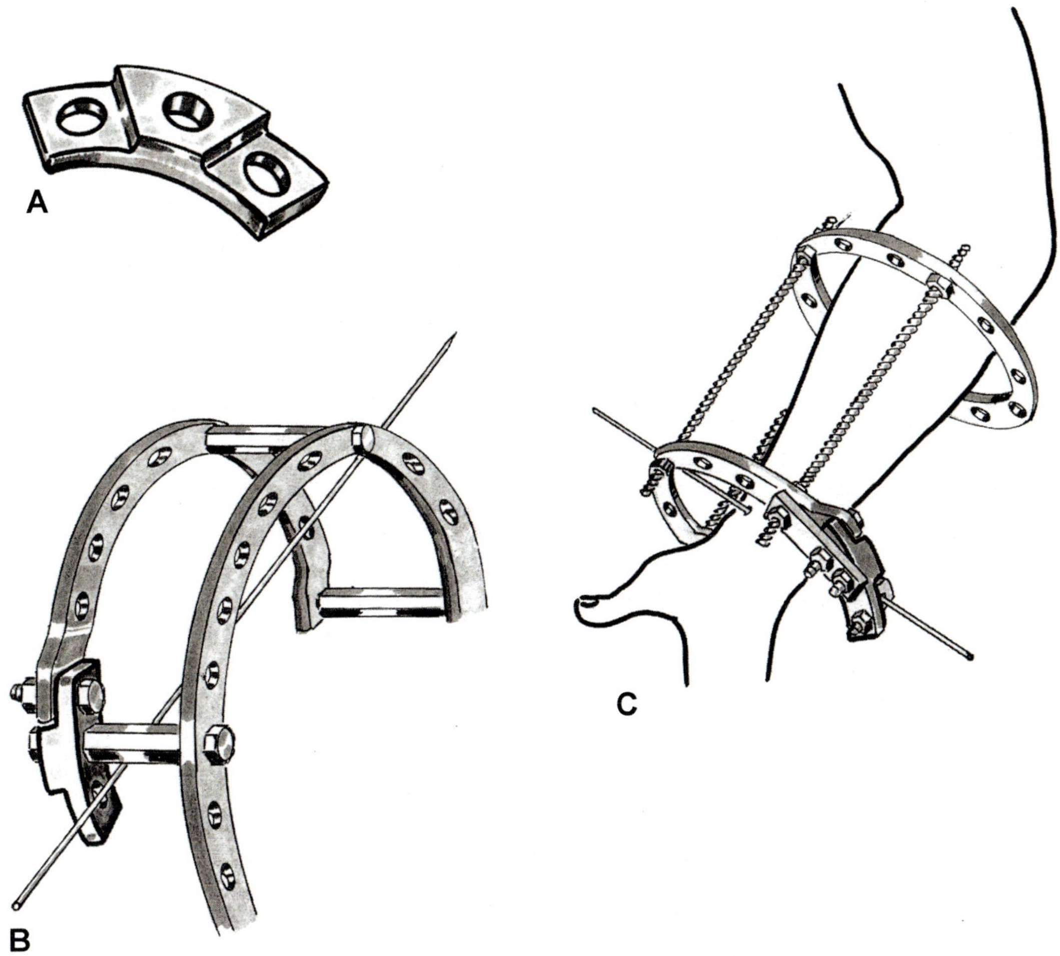

Figure 9.21: Curved plate and its utilization. A, three-hole curved plate is used to increase the half-ring circumference and to connect two half-rings. It can be introduced in places where a straight connector cannot fit. B, partial view of the frame component consisting of one full ring and one half-ring, connected to each other, and the wire introduced obliquely. In this case the curved plate is used to increase the half-ring circumference for the purpose of wire fixation. To reinforce the curved plate connection to the half-ring, it is also connected to the ring by a threaded socket. C, two-ring frame for a forearm. The half-ring is used distally. In this case the curved plate increases its circumference. A short straight plate is introduced to reinforce its connection to the half-ring

The surgeon must bear in mind that, despite its solid connection, a curved plate still may yield to wire tension and become displaced. Therefore, to ensure firm positioning it must be reinforced with an additional short plate or with a threaded rod fixed with posts and hinges (Figs 9.21B and C).

THREADED SOCKETS AND BUSHINGS

The threaded rods can be reinforced and lengthened by adding two types of connectors: a threaded socket and a bushing. Both of these components can serve many purposes, but they mainly function as auxiliary connectors between two rods. Both of these parts are cylindrical with a hollow vertical canal, and both have a perpendicular, threaded hole running through the center from side-to-side. But they differ in other features, and chiefly in their function in the frame.

Threaded Sockets

Threaded sockets can be 20 or 40 mm long. They are hexagonal, with a diameter exactly corresponding to that

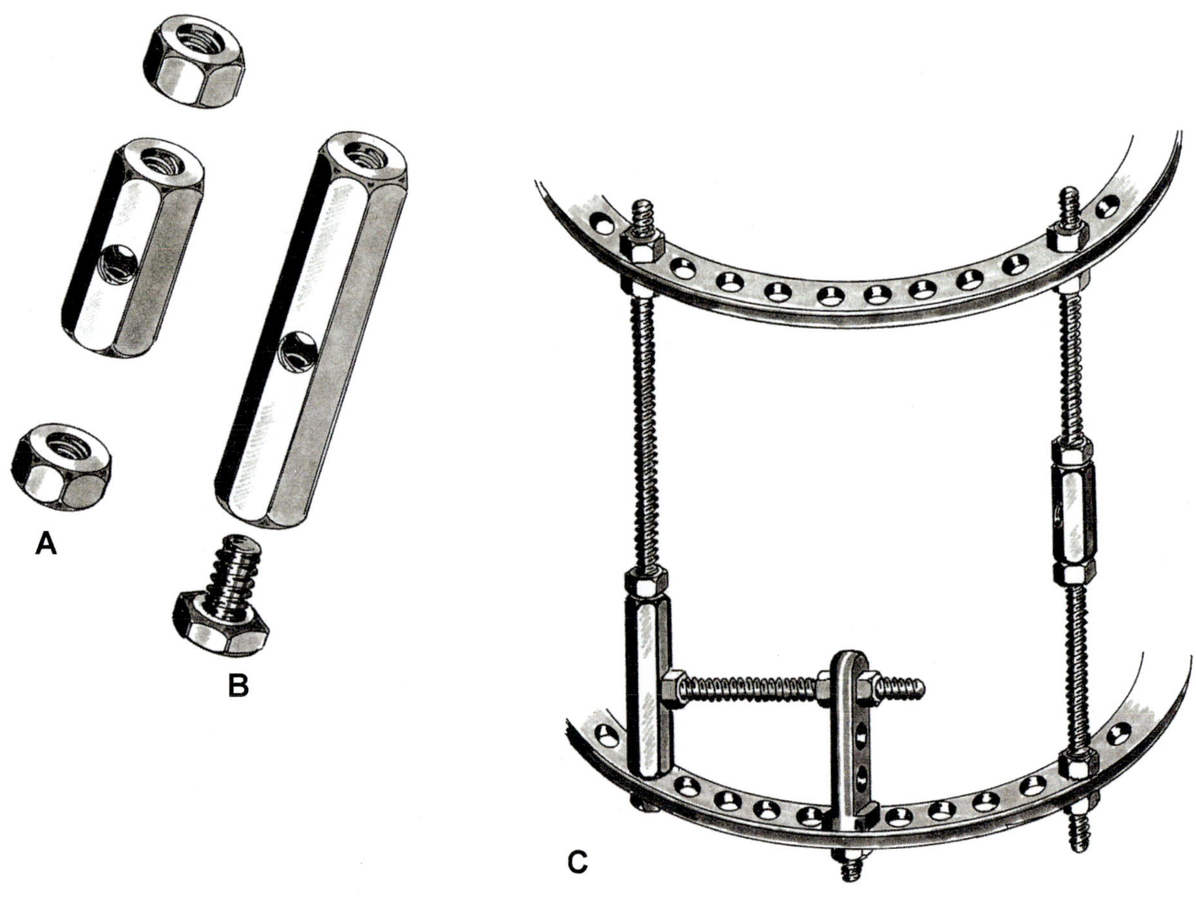

Figure 9.22: Threaded sockets and their use. A, small, 20-mm threaded socket with two nuts. B, large, 40-mm threaded socket with a bolt. Note that all apertures are threaded. C, in a section of the frame shown, two threaded sockets are used for construction reinforcement. The large socket connects a threaded rod to a ring and also is connected by another rod to a male support. The small socket connects two threaded rods and thereby makes these rods much stronger connectors. Note that in all cases the threaded sockets are securely connected to the rods with nuts

of a no. 10 (10 mm) nut, which makes it convenient to adjust with the standard no. 10 wrench.

Both ends of the socket canal are threaded for fixation to the bolts or to the threaded rods. There also are two perpendicular threaded holes through the center of two opposite sides. These holes may be used for connections to bolts and rods (Fig. 9.22). Threaded sockets of both sizes are used as extensions of threaded rods (Fig. 9.22C) and for connecting a half-ring or a five-eighths ring to the full ring in the metaphyseal component of a frame. At least three threaded sockets of the same size must be used to connect the ring to the half-ring.

In some cases it may be necessary to reinforce the full ring by positioning it parallel and close to the second ring. In such situations four threaded sockets (20 mm long) are the best connectors. They must be placed equidistant to one another (see Fig. 8-14). To attach the

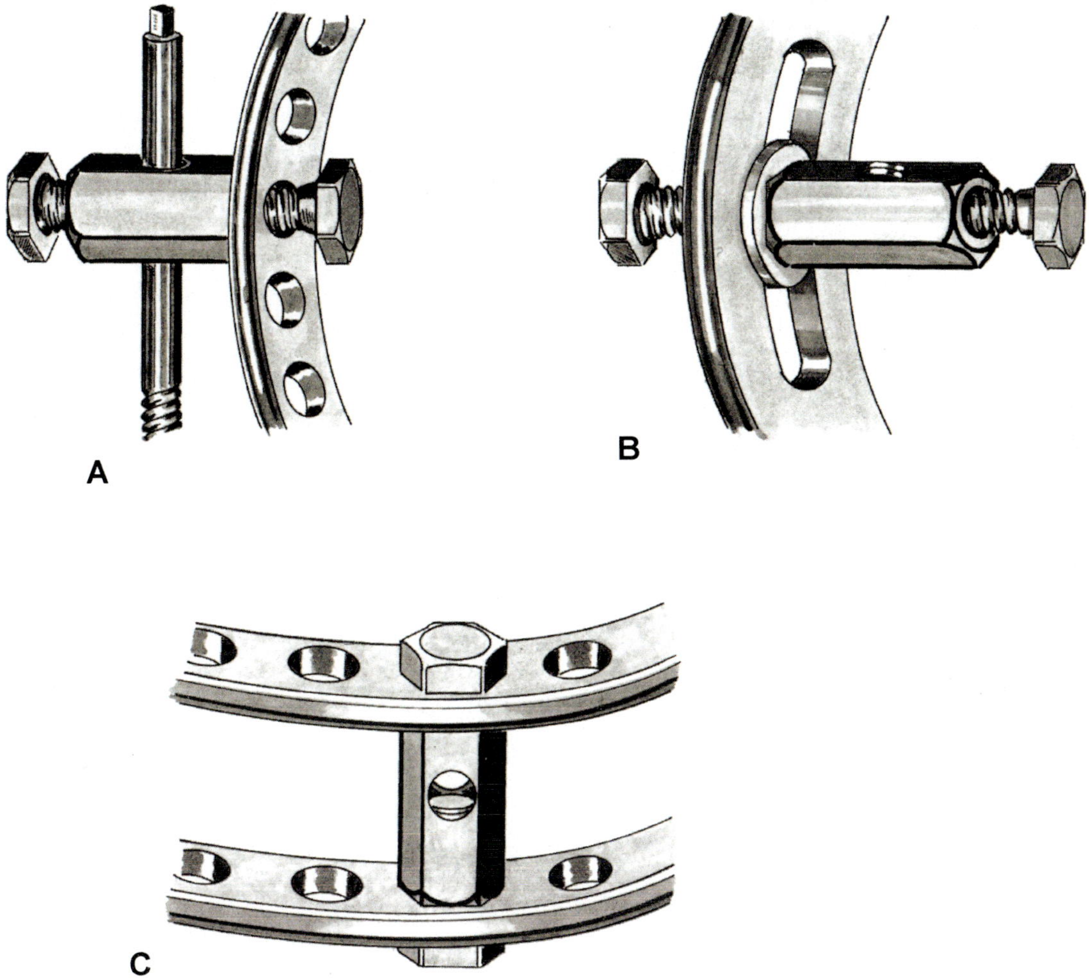

Figure 9.23: Use of threaded sockets. A, in a section of the frame shown, the small threaded socket is used for support of a half-pin. Note that one bolt tightens the socket to the ring, and the other bolt fastens the half-pin in the socket. B, a small socket is fastened to the arch. Note the washer between them, necessary because the arch slot is wider than the socket diameter. A bushing can be used for the same purpose. C, two parallel rings are connected by a small socket. Note that three to four sockets are necessary to connect two rings

threaded sockets to the rings, 10-mm bolts must be used (Fig. 9.23).

Bushing

The bushing is a short (12 mm) cylinder with a smooth, unthreaded aperture (7 mm in diameter) running through it (Fig. 9.24). It is 1 mm wider than a threaded rod, which makes it easy to place on the rod. To stabilize the bushing while it is on the rod, nuts must be fastened on both ends, above and below. A perpendicular threaded hole dissects the center of the bushing, which serves different purposes but is particularly useful for the attachment of additional frame components. In some cases two or more bushings placed over one another can be put on one rod, usually to reinforce the rod.

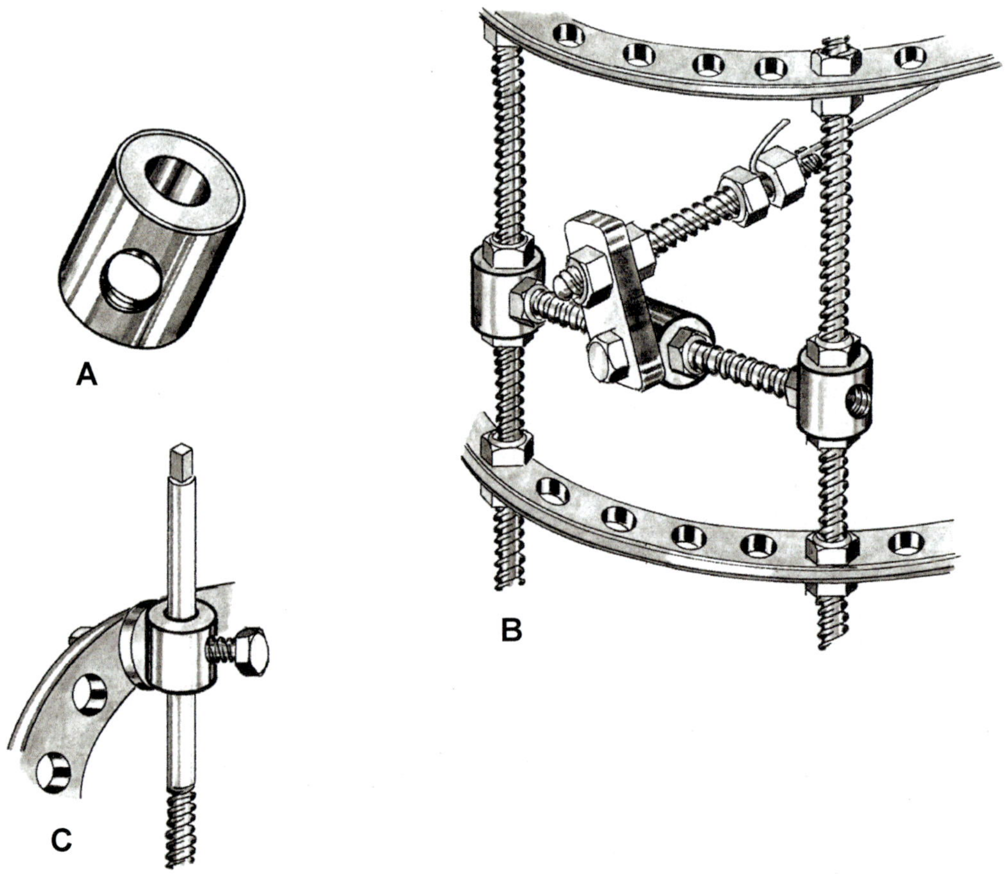

Figure 9.24: A, a bushing is a round cylinder with a smooth aperture and two perpendicular threaded holes. In this view only one of the holes is shown; that on the opposite side is hidden. B, in the frame section shown, three bushings are used to support the pulling device. Two bushings are attached to the connecting threaded rods, and are secured by the nuts. These two bushings are connected to each other by the threaded rod placed as a cross beam. The third bushing is attached to the middle of this rod and is secured by nuts. This bushing supports the sloped two-hole plate, which is fixed by a bolt to the bushing's threaded hole. The sloped, threaded rod with a slotted end is fastened to the top hole of the plate and secured with two 6-mm nuts, which will permit rod movement. The bent K-wire is fixed firmly at the slotted end of this rod with two 5-mm nuts. Note that this represents another type of pushing-pulling device. C, in the frame section shown, a bushing is used to support a half-pin. The bushing is connected to the ring with a bolt. Note that a washer is introduced between the bushing and the ring, which is necessary for a secure, tight connection. The half-pin is secured by a bolt into the bushing hole. The threaded socket also may be used for this purpose.

SUPPORTS AND POSTS, AND HALF-HINGES

Posts, supports, and half-hinges are auxiliary parts of great importance because they facilitate a variety of frame constructions. Their main advantages are that (i) they can be placed virtually at any location, (ii) they can be turned 360 degrees around their axis, and (iii) they can be fixed in any desirable position. They also serve as additional reinforcement for many components. When connected to each other, half-hinges allow parts to be situated at an angle (sloped) to each other.

Supports and Posts

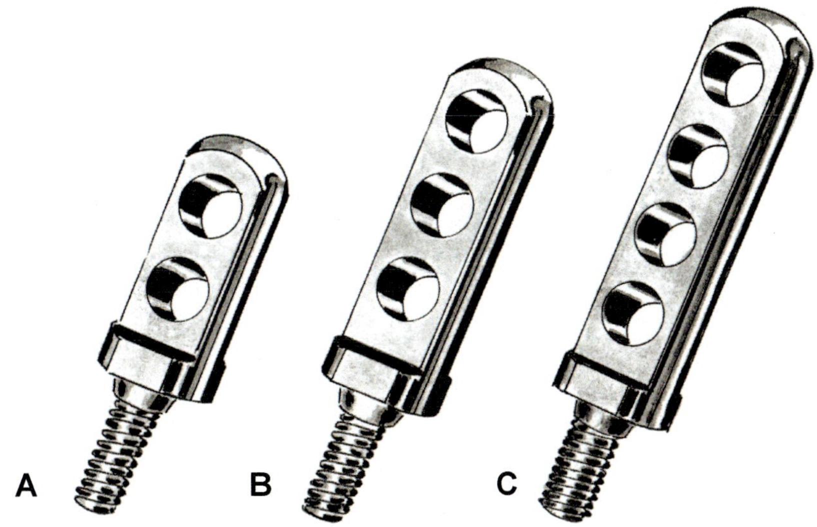

Figure 9.25: A, two-hole male support. B, three-hole male support. C, four-hole male support

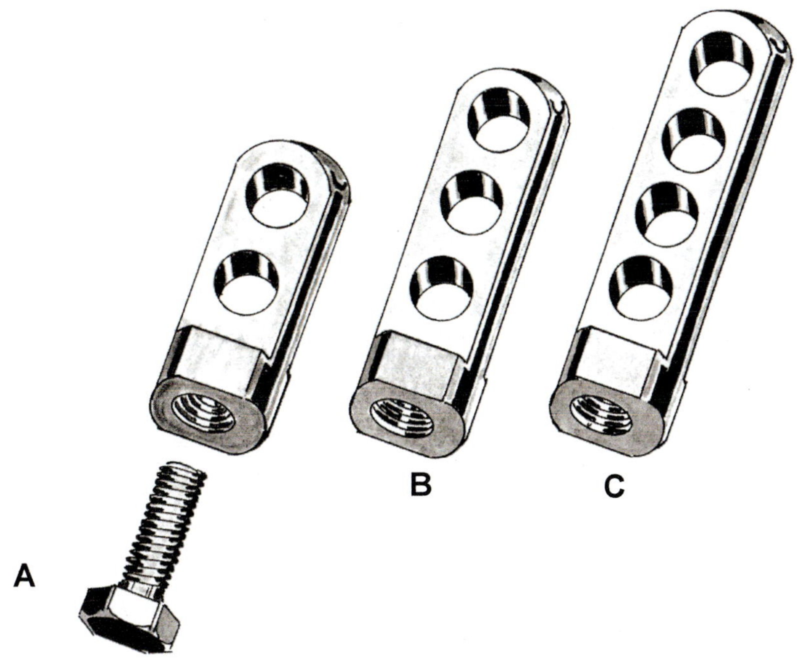

Figure 9.26: A, two-hole female post, with a bolt. B, three-hole female post. C, four-hole female post. Note that the bases of these posts are thicker than that of the supports and that they have an aperture for the bolt

Supports and posts differ from half-hinges in thickness and in the number of standard 7-mm holes. There are two types of posts and supports in the Ilizarov set:

1. The male support has a 13-mm long standard threaded leg protruding from the butt end (Fig. 9.25). This "leg" serves as a connection to other components.
2. The female post has no protruding rod, but a 10-mm deep threaded hole at the butt end. This hole serves to connect bolts or rods (Fig. 9.26).

The male support is 4 mm high at its base, and the female post 6 mm. This difference permits the solid insertion of the bolt or rod into the post hole.

The supports and posts are thicker than other parts because they bear tremendous loads. The supports are available in the following sizes: 28 mm with two holes, 38 mm with three holes, and 48 mm with four holes. Posts are available as 30 mm with two holes, 40 mm with three holes, and 50 mm with four holes.

Half-Hinges

The half-hinges have a supporting base with two flat surfaces matching the standard 10-mm wrench. They differ from the posts in that the flange has only one hole and is only 4 mm thick, with a standard threaded leg. There are two types of half-hinges:

1. The male half-hinge (Fig. 9.27A) has a standard threaded leg protruding from the base. This leg connects it to other components.
2. The female half-hinge (Fig. 9.27B) has no leg, but a threaded hole at the base. This hole connects it to a bolt or rod.

Despite the relatively small size of the regular half-hinges, they are far too large to be used as multiplanar hinges. Therefore there is a smaller half-hinge in a set. Its

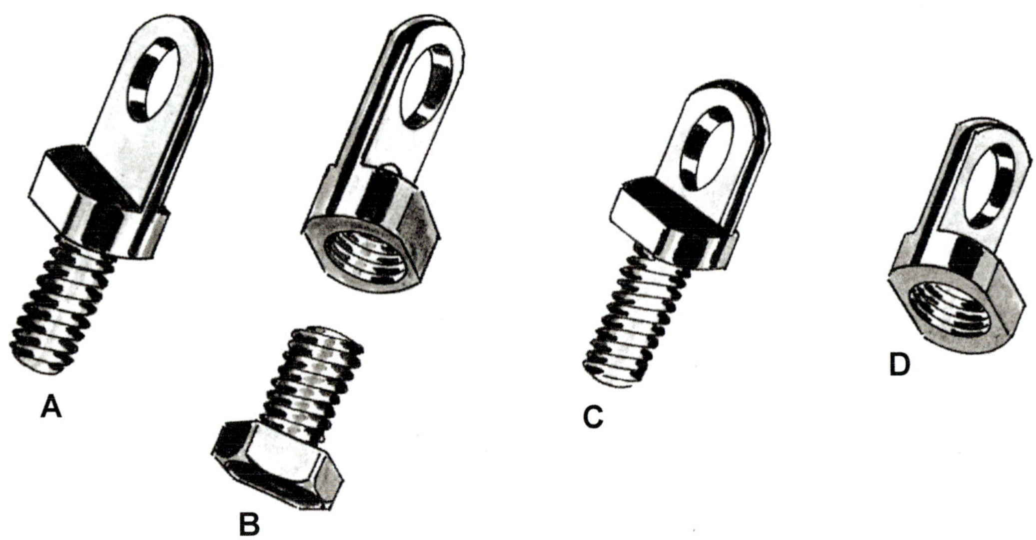

Figure 9.27: A, regular male half-hinge. B, regular female half-hinge. C, small male half-hinge. D, small female half-hinge. Note that the base of the small half-hinge is thinner and smaller than that on a regular hinge

flange is 13-mm high, with a base of 3 mm (Figs 9.27C and D). The difference in size may not seem dramatic, but it affords noticeable improvement in hinge function. The small half-hinges have either male or female ends.

Both types of half-hinges have flanges at one side of the base. Connected to each other and fixed by the bolt-nut system, the two half-hinges form a low-profile hinge.

The proper use of hinges in frame assembly is essential, and is described in Chapter 13. In some cases two-axis and even three-axis hinges are used for special-purpose frames. For such frames, three or four half-hinges can be used (Fig. 9.28A).

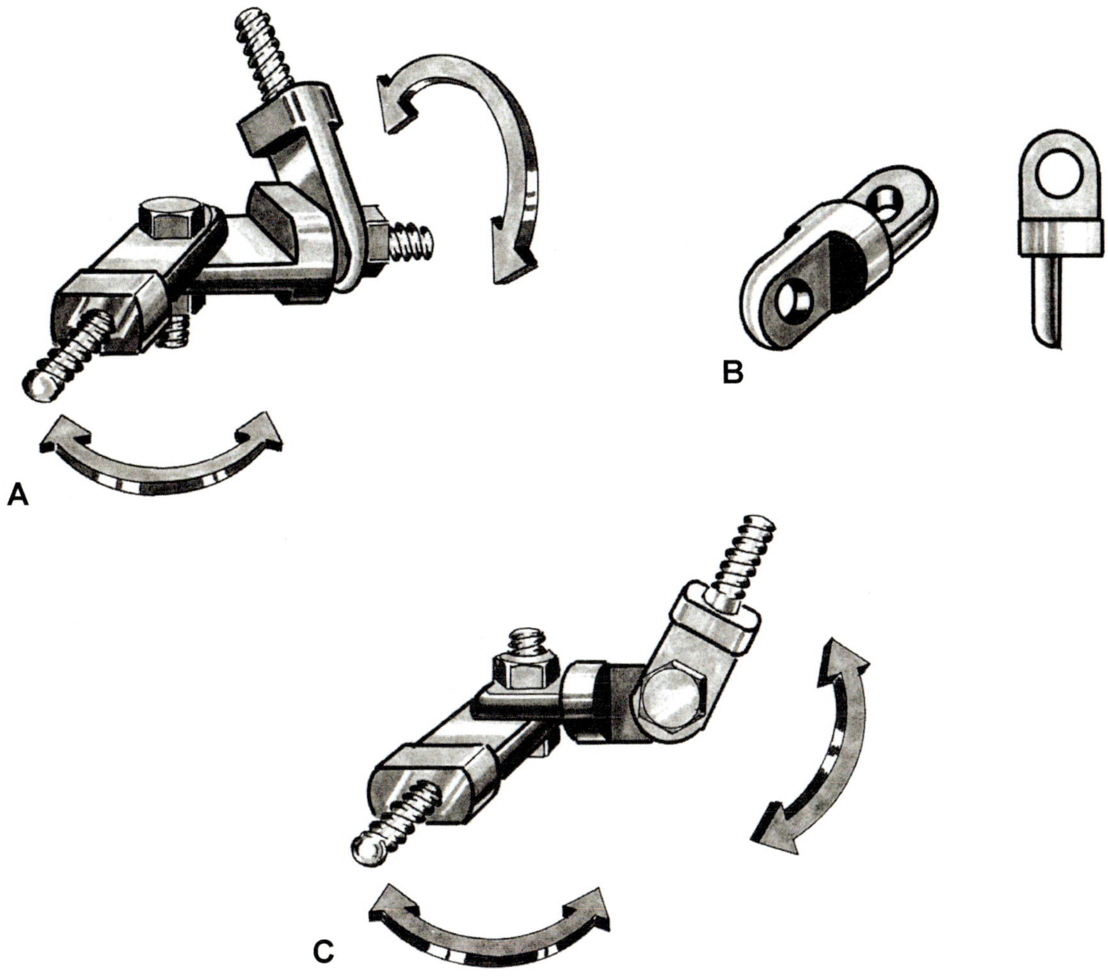

Figure 9.28: A, two-axis hinge. *Arrow* indicates the directions in which the hinge turns. B, two-axis hinge. The middle part of this construction is a combined-type hinge. C, combined-type hinge shown in diagonal and side views. Note that this hinge has a small common base for two flanges at 90 degrees to each other. Arrows indicate the directions in which the hinge turns

The Richards Medical Company also developed a new type of combined half-hinge, which is one piece with two flanges positioned at 90 degrees to the long axis, each with the standard holes (Fig. 9.28B). The two flanges have one common base. Thus this type of hinge can be used only as a middle component of a two-axis hinge (Fig. 9.28C).

WIRE-FIXATION BOLTS

The Ilizarov set contains bolts specially designed to fasten K-wires to the flat surface of the ring. The strength of this fastening determines the stability of the bone fragment to which the wire is introduced (see Chapter 11). The range of this wire stiffness is between 200 and 300 kg. To maintain a strong wire fixation, two special bolts are used: the cannulated wire-fixation bolt and the slotted wire-fixation bolt (Fig. 9.29). Both bolts are 6 mm in diameter at the head, with 18-mm threaded legs. Near the base, where the leg meets the head, is a 3-mm smooth band, which conforms to the ring hole.

The slotted wire-fixation bolt has an oblique slot just below the bottom of the head (Fig. 9.29A). The cannulated wire-fixation bolt has a 2-mm hole through it, just below the bottom of the head (Fig. 9.29B). Along with this hole is a 0.5 mm groove, to accommodate the K-wire.

Both types of wire-fixation bolt permit introduction of a K-wire into a hole or slot and also the fixation of a K-wire between the ring wall and the bolt head. To

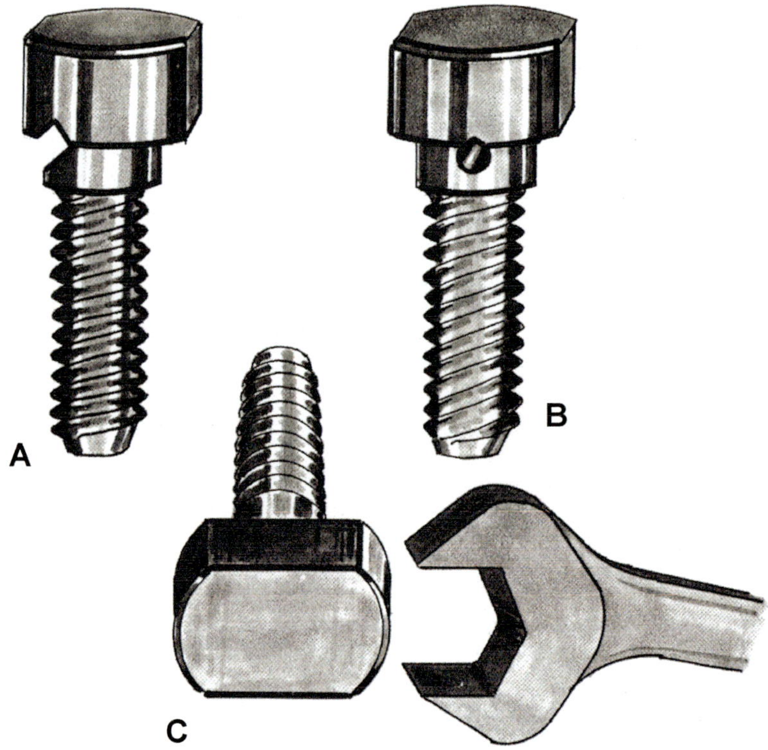

Figure 9.29: A, wire-fixation bolt, slotted. B, wire-fixation bolt, cannulated. C, head of the wire-fixation bolt, with a wrench

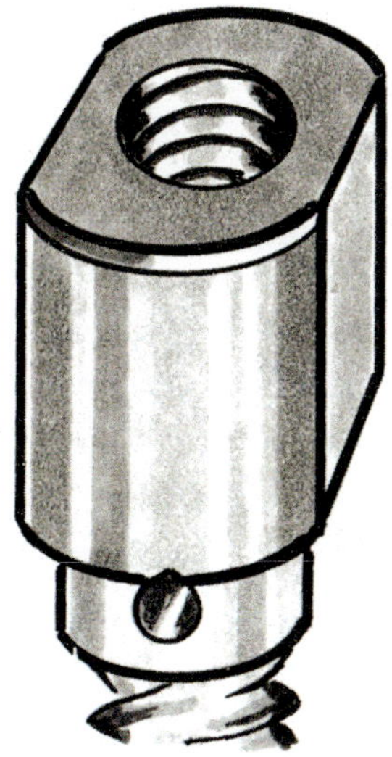

Figure 9.30: Partial view of the wire-fixation bolt head with a threaded aperture

achieve secure wire fixation, the bolt head has a special shape: 14 × 10 mm oval, with two flat cuts on both sides for a 10-mm wrench (Fig. 9.29C). The length of the bolt head corresponds to the 14-mm width of the ring, providing the tensioned wire with a maximum area of surface-to-surface tightening (Fig. 9.30). The 10-mm width of the head allows easy introduction of any standard bolt or nut into the next hole on the ring.

The 6-mm height of the wire-fixation bolt head is twice that of a regular bolt head, and is slightly larger in height than a regular nut. This has a special purpose. If the ring hole next to it is occupied by a lower nut or regular bolt, it is much easier to turn the head of the wire-fixation bolt.

In some cases there is not enough space to introduce components onto the ring because all the adjacent holes are occupied. Therefore there is one special type of wire-fixation cannulated bolt with an 11-mm head (Fig. 9.31). center

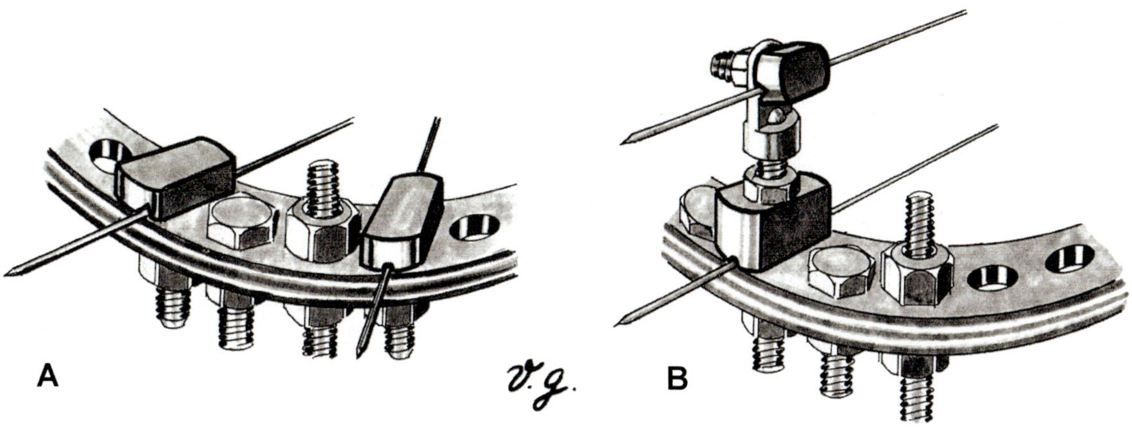

Figure 9.31: A, in a segment of a ring two wire-fixation bolts fasten the K-wires. To the left is a slotted bolt, and to the right a cannulated bolt. Note that the heads of these bolts are higher than that of the regular nut and bolt. B, in a segment of a ring a combination of two wire-fixation bolts is shown. Note that to be able to fasten an additional K-wire situated above the ring level the second wire-fixation bolt is secured on top of one with a head with threaded aperture. A half-hinge supports the second wire-fixation bolt

of the head top. It permits bolt or rod introduction, and saves a great deal of space (Fig. 9.30).

Because both types of bolts have equal ability to fix the wire to the ring wall, there is always the question of which is better. As a rule, the 1.5-mm wire is more securely fixed with the cannulated bolt, and the 1.8-mm wire with the slotted bolt. The slot on the head is situated 1.5 mm deeper than the hole, and squeezing the thinner wire is more difficult with the slotted bolt.

For optimal tightening, use of a regular 5-mm nut is recommended. Both types of bolts can be made extremely tight, which may cause metal fatigue near the base of the threaded leg. Thus, again we state the rule that a wire-fixation bolt, a threaded part, never can be used twice.

WIRE-FIXATION BUCKLES

Wire-fixation buckles are used primarily to affix K-wires to the rings, but also are used for multiple purposes during frame construction. Their principal advantage is that they can be used in ring locations where there are no accessible holes. For example, they may be placed over the junction of two half-rings or between two holes. In

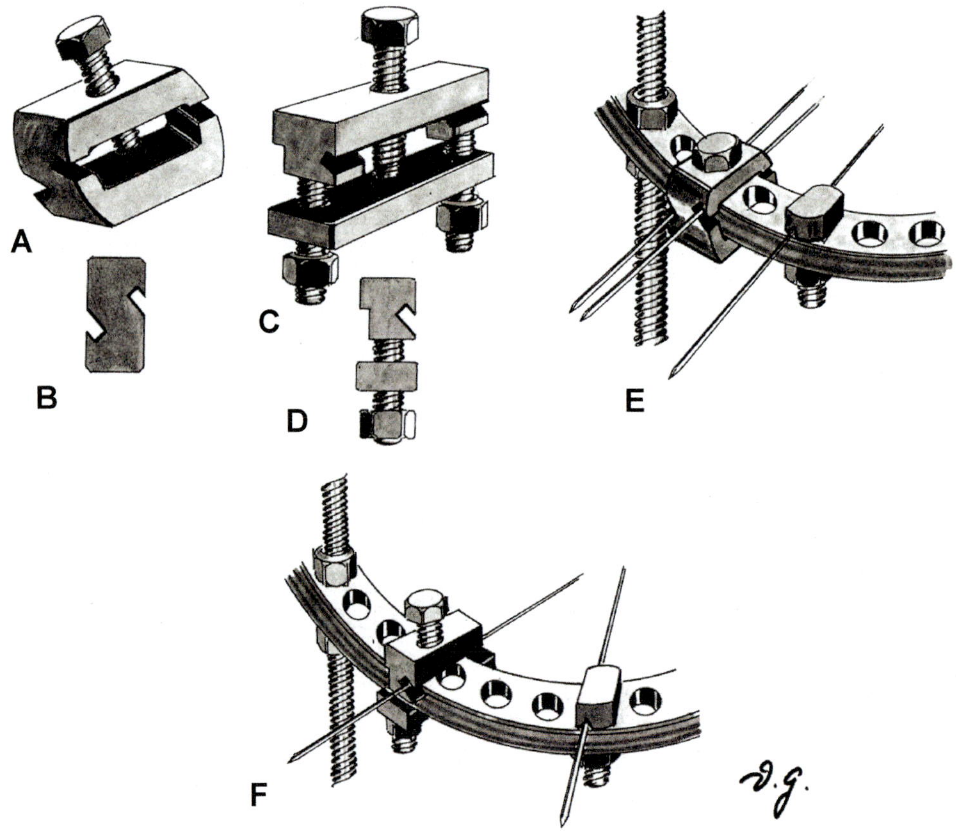

Figure 9.32: Wire-fixation buckles. A, dual-sided wire-fixation buckle, assembled. B, side view of the dual-sided buckle shows two indentations for K-wires. Note that the indentations face opposite (top and bottom) surfaces of the buckle. They fasten the K-wires to the ring walls when the buckle is tightened. C, detachable wire-fixation buckle, assembled. D, side view of the detachable buckle with an indentation on one side. A second rectangular base is attached by the threaded leg and nut to the top piece. E, in a ring section, a dual-sided wire-fixation buckle is attached between two holes. Two K-wires are fixed to the two opposite walls of the ring. A slotted wire fixation bolt is shown for comparison to the buckle. F, in a ring section, a detachable wire-fixation buckle is attached between two holes. A K-wire is fixed to the upper side of the ring, and a slotted wire fixation bolt is shown for comparison to the buckle

contrast to all other parts, wire-fixation buckles are not fixed to the ring holes but to the flat surfaces of the ring, with nuts and bolts.

The Ilizarov set contains two types of wire-fixation buckles: the dual-sided wire-fixation buckle and the detachable wire-fixation buckle (Figs 9.32A to D). Both buckles clamp to the ring, but one has the ring threaded through it and the other buckles (in two parts) over the ring. The dual-sided buckle has two grooves in it to affix the K-wires to the ring. When fully tightened these grooves are flush with both the top and bottom surfaces of the ring. The K-wires thus are squeezed and fixed firmly to the ring (Fig. 9.32E). The great advantage of this wire-fixation buckle is that it can hold two K-wires, situated on two different planes. The disadvantage is that it must be threaded onto the ring in advance, in the exact location where it will be tightened. For this reason it is easier to use the detachable wire-fixation buckle.

The detachable wire-fixation buckle consists of two parts: a top piece with a hole in it and two small bolts protruding from it, and a small bottom plate that affixes the buckle to the ring with nuts (Figs 9.32C and D). It also has a groove cut into the upper part of the buckle, for K-wire fixation. When assembled and locked down with nuts, this detachable wire-fixation buckle stays firmly on the ring, and even can be used for connecting two half-rings. Moreover, the hole in the buckle head

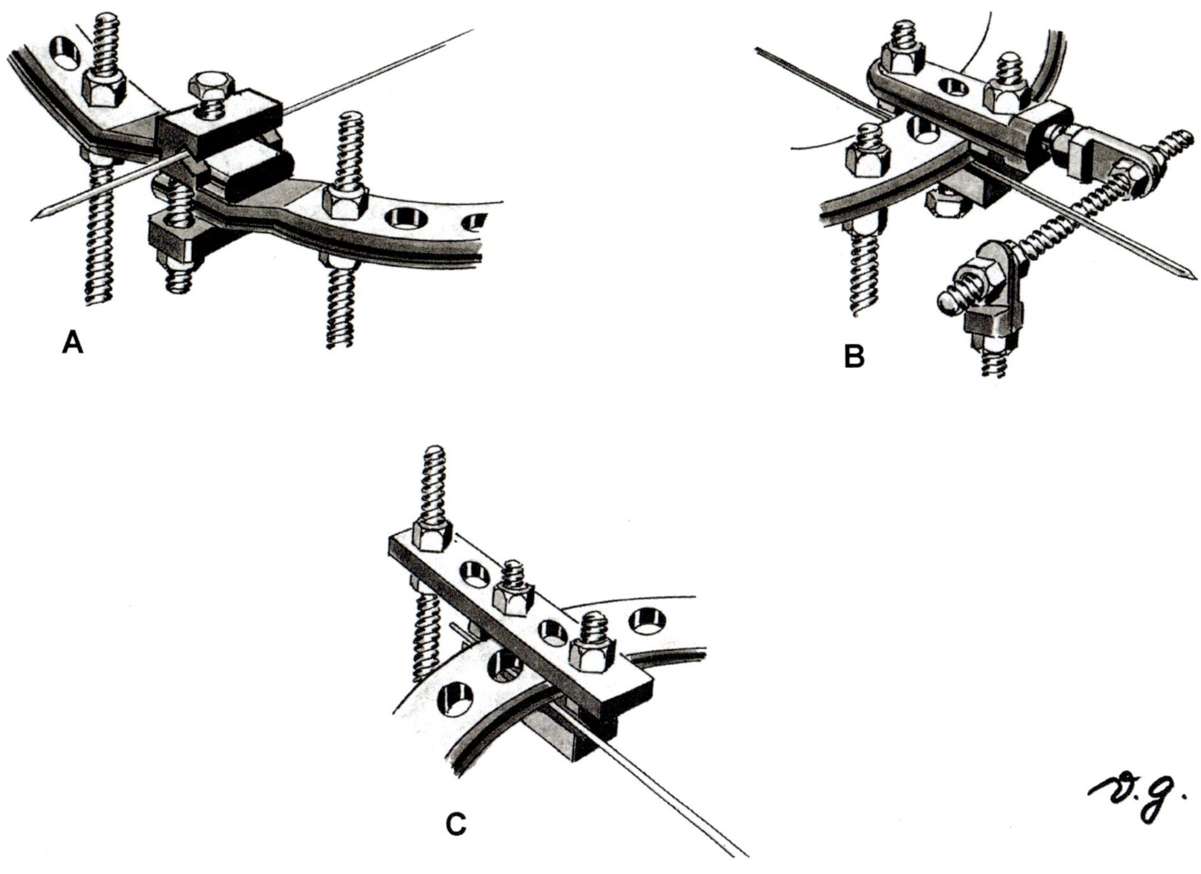

Figure 9.33: Use of wire-fixation buckles. A, in a ring section, a detachable buckle is shown at the site of a two half-rings connection. Note that the buckle serves two purposes: K-wire fixation to the ring and strengthening of the two half-rings connection. B, in a ring section, a construction combining one part of a detachable buckle with a three-hole post is shown. Note that in this case the buckle serves two purposes: K-wire fixation to the ring wall and support of the post. This post supports the construction of an external derotational device, consisting of two half-hinges and a threaded rod. C, in a ring section a construction that combines one part of a detachable buckle with a five-hole plate is shown

accommodates either a bolt or a threaded rod, which when tightened all the way down to the ring, squeezes and affixes the K-wire (Fig. 9.32F).

The advantage of the detachable buckle is that it can be assembled and used at any ring position without being placed in advance. And the top part of the buckle may be used independently to connect two half-rings (Fig. 9.33A), or as frame reinforcement if connected to a post (Fig. 9.33B) or to a connecting plate (Fig. 9.33C).

WASHERS

Washers, although they may seem inconsequential, fill the space between the various parts and the rings and provide lock-tight fastening. The washers differ in thickness and diameter, but all have a 7-mm hole in the center. Six types of washers are included in the Ilizarov set (Fig. 9.34):

1. The 1.5-mm thick, 12-mm diameter washer with two flat surfaces. The diameter of this washer is equal to that of the nut and bolt head, enabling its use on ring holes situated next to each other (Fig. 9.34A). Since two of these washers easily fit within the space between two holes, they do not prevent tightening. This washer, however, is not recommended for securing the wire-fixation bolt. This washer is too small for fastening a K-wire; thus the wire can slide out under some pushing force or impact.
2. The 2-mm thick, 14-mm diameter washer with two flat surfaces (Fig. 9.34B). This washer is used mostly with the wire-fixation bolts and for support-post pairs adjustment. The larger diameter of this washer (it protrudes 2 mm beyond the fixation bolt head) guarantees that the fixed K-wire will not slide out under any circumstances. In support-post pair adjustment it helps to fix these parts in the same axial plane. This washer can be used with all other parts,

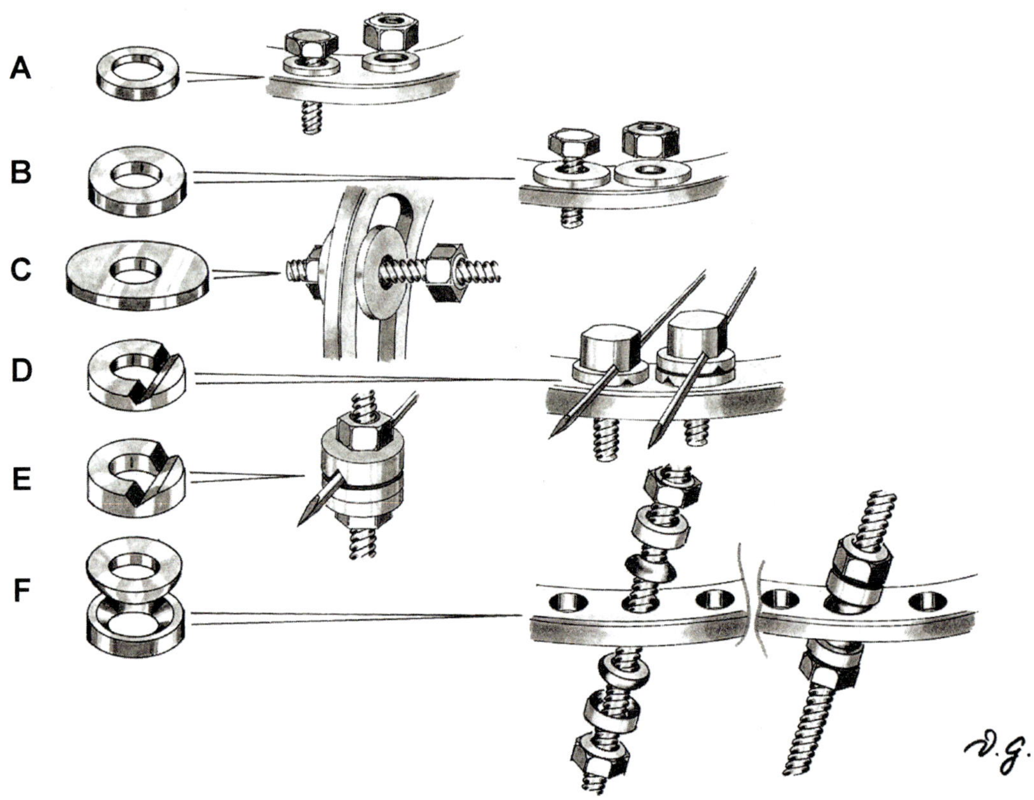

Figure 9.34: Washers used in construction of the Ilizarov fixator. A, 1.5-mm washer. B, 2.0-mm washer. C, 2.0-mm "wide" washer, used only for femoral arch-threaded rod interface. D, 3.0-mm washer. E, 4.0-mm washer. F, conical washer-couple, used for positioning with angulation

with the important exception that it cannot be placed on ring holes situated next to each other because this washer takes up the entire space on both sides of the hole, thus preventing secure tightening.

3. The 2-mm thick, 20-mm diameter washer with two flat surfaces (Fig. 9.34C). This washer is used only for adjustment of a threaded rod to the femoral arch. Its diameter is larger than the width of a regular ring. The width of the arch is 30 mm, and the width of its slot is 9 mm. To fix the 6-mm threaded rod into this slot, two of these washers must be used, one on either side of the arch (Fig. 9.34C).
4. The 3-mm thick, 14-mm diameter washer with one flat and one slotted surface (Fig. 9.34D). Often this washer is used to adjust the wire-fixation bolt to the plane of an introduced K-wire. If there is a gap of 3 mm or larger in the wire-ring alignment, one or two of these washers can be introduced between the ring and the fixation bolt head. In this situation the flat surface of the washer must face the bolt's slotted or cannulated head surface. The opposite surface of this washer has a 1-mm deep groove on one side. This groove permits the use of the slotted washer for wire fixation without using a wire-fixation bolt. For this purpose the slotted washer can be connected to the regular bolt (Fig. 9.34D) or to the threaded rod (Fig. 9.34E).
5. The 4-mm thick, 14-mm diameter washer with one flat surface and one slotted surface (Fig. 9. 34E). This is essentially the same washer as in Figure 9.34D, but is 1 mm thicker.
6. The 3-mm thick, 12-mm diameter conical washer-couple (Fig. 9.34F). This washer has a particular purpose, which is to adjust parts positioned in an angulation of up to 15 degrees. The conical washer-couple consists of the exterior piece, which is a kind of hollowed-out base, and the interior piece, which fits

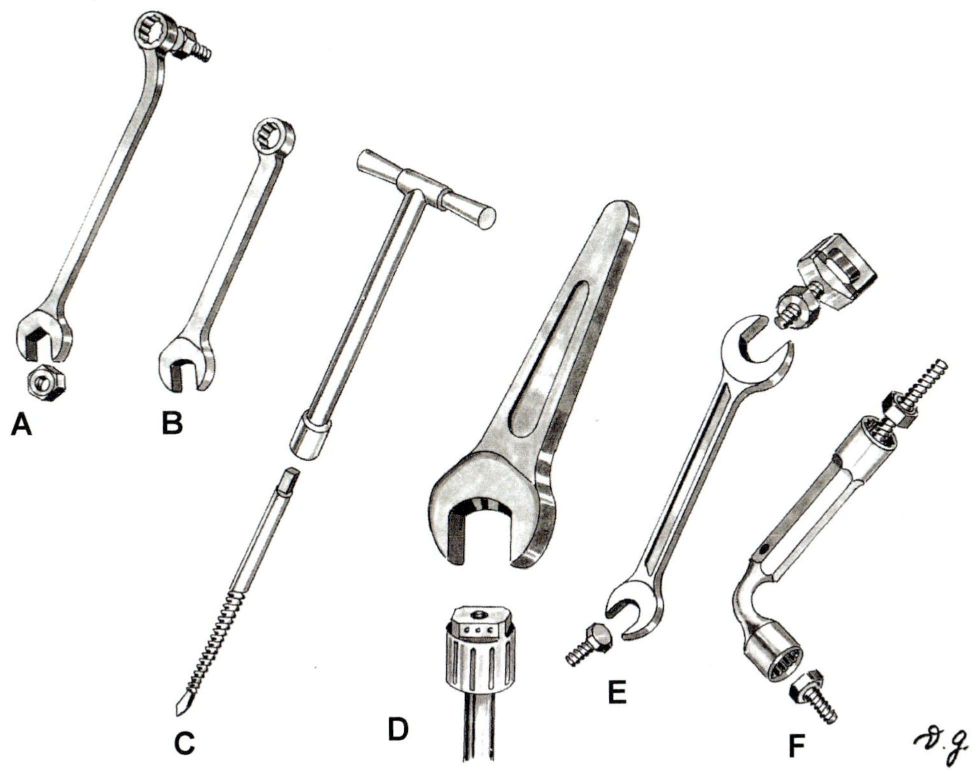

Figure 9.35: Wrenches used for the Ilizarov fixator. A, 10-mm (long) wrench with open and circular ends. Note that circular end is angulated. B, 10-mm (short) wrench with open and circular ends. C, T-shaped wrench for half pins (with half pin shown). D, 19-mm wrench for telescopic rod (the head of the telescopic rod shown). E, combined 13-mm and 10-mm wrench with open ends (shown with a pin fixation bolt and a regular bolt). F, 10-mm tubular angulated wrench, shown with a threaded rod introduced into the long leg and a regular bolt in the short leg

into the exterior base. The interior piece can be turned inside the base to 15 degrees without displacement of the central holes. If it is locked in angulation by the nuts, it will remain stable. The conical washers can be used on one or both surfaces of the ring, but the interior piece must face the stable surface, in most cases the ring surface.

WRENCHES

Nut-bolt and nut-ring tightening is performed with various types of wrenches (Fig. 9.35).

It is important to emphasize that tightening always must be performed simultaneously with two wrenches. One wrench is attached to a motionless part (e.g. the head of a bolt), and the second is attached to the part being tightened (e.g. a nut). This maneuver makes it much easier to produce the necessary tightening force, as much as 200 kg.

Occasionally it is difficult to attach the wrench to the nuts and bolts because adjacent parts are in the way. An attempt must be made to approach the part from the other side. If this also is impossible, a tightened adjacent part must be loosened, the desired tightening must be performed, and the loosened part must be retightened. This practical tip is described in detail in Chapter 11.

10 Chapter
Frame Assemblage

GENERAL CONSIDERATIONS

In constructing any type of Ilizarov frame, the major considerations are:

1. The stability of the fixation of the frame to the bone
2. The prevention of gross bone fragment motion
3. The ability to manipulate bone and to perform necessary fragment movements such as straightening, bending, distraction, compression, rotation, and combinations of these movements.

There are two methods of Ilizarov frame construction. The first is to construct the required frame in advance, assembling all the parts, then placing the sterilized frame as a whole over the limb during surgery, and transfixing the rings to the bone with the K-wires (Fig. 10.1).

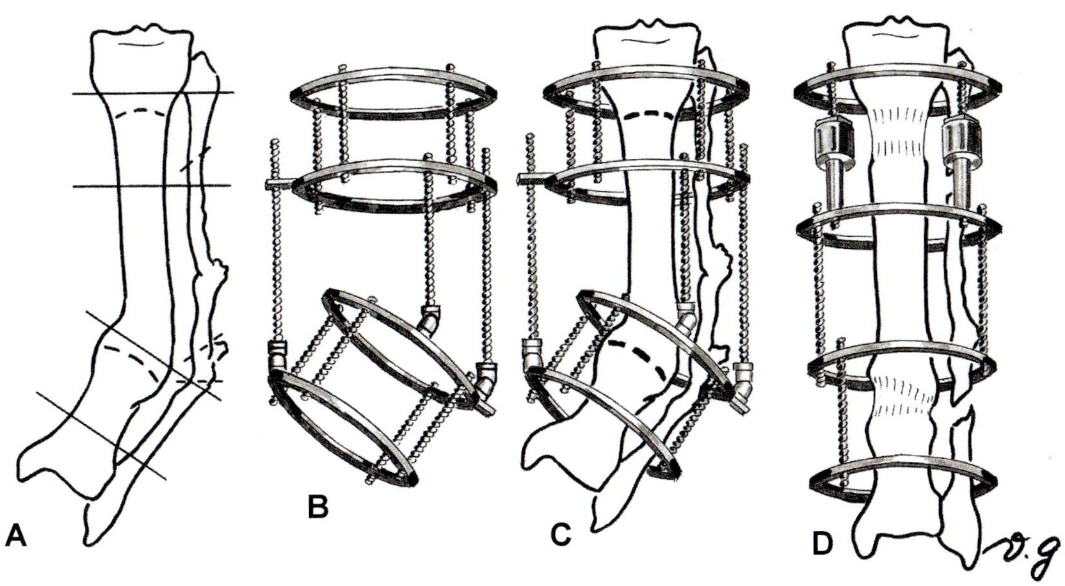

Figure 10.1: Schematic representation of preassembled method of application of the frame. A, bony outline of a roentgenogram of tibia-fibula malunion with shortness and severe varus deformity (posteroanterior view). Positioning of the rings is indicated by *uninterrupted lines,* the sites of the bone osteotomies by *interrupted lines*. B, preassembled frame according to the marked indications in A. Note that the ring angulation is supported by three hinges *(thick lines)*. C, preassembled frame in B is applied to the limb, matching the marked levels. Note that proximal and distal pairs of rings are positioned perpendicular to the long bone axis. D, projected appearance of the bones in A and C after lengthening at the site of proximal osteotomy, and correction at the site of distal osteotomy. The newly regenerated bone is marked. Note that all four rings now are positioned parallel to each other. (Details of the distraction and correction techniques are described in Chapter 14)

The second method is to construct the frame during surgery, assembling it piece-by-piece over the limb. To do this the K-wires first have to be introduced into the bone, then the rings and other parts connected to them, until the entire frame is built (Fig. 10.2).

The main advantage of the first method of frame assembly is that it saves time during the surgical procedure. Frame preassembly also gives a surgeon the latitude to try some component variations. The disadvantage of a preassembled frame is that it may require adjustments during the surgical procedure, because it is impossible to foresee all necessary modifications, especially in complicated cases.

The chief advantage of the second method of frame assembly is that it affords the surgeon greater experience in practical frame construction details and may help the surgeon avoid having to make corrections during surgery. The primary disadvantage is that piece-by-piece frame assembly requires a great deal of time, adding to an already lengthy surgical procedure.

Some surgeons who are experienced in the Ilizarov technique recommend the first method, and some recommend the second. Professor Ilizarov prefers to construct the frame in advance. We found the intraoperative frame assembly method to be more effective in terms of learning the Ilizarov technique, because it is learned through actual surgical experience. Once the physician has adequate experience, however, the use of a preassembled frame is far more advantageous.

No matter which method is chosen, the surgeon must have a clear idea in each case of the number and sizes of rings required, at what levels and positions these rings must be placed, the types and sizes of ring connectors, and all auxiliary parts that will be used. To formulate all of these frame considerations as clearly as possible, it is useful to trace the radiographic bony outline and draw the frame design on paper or directly on the film.

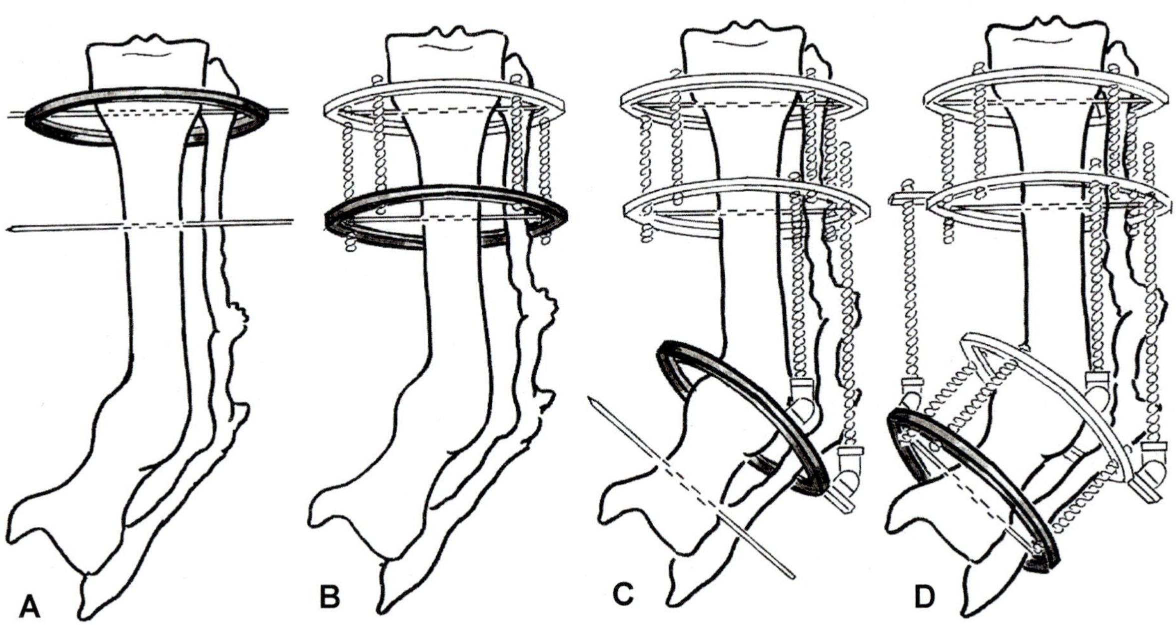

Figure 10.2: Intraoperative method of frame assembly, piece-by-piece during surgery. The tibia-fibula malunion is essentially the same as in Figure 10.1, and positioning of the rings is the same. A, in the first stage a K-wire is introduced at the site of the proximal ring, and the ring itself is placed over the limb and fixed with a wire. Before the second ring is applied, the K-wire is introduced at the level of this ring. B, in the second stage, the next ring *(shaded)* is applied and fixed with the wire. Both rings are then connected by threaded rods. C, in the third stage, the third ring *(shaded)* is applied over and connected to the previous ring with threaded rods with hinges. Note that this ring has no transfixing wire because it is positioned at the apex of angulation over the site of osteotomy. However, a wire is introduced for distal ring fixation. D, in the fourth stage the distal ring is placed over the wire and fixed to the wire and the rods. Note that the frame configuration is essentially the same as in Figures 10.1B and C. The projected appearance of the bones will be the same as in Figure 10.1D

RING POSITIONING

The rings are the chief components of any Ilizarov frame configuration. They serve three main purposes: K-wire support, frame formation, and supplementary part support. There are several ring types.

The *main proximal frame supporting ring* (Fig. 10.3A) is stationary and always located at the base of the frame. It bears the weight of the entire construction. In a femoral frame it is replaced by the supporting arch; in the humeral frame it is replaced by the half-ring with extremities.

The *stabilizing frame supporting ring* (Fig. 10.3B) always is located most distally. It can be stationary or movable, depending on frame purpose.

The *pusher-puller ring* (Fig. 10.3C) is a movable ring used for application of distraction-compression forces. It is located distal to the fracture-osteotomy-nonunion site. Depending on frame size, there may be two puller-pusher rings acting simultaneously or in opposite directions.

The *reference ring* (Fig. 10.3D) is medially located ring and used as a reference for the supporting rings or distraction-compression rings; it can be stationary or movable, depending on location.

The ring with combined functional significance is used for such multiple purposes as a pusher-puller ring and a reference ring simultaneously (for angulation correction and pseudoarthrosis distraction-compression).

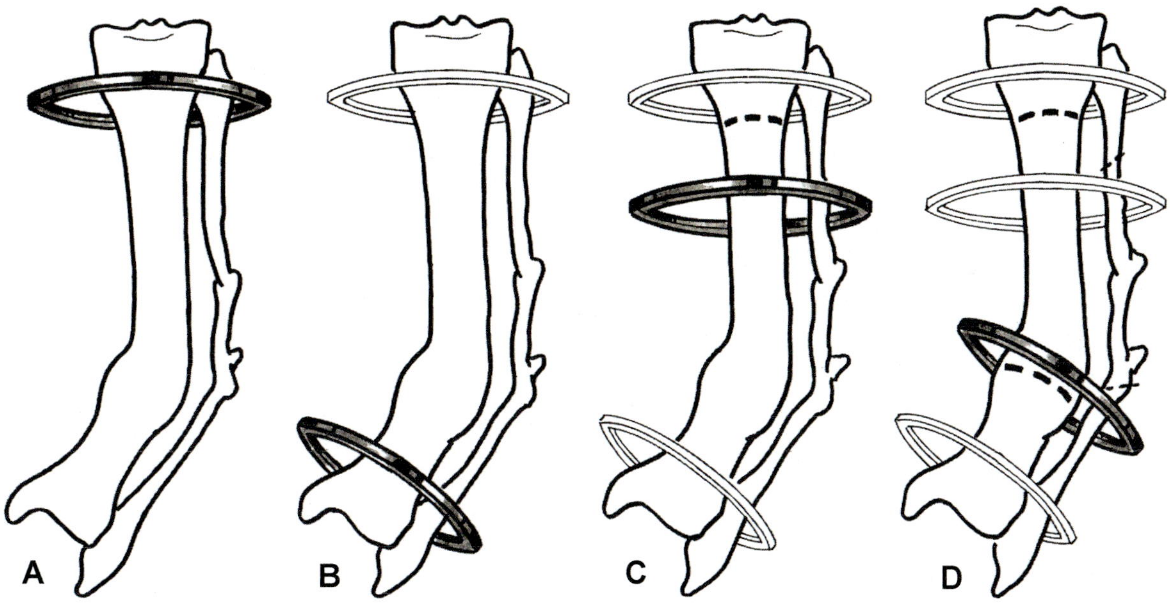

Figure 10.3: Schematic representation of intraoperative frame construction assembled piece-by-piece (during surgery) over the same type of malunion of the tibia and fibula as in Figure 10.1. A, stage I: the main frame-supporting ring *(shaded)* is applied to the proximal tibia metaepiphysis at the site of the frame base. This is the stationary ring. B, stage 2: The stabilizing frame-supporting ring *(shaded)* is applied to the distal tibial metaepiphysis. Note that it is positioned in angulation to the main supporting ring. Because its position gradually changes as the process of correction of the varus deformity progresses, this ring is considered the "movable" ring. C, stage 3: the pushing-pulling ring *(shaded)* is applied distal to the site of a planned osteotomy *(interrupted line)*. Note that it is applied parallel to the proximal main ring. This is the movable ring. D, stage 4: the reference ring *(shaded)* is applied to the site of tibia angulation deformity at the level of the planned osteotomy *(bottom interrupted line)*. Note that it is applied parallel to the distal stabilizing ring. Because its position will change with correction of the varus deformity, it also is a movable ring. Also, since it is not recommended that K-wires be introduced at the apex of a deformity, this ring can be left without wire fixation. Nevertheless, this ring will be transfixed by the offset (drop) wires as soon as the deformity is corrected, and will be used as pushing-pulling ring for the distal osteotomy. Thus this ring is considered to have combined functional significance

An additional, correcting ring is used for the application of special forces in transverse or oblique directions. Two or three such rings may be used on some frames.

Each ring must be positioned exactly and meticulously around the patient's limb at a particular level and in a correct inclination perpendicular to the bone, on both frontal and sagittal planes.

RING LEVEL

Choice of ring level determines distribution of the forces applied to the ring. The motionless, main supporting ring supports the primary frame stabilization forces; thus it must be located on the strongest and widest part of the bone. Anatomically this is the proximal metaepiphysis, and in most cases the main supporting ring level will be located at the proximal end of the bone. When considering the preservation of the range of motion of the adjacent joint this ring level is located 3 to 5 cm distal to the joint space. In the case of a short frame located distally, the level of this ring is translated distally to the diaphyseal portion of the bone (Fig. 10.4A).

The stabilizing frame supporting ring determines the forces of stabilization and balance located at the frame end opposite the main supporting ring. Depending on frame length, the level of this ring would be located at the distal metaepiphysis (3 to 5 cm from the joint), or transfixed to the diaphysis (Fig. 10.4B).

The pushing-pulling ring determines the direction of the forces of distraction-compression. To act most effectively, these forces must be applied close to the site of the osteotomy, fracture, or nonunion, with consideration of the general principle of preservation of the bone fragment ends; that is, a distance at least 3 to 5 cm must remain.

Depending on the osteotomy, fracture, or nonunion site and the chosen direction of distraction-compression, the pushing-pulling ring may be placed at a level closer to either the proximal or distal supporting rings.

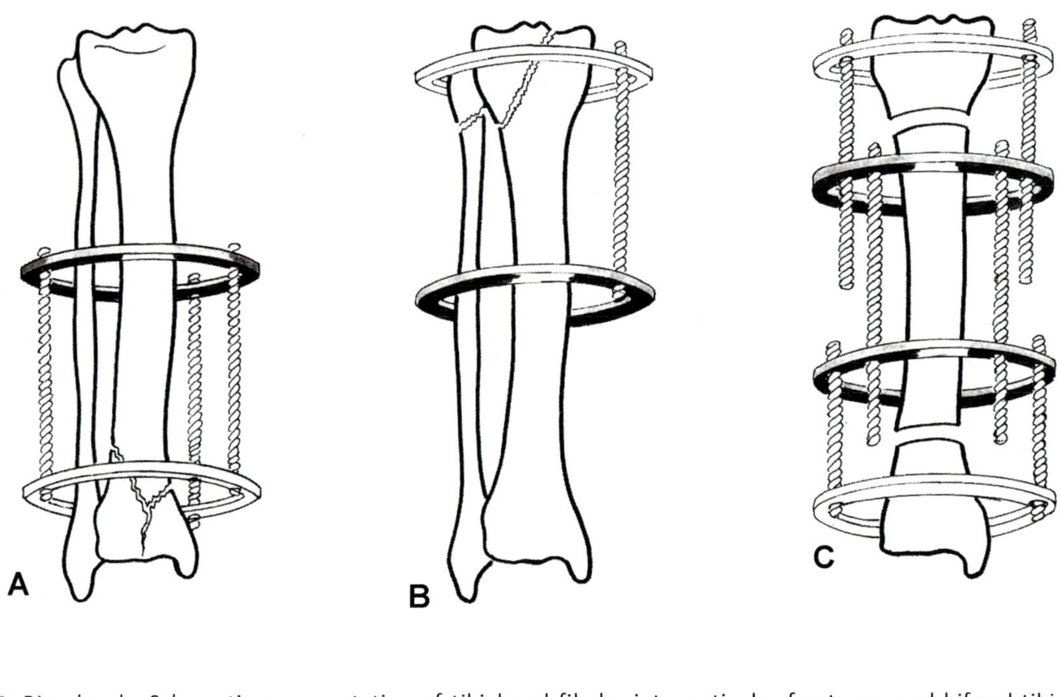

Figure 10.4: Ring levels. Schematic representation of tibial and fibular intra-articular fractures, and bifocal tibial corticotomy, showing various ring levels. A, with an Intra-articular fracture of the distal tibia the supporting ring *(shaded)* is in the middle portion of the limb. B, with a fracture in the proximal tibia the supporting ring again is in the middle of the limb. C, with a bifocal corticotomy the most proximal and distal rings are both supporting rings, whereas the two rings *(shaded)* in the middle area are movable rings that transport the bone fragments

Correspondingly, it is placed either distal or proximal to the osteotomy gap (Fig. 10.4C). In some cases two pulling-pushing rings are used in one frame, placed near both the proximal and distal supporting rings.

The reference ring (so-called free ring) determines the distribution of the translational forces along the limb, and thus must be placed at the level of the intersection of these forces (Fig. 10.5). In most cases this corresponds to the apex of the bone angulation. Because it is not practical to introduce the K-wires at the apex, the reference ring remains without any wire fixation.

The correcting ring determines the distribution of forces in transverse or oblique directions. For example,

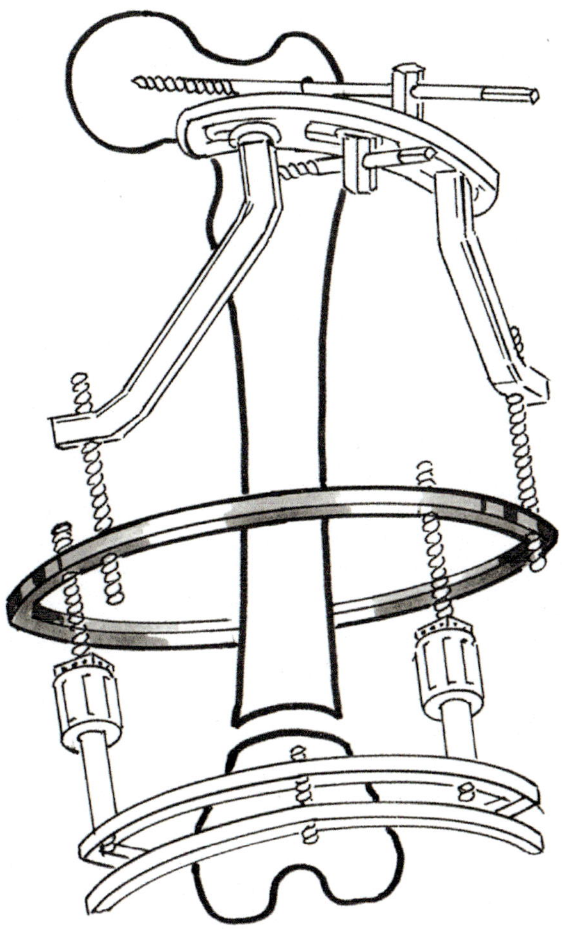

Figure 10.5: Reference or "free" ring *(shaded)*, shown in a schematic diagram of a frame used for femur osteotomy and lengthening

for the correction of shearing displacement it is necessary to connect two rings with two translational devices. The level of this kind of ring must correspond to the location of corrected segment, leaving a 2- to 3-cm space from the fragment end (Fig. 10.6A).

The ring with combined functional significance determines distribution of forces in multiple directions. For example, if there is need for distraction and derotation, the ring must work simultaneously as a pulling and correcting ring. The location of the ring corresponds to the focal point of the application of these combined forces (Fig. 10.6B).

RING INCLINATION

The choice of the ring inclination determines the direction of the forces applied to the ring. At any chosen level, each ring has to be set in a position of correct inclination in regard to the bone axis. In most cases this inclination is perpendicular to the bone segment-fragment at this level (Fig. 10.7A).

A 90-degree angle of ring inclination is ideal. An angle of 100 degrees would, for example, derange the attachment to the other connected rings. The resultant angle the would place one side of the distal rings too close to the skin or soft tissue, exerting forces that act

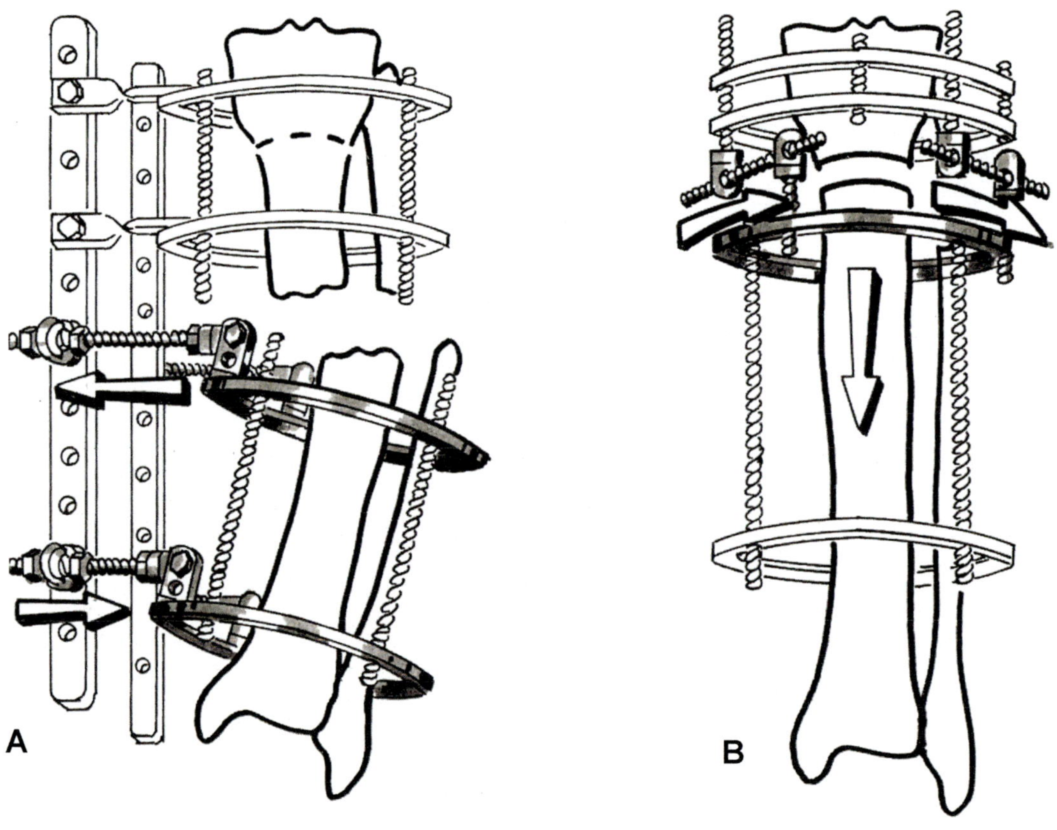

Figure 10.6: A, correcting rings *(shaded).* **B,** ring with combined functional significance *(shaded)*

under inclination and deforming the limb in the direction of this incorrect angle (Figs 10.7B and C).

To position the ring the surgeon must take into account the surrounding soft tissues, particularly muscle and subcutaneous fat. The ring is not positioned around the exact geometric center, but around the anatomic bony center of fixation. The muscle or fat mass may, however, confound ring inclination. In addition, in some cases there may be soft tissue defects or deep scars. This may confuse even more the determination of correct ring inclination. The only way for the surgeon to determine correct ring inclination is by taking into consideration the bone shape and position on the anteroposterior and lateral radiographic views.

During limb lengthening, muscle tension can influence some deviation in the distracted bone fragment. This possible influence must be taken into account when setting the inclination of the proximal main supporting ring, to ensure prevention of development of deformity, especially in the case of extensive leg lengthening.

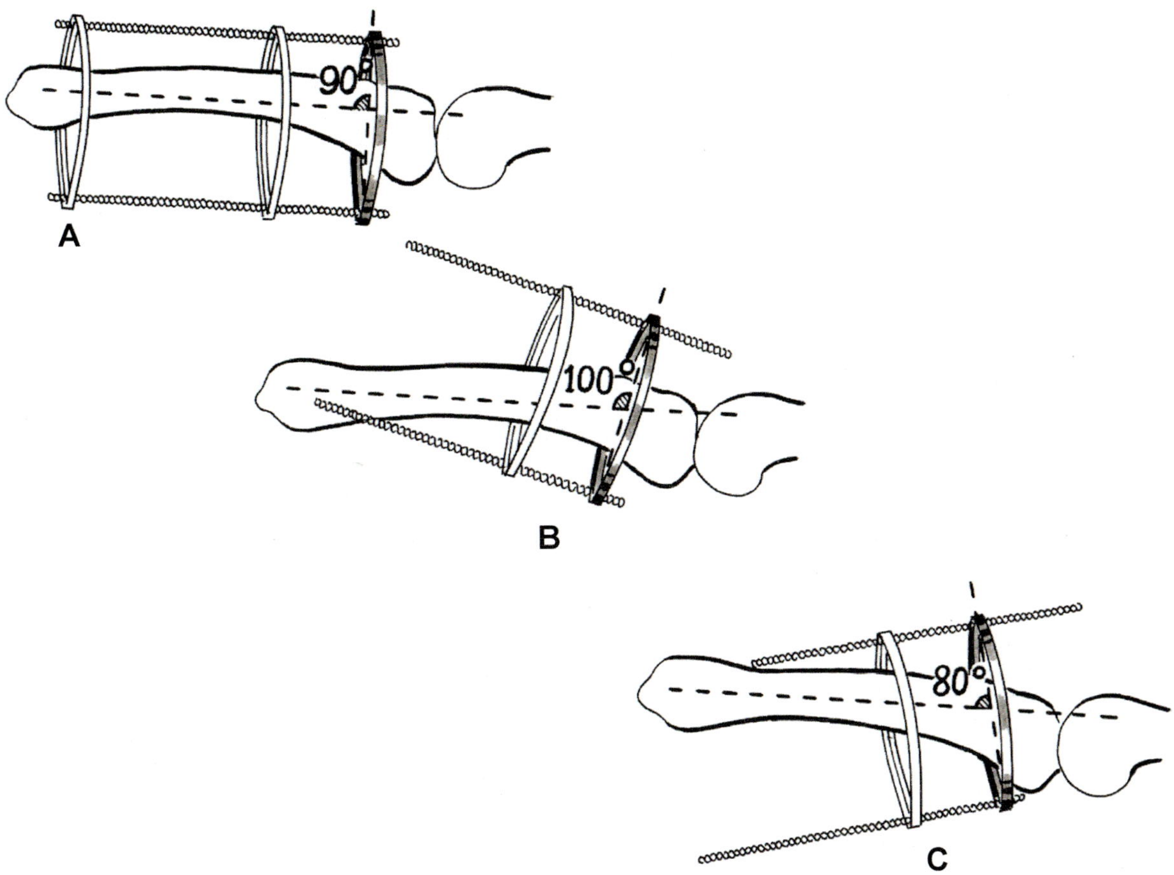

Figure 10.7: Ring inclination in three situations. Lateral view of tibia is represented, with *broken lines* showing the long bone axis and the ring inclination. **A,** main supporting ring *(shaded)* is in a position of 90-degree inclination to the bone axis. The resultant angle is the same for all rings of the frame. **B,** main-supporting ring *(shaded)* is in a position of 100-degree inclination to the bone axis. The resultant angle puts the middle ring too close to the bone at the posterior side and totally deranges the attachment of the distal stabilizing frame supporting ring. **C,** main supporting ring *(shaded)* is in a position of 80-degree inclination to the bone axis. The resultant angle puts the middle ring too close to the bone at the anterior side and again totally deranges the attachment of the distal stabilizing frame supporting ring

Experience shows that the lateral leg muscles, in particular the tibialis anterior, extensor digitorum longus, and extensor hallucis longus muscles, tend to drag a distal fragment laterally, and the posterior muscles, in particular the soleus, gastrocnemius, and tibialis posterior muscles, tend to drag it posteriorly. In such a situation, these forces can put the distracted leg in a position of valgus deformity and antecurvation.

To prevent the development of this deformity, it is recommended that the proximal ring be tilted. Five degrees of recurvation of this main supporting ring will bring correct positioning of the distracted leg (Fig. 10.8). It is important to remember that in this type of ring inclination an average of 1 cm of difference medially vs. laterally, and anteriorly vs. posteriorly, will produce the 5-degree tilt necessary to lengthen the leg in the correct direction.

In planning femoral lengthening at the proximal osteotomy (corticotomy) site, it is recommended that the proximal main supporting arch be tilted. The tension of the adductor group (the adductor brevis, longus, and magnus muscles) tends to drag a distal fragment medially. Tension of the posterior muscles (particularly the biceps femoral muscle) tends to drag a distal fragment posteriorly. In such a situation, these forces would set the distal femur in a position with a varus and posterior bending deformity.

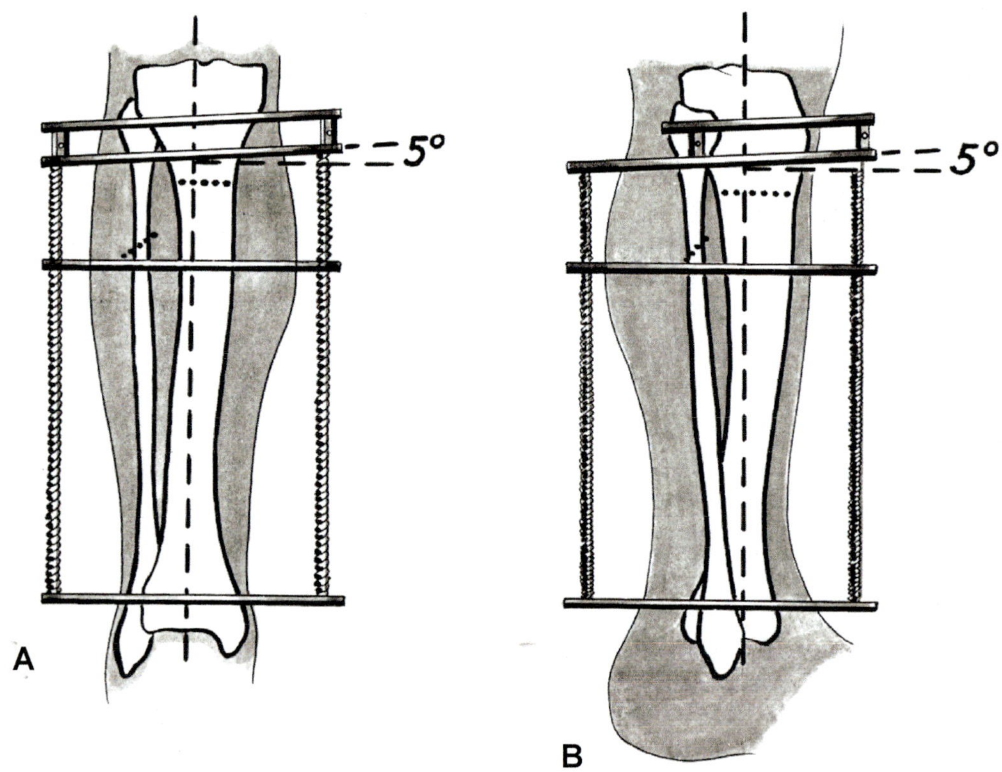

Figure 10.8: Ring positioning in the tibial lengthening frame, anteroposterior (A) and lateral (B) views. Dotted lines show osteotomy sites; *interrupted lines* show long bone axis. A, in anticipation of the osteotomized bone lateral deviation, the main supporting ring is placed in a position of 5 degrees varus inclination. Note that this ring is reinforced by the half-ring. B, in anticipation of the osteotomized bone posterior deviation (antecurvation), the main supporting ring together with the reinforcing half-ring is placed in a position of 5 degrees of recurvation inclination

Seven to 10 degrees of abduction and 5 to 7 degrees of anterior elevation of the main supporting arch will help to achieve the correct positioning of the distal frame (Fig. 10.9A).

In planning an upper arm lengthening at the site of a proximal osteotomy, the proximal main supporting half-ring with curved extremities has to be tilted. Tension of the coracobrachialis muscle and of the triceps brachii muscle (medial head) tends to drag a distal fragment medially. Such a result would set the distal humerus in a position of varus deformity. Five to 7 degrees of abduction of the supporting half-ring will help to achieve correct positioning of the distal humerus (Fig. 10.9B).

There is no need to tilt the rings when considering an osteotomy of the distal site. The reason for this is that muscle tension diminishes at the sites of distal attachment to the bone. Moreover, the frame's proximal component above this level always is stable enough to be able to resist any tendency to drag a distal fragment.

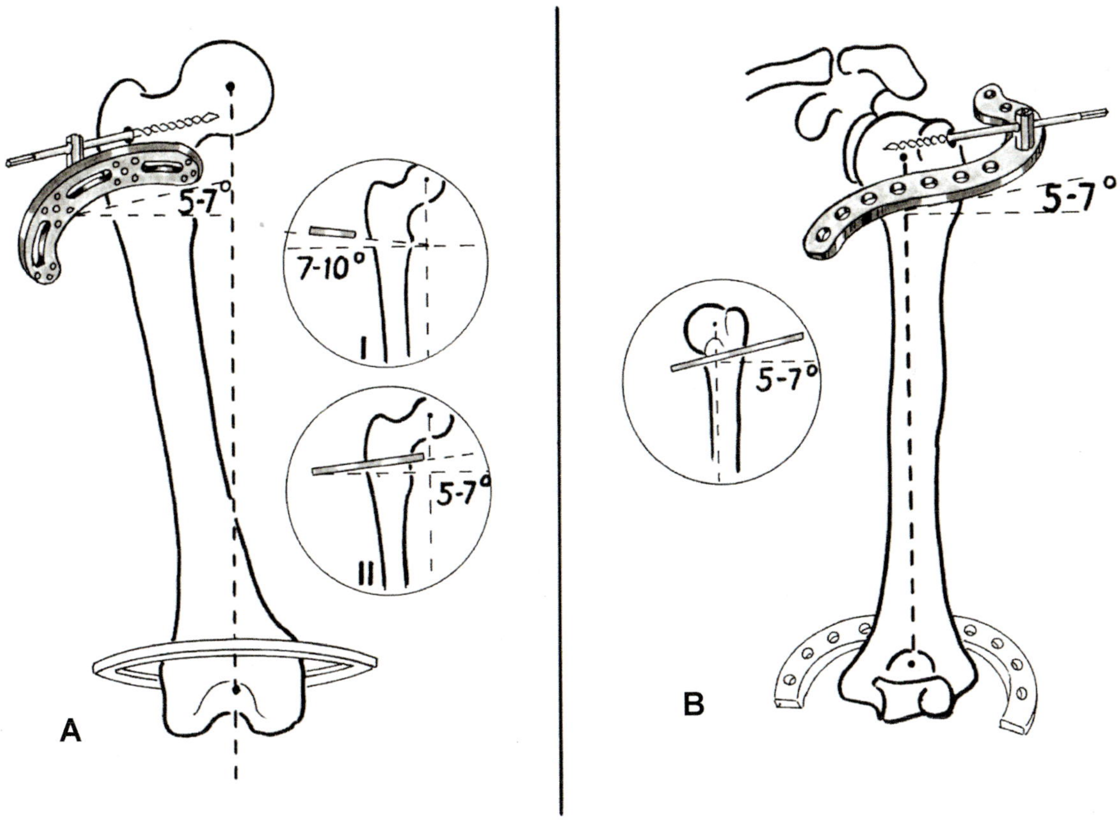

Figure 10.9: Ring inclination in the frames for femoral and humeral lengthening. A, femoral bone with the attached main supporting arch *(shaded)* and pulling ring. *Insets,* partial views of the same arch in a position of 7 to 10 degrees of abduction *(I)*, and 5 to 7 degrees of anterior elevation *(II)*. B, humeral bone with the attached main supporting half-ring with curved arms *(shaded)* and five-eighths pulling ring. *Inset,* partial view of the same half-ring in a position of 5 to 7 degrees of abduction

SPACE BETWEEN SKIN AND RING

Independent of the level and angle of any rings, a space, as a rule, at least 3 cm, should be maintained between the inner curve of the ring and the skin. Because the breadth of an extremity varies at different levels, this space also will vary. It is calculated, however, at its narrowest gap. In other areas, this space can extend to 4, 5, and sometimes even 6 cm.

The space between the skin and ring gives the surgeon freedom to manipulate the bolts and nuts, to introduce the threaded rods into the ring holes, and to attach all necessary additional parts. This gap also is important in protecting the skin and soft tissues if swelling occurs, and it permits wire tract care during the duration of the treatment. There are three ways to ensure an adequate skin-ring gap.

The first method is to measure the width of the limb at the anticipated levels of rings. This measurement is performed in centimeters with a measuring tape before frame assembly. The measurement is taken in both frontal and sagittal planes, and only the largest figure is taken into consideration. Adding 6 cm to this figure provides a necessary internal ring diameter, with a secure 3-cm space between ring and skin (Fig. 10.10A).

The second method is to attach the ring of anticipated size over the limb where the surgeon expects to attach it and to ensure a minimum 3-cm gap at its most narrow section. This is a more suitable way of measurement if the frame is being assembled part by part intraoperatively (Fig. 10.10B).

The third method is to introduce standard plastic templates over the limb at the presumed ring levels and to determine at each level which rings provide the necessary skin-ring gap. These templates have been introduced by the Smith and Nephew Richards Company, and can be used before frame assembly or during the procedure (Fig. 10.10C).

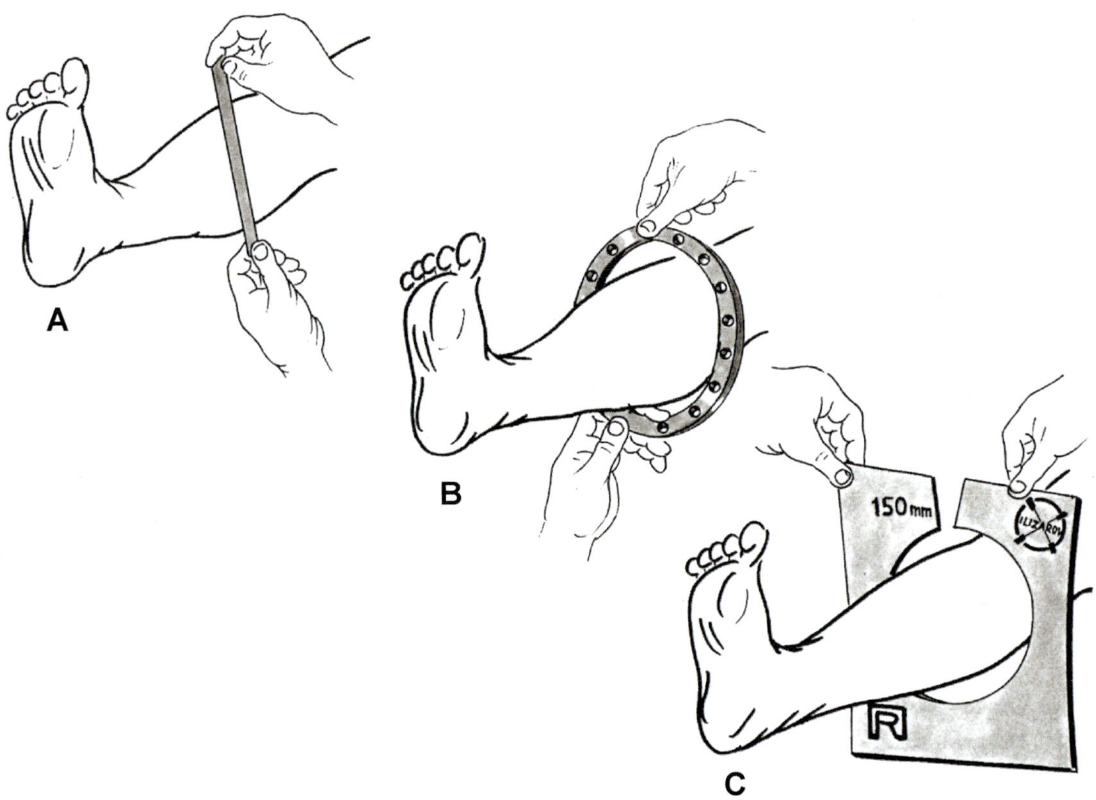

Figure 10.10: Three ways to select a ring of proper size for the leg are shown. A, measure the widest part of the leg with the measuring tape and add 6 cm to the obtained figure. B, try the proper size ring in advance. C, apply a Smith and Nephew Richards special template

TECHNICAL HINT

TWO-FINGERS BREADTH RULE

An easy technical tip to determine that enough space has been maintained between the ring and the skin is the two-fingers breadth rule. Ensure that the gap between the ring and the skin is at least the width of two fingers by inserting your fingers in this space (Fig. 10.11).

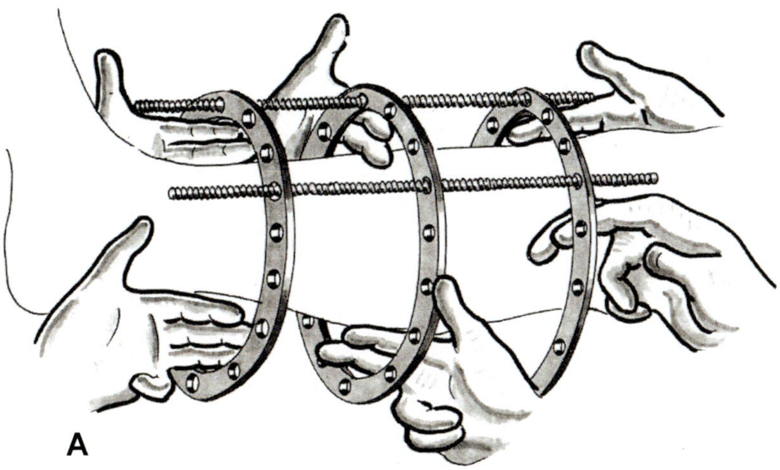

A

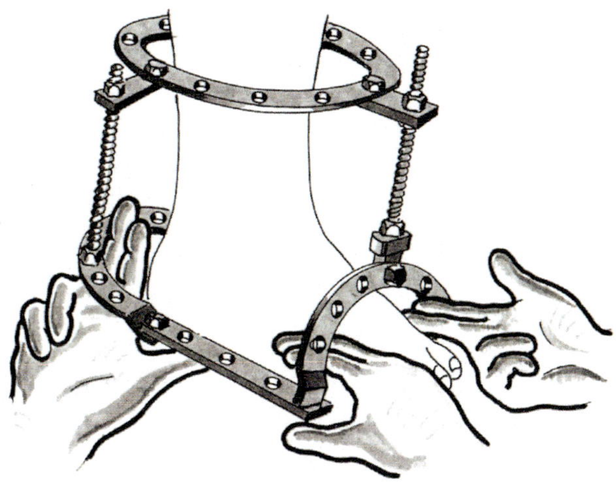

B

Figure 10.11: A, three-ring frame applied to the leg. At the level of each ring the surgeon's fingers are in the space between skin and ring. Normally this space should be at least two fingers wide. Only at the level of the proximal metaepiphysis on the anterior surface can it be smaller, because not much soft tissue is found there. At the distal site it can be larger. B, three-ring frame applied to the foot. Note a two-fingers breadth space between skin and ring

RING POSITIONING AT OSTEOTOMY/CORTICOTOMY, NONUNION AND/OR FRACTURE SITES

At the sites of osteotomy, nonunion, or fracture with displacement there are always free bone fragment ends. With application of the Ilizarov frame, stability of this free end depends much on the level and positioning of the pusher-puller ring. Considering any forthcoming distraction, compression, bone straightening, or derotation, the closer the ring is placed to the tip of free bone fragment end the more stable this fragment is during all necessary bone movements. At the same time, the bone fragment end structure almost always is weakened by the net of microfractures developed with the bone split during osteotomy or fracture (Fig. 10.12). In the case of nonunion, the free bone fragment structure also is weakened by regional osteoporosis, and sometimes may be icicle shaped. In all of these situations there is a need for the free-fragment-end structure preservation. Hence the pusher-puller ring is placed at some distance from the tip of the free bone end.

Consequently there is something of a contradiction in these recommendations. The ring must be close to the tip of the bone, but also must be distant enough to permit access to the frame parts. In choosing the proper ring level in relation to the free bone fragment end, the surgeon must consider all of these aspects and find a

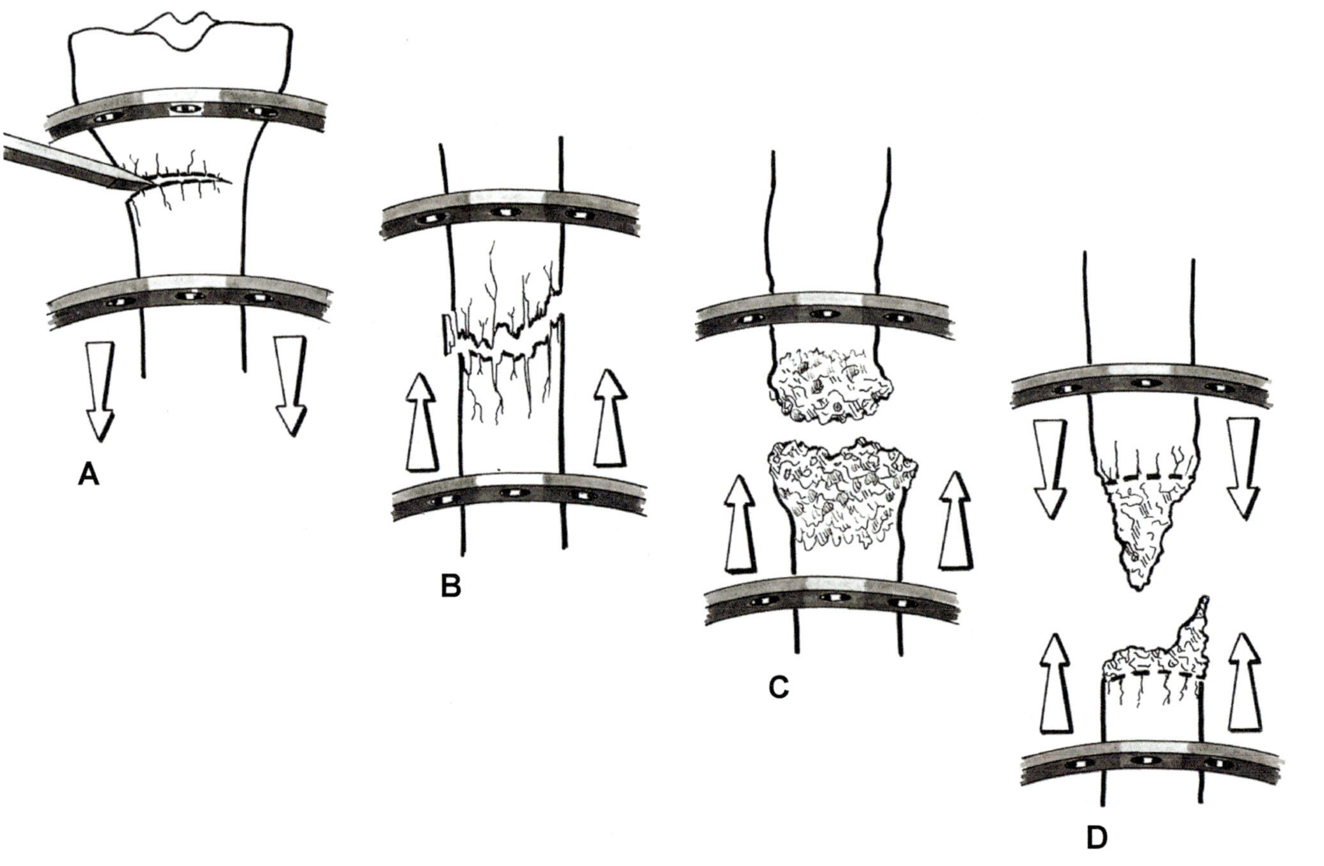

Figure 10.12: Four sectional views of the bone and rings positioned above and below an osteotomy, fracture, and nonunion. *Arrows* show the direction of the bone fragment movement. A, performance of osteotomy (corticotomy) by the narrow osteotome and the net of microfractures developed at the bone fragment ends. The rings are positioned close to the osteotomy site but far enough from the microfractures. B, fresh bone fracture creates a more significant microfracture net. The rings are positioned slightly farther from the fragment ends than in A. C, bone nonunion with regional osteoporosis. The rings are positioned just to the side of the osteoporotic areas. D, bone nonunion with the icicle-shaped osteoporotic free ends. *Broken lines* show bone resection sites. The net of microfractures is expected to appear as a result of resection. The rings are positioned with consideration of the bone resection and microfractures, and thus are placed far to the side of the nonunion

suitable solution for each case. As a rule, the pusher-puller ring should be situated no closer than 2 cm and no further than 4 to 5 cm from the tip of the fragment end.

RING ORIENTATION

Regardless of the level, inclination, or angulation at which different rings of the same frame are positioned, they all must be aligned in a configuration in which the connecting parts of the half-rings are situated along the same straight line (Fig. 10.13A). This orientation puts the corresponding holes of all rings along the same straight lines, thus making ring connection, especially with the threaded rods, relatively easy. More important, this manner of ring orientation establishes the positioning of the rings in relation to the long bone axis. For example, in the case of rotational deformity correction this parallel ring alignment contributes to the control of derotation. By following the two neighboring half-ring connections above and below the rotation level, a degree of derotation can be established (Fig. 10.13B).

As soon as the ring level, inclination, skin surface relation, and orientation are established and reconfirmed, the rings should be transfixed to the bone with K-wires.

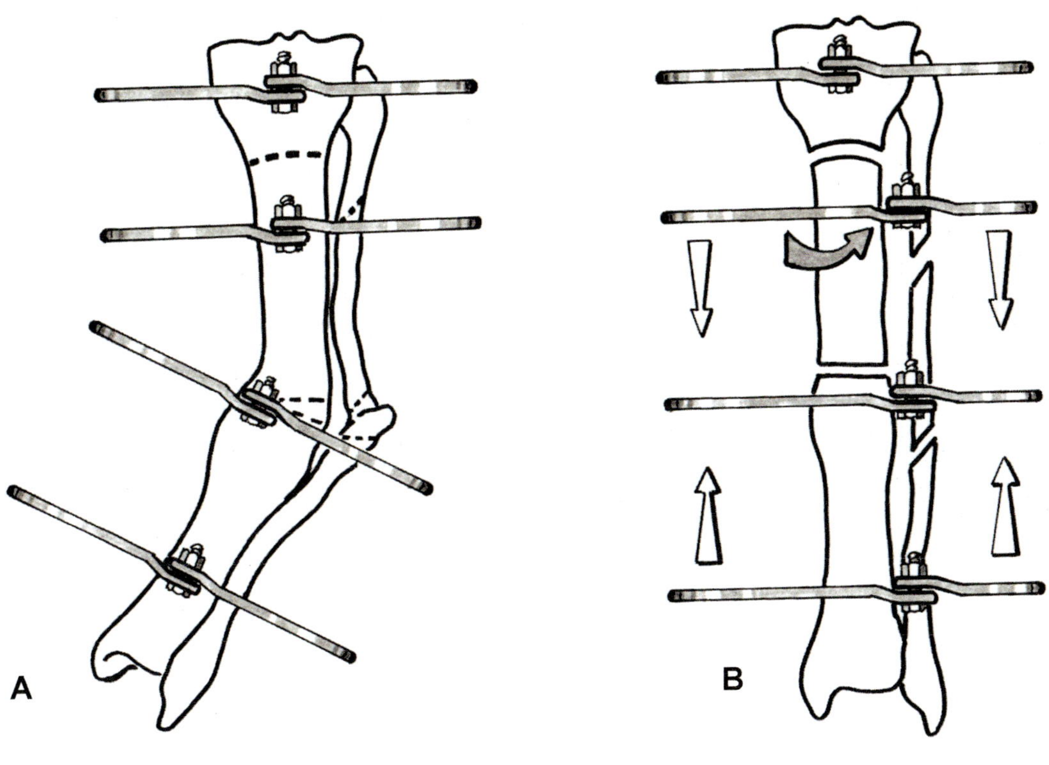

Figure 10.13: Ring orientation is shown in a schematic representation of tibia-fibula varus and rotational deformity with a four-ring frame. A, rings at different levels and in different inclinations all are oriented so that the connections of the half-rings are aligned on the same straight line, over the tibial anterior border. Sites of osteotomy are shown by *broken lines*. B, after varus and rotational deformity correction, all rings are parallel to each other, and bone fragments are in good alignment. *Arrows* show the direction of distraction, compression, and derotation. Note that the orientation of the proximal main stabilizing ring and the pulling ring next to it is now different: the half-rings connection to the pulling ring is rotated externally *(shaded arrow)*. Other rings are in the same orientation as the pulling ring

11 Chapter

Wires: Types and Utilization

GENERAL CONSIDERATIONS

The smooth nonthreaded wire originally was introduced in 1909 by the German surgeon Martin Kirshner for skeletal traction. It gradually lost favor to the thicker and stiffer Steinman pin. During the late 1940s and early 1950s, when Dr. Ilizarov began his pioneering clinical research, the K-wire still was used widely, and in a special way in backward Russia. Despite its unimpressive appearance, the Kirschner wire has important advantages:

1. When drilled into tissue, it destroys very little compact bone and bone marrow.
2. If tensioned properly, it dampens vibration and prevents soft tissue and bony destruction because of its elasticity.
3. After removal, penetration holes are very small.
4. Its small-diameter hole permits minimum external contamination.

What the wire lacks in comparison with the pin is stiffness. This is overcome partially by the way in which the wires are situated in the bone and fixed to the ring. Insertion of two or three wires on the same plane and in multiple directions replaces the linear force of a stiff pin with the wire forces acting along this plane. Fixation of each of the wires at both ends under great tension augments their combined stiffness. Elasticity is largely sacrificed, but some remains. This combination of strong tensioning and elasticity is the principal advantage of wire transfixation.

The availability of K-wires dictated Dr. Ilizarov's use of them for his fixator. Soon afterward, Ilizarov discovered that the limited-elasticity type of fixation from the wires had a particular advantage: it generated more rapid callus formation and maturation.

Further research showed that the restricted elasticity of the tensioned wires activated the piezoelectric phenomena in the cells of bone marrow, in compact bone, and in the newly developed regenerate.

Membrane potential differs in the electrical charges within and outside a cell. It has been demonstrated that electrical current in the cell can stimulate ion channels selectively. If the tissues are stimulated by the elastic micromotion the nerve impulses are activated. The nerve impulses help control the passage of electrically charged ions through the cells activating these ion channels. The exact mechanism of the elastic micromotion—cellular development interaction is not clear, however. Dr. Ilizarov considered it an analog to the mechanism of the fetal growth plate. He coined the term "tension stress" for this mechanism (Fig. 11.1).

It may seem puzzling that the thin K-wires can withhold the enormous stress of axial loading over a course of several months of treatment and also can bear the forces of distraction-compression without breaking or

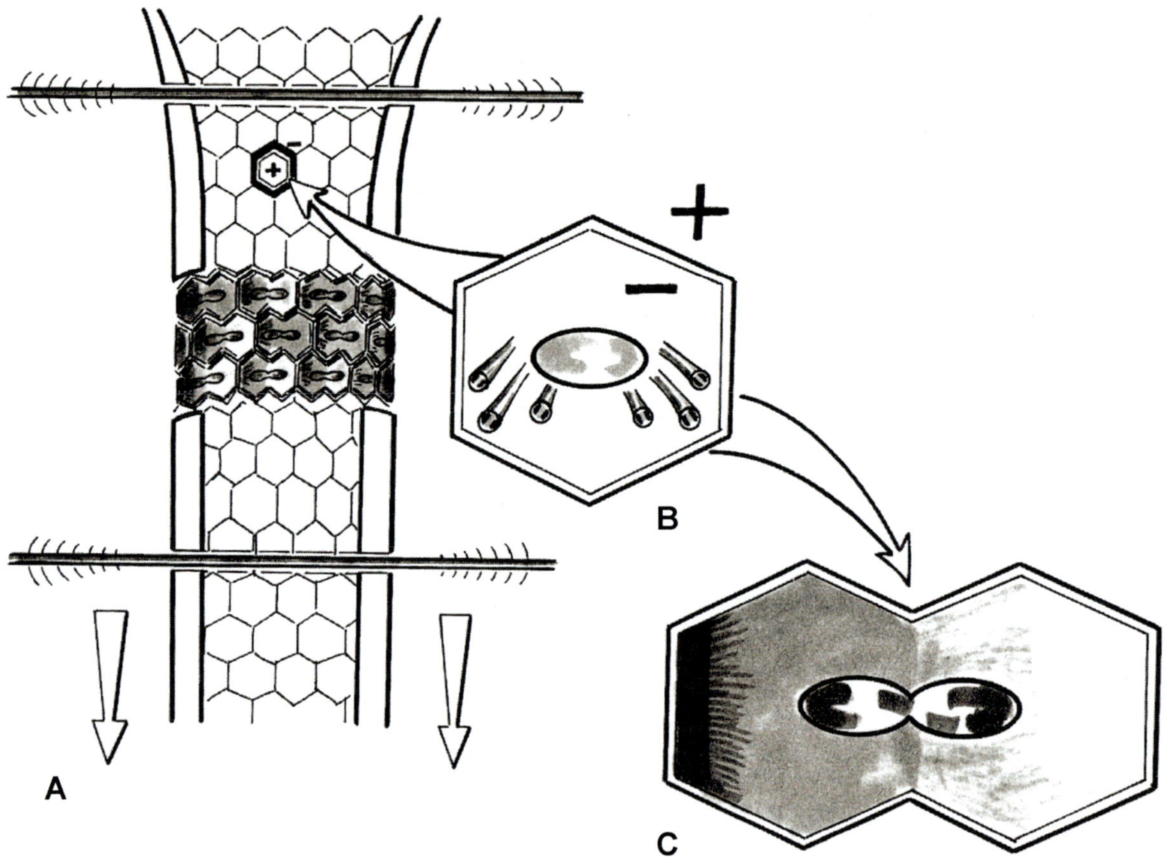

Figure 11.1: Schematic representation of the elastic micromotion stimulating effect of the wires on the ion channels of the bone cells and the resulting rapid cellular mitosis during bone distraction. A, bone segment with two transfixing wires in a state of vibration. The bone marrow cells are shown as hexagons. Interruption of the cortex showing the site of osteotomy; *arrows* show the direction of distraction. *Shaded figures* represent doubled cells in the telophase state of mitosis. A cell (distinguished by *heavy outline*) is shown in a polarized state. B, magnified representation of a bone marrow depolarized cell with the selectively stimulated microtubes and nucleolus *(shaded)*. The microtubes are the ion channels in a state of activation. C, same cell as in B, shown in telophase of mitosis with doubled nucleolus and cytoplasm

cutting bone tissue. The unique wire-ring combinations in the Ilizarov apparatus produces a much lower axial stiffness and axial loading force, which distributes load to all parts of the frame, than do the uniplanar and biplanar fixators that use much heavier pins. At the same time it shows higher axial stiffness against loading from bending forces (Fig. 11.2).

The wires combined with the rings endow the Ilizarov fixator with the optimal biomechanical characteristics for bone fragment stabilization. In addition to serving as a structurally supportive network, the wires translate distraction-compression forces and execute bone fragment alignment along with all the other necessary fragment position corrections.

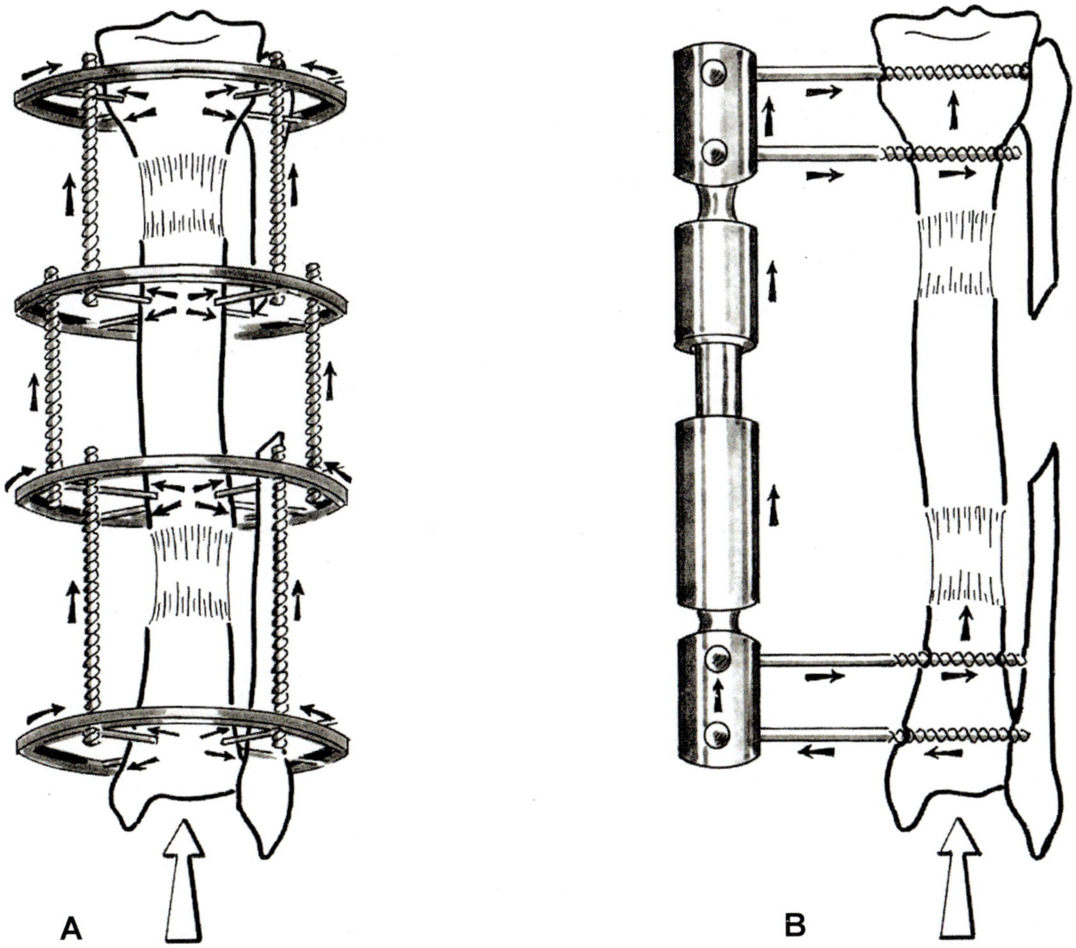

Figure 11.2: Schematic representation of the axial loading distribution in the Ilizarov apparatus (A) and in the unipolar dynamic axial external fixator during a tibia-fibula bifocal distraction. (B) *Large arrows* show direction of axial loading; *small arrows* show direction of loading distribution. A, balanced, circular forces mimic the dynamic loading and biomechanical function of the bone. B, uniplanar forces place stress at right angles, at two sites on this apparatus

In essence, the wire is the part of the Ilizarov apparatus that determines how the treatment proceeds, and the result. Dr. Ilizarov modified the original K-wires for use with his apparatus by making them in two, more useful diameters: 1.8-mm wires for use in adult patients and 1.5-mm wires for use in children (in some situations they can be cross-used).

For cortical bone drilling there are wires with bayonet point tips, and for cancellous bone drilling there are wires with the trocar point tip. To ensure ring stabilization there are wires with olive-type stoppers, which are made from one piece of metal. All types of wires are made in three lengths: 300, 370, and 400 mm, which enables them to be used with the differently sized rings (Fig. 11.3).

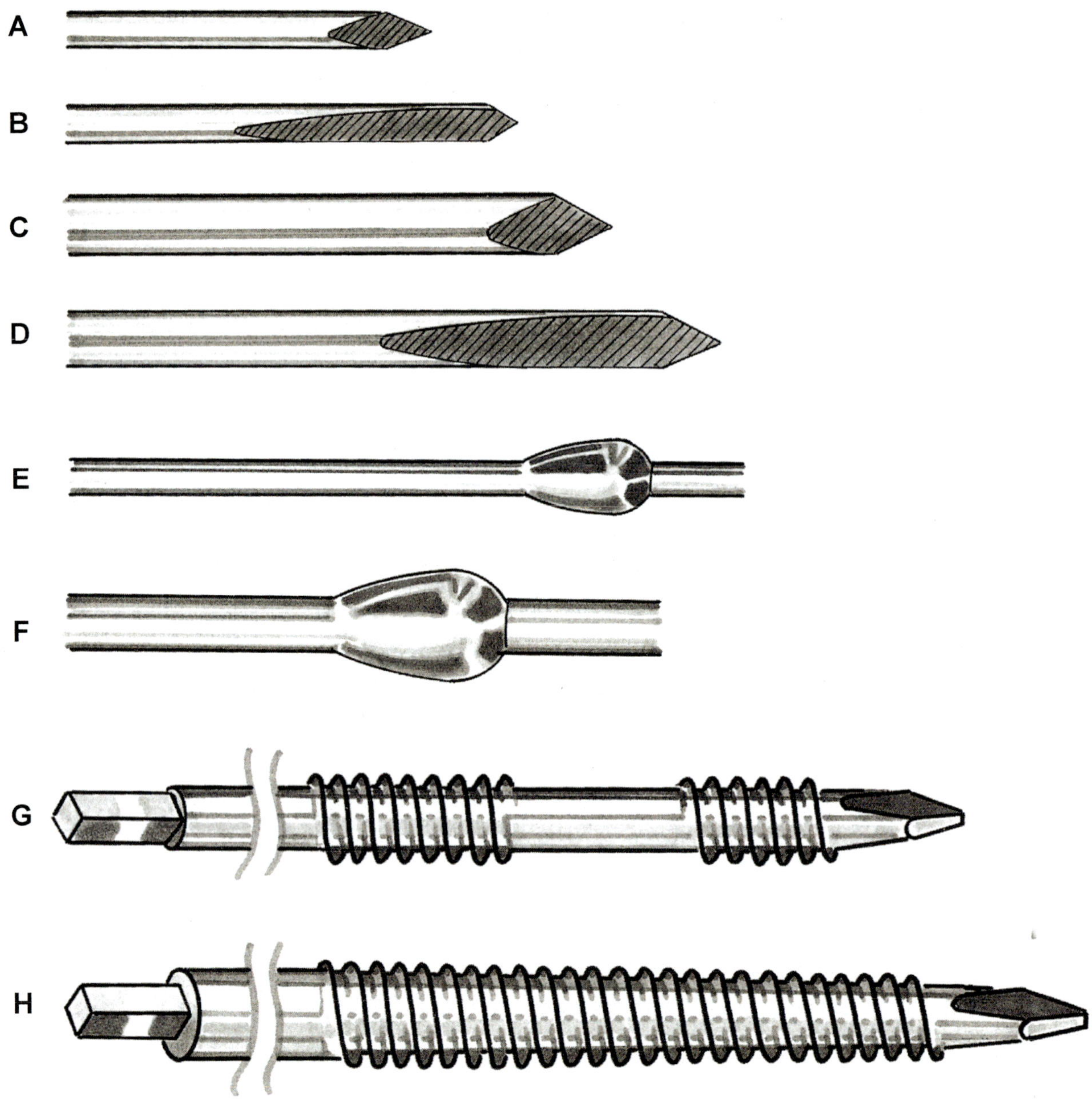

Figure 11.3: Wires and pins used in the Ilizarov system. A, 1.5-mm trochar-pointed wire. B, 1.5-mm bayonet-pointed wire. C, 1.8-mm trochar-pointed wire. D, 1.8-mm bayonet-pointed wire. E, 1.5-mm olive (stopper) wire. F, 1.8-mm olive wire. G, 4-mm half-pin with interrupted threaded section. H, 5-mm half-pin with continuous threaded end

TECHNIQUE OF K-WIRE INTRODUCTION

Principles

The introduction of K-wires for the fixation of bone is a key technique in the Ilizarov apparatus application. Wire introduction must be performed with precision because it determines both the positioning and stability of the rings. Moreover, during wire introduction the wire's sharp tip penetrates tissues of different density and type, hidden from the surgeon's eye. These tissue characteristics can change the wire's trajectory, causing possible injury to structures of vital importance (e.g. vessels, nerves). To perform wire introduction properly, and thereby avoid damage to vital neurovascular structures, several rules must be followed:

1. The wire entrance and exit sites are predetermined by the surgeon. While the surgeon is positioned at the wire entrance site, preparing to drill the wire through the opposite side of the extremity, an assistant should point to the expected exit site with a finger or an instrument so that the surgeon can direct the wire exactly toward that visual marker (Fig. 11.4).
2. The entrance and exit points of the K-wire must be located at least 1.5 to 2.0 cm from the major blood vessels and nerves; this helps to avoid any penetration and/or later development of pseudoaneurysm and neuroma resulting from wire contact. To achieve this distance, the surgeon should mark the projection of a pulsating artery on the skin with a pen. The major veins and nerves usually are located near the artery within the intermuscular septum layers and are easily movable within the range of 0.5 to 1.0 cm (Fig. 11.5).
3. Any K-wire has to be positioned according to the ring plane, and preferably across only one side of the ring wall, either proximal-to-proximal or distal-to-distal. A guidance system, particularly the slotted fixation bolt, is useful in K-wire positioning. Once the proper ring hole has been chosen for this bolt, proximate to the wire entrance, the wire can be placed in the groove of the bolt head and directed parallel to the ring wall (Fig. 11.6).

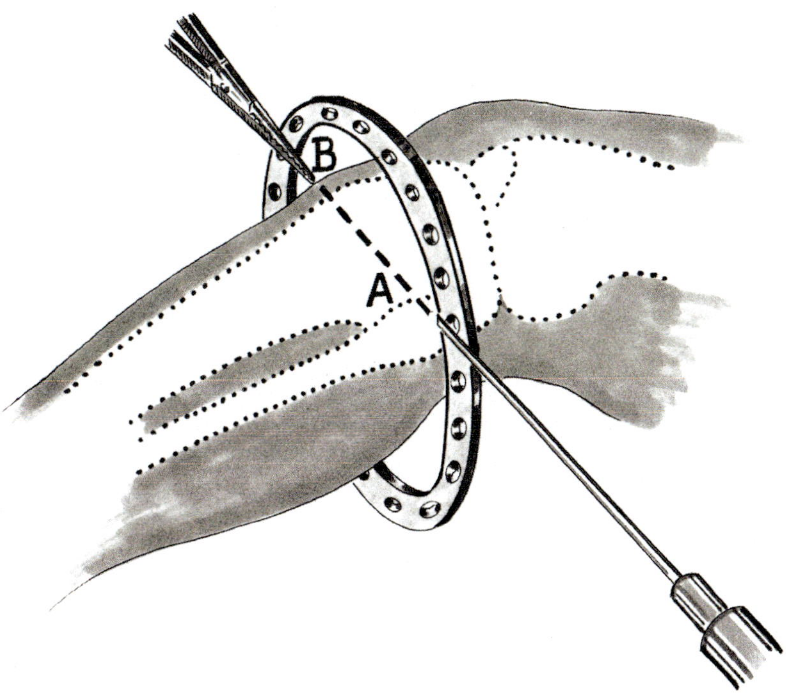

Figure 11.4: Direction in which the K-wire is inserted in the proximal tibia. Before the wire tip is introduced into the skin, entrance (A) and exit (B) drilling sites must be determined. Exit site is pointed to by a tip of clamp. Correct wire direction is indicated by the *dashed line*. In this situation the surgeon must ensure that the wire passes through the head of the fibula

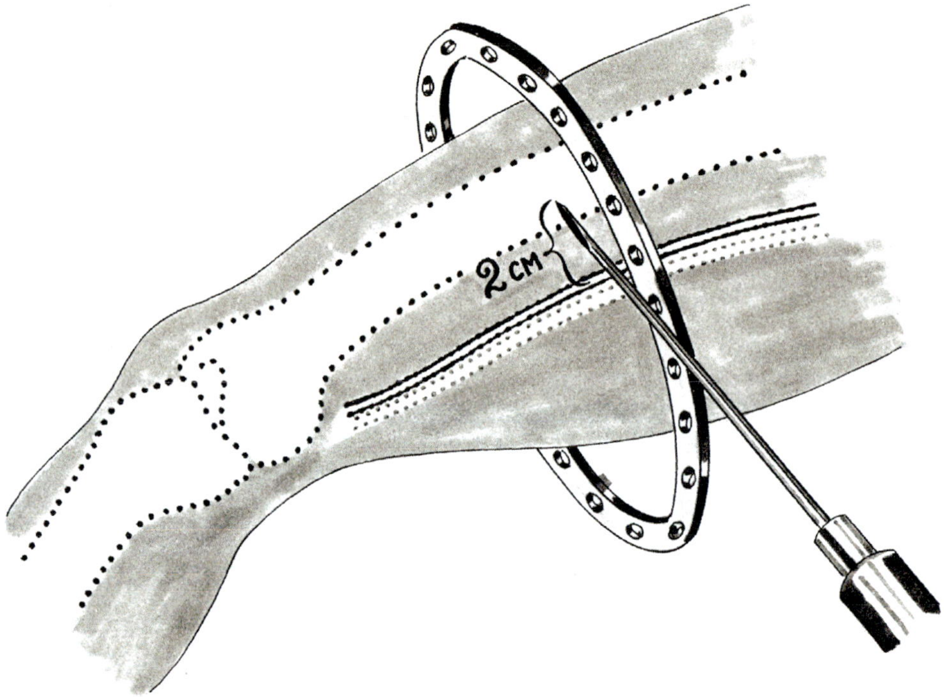

Figure 11.5: Introduction of the K-wire into the medial side of a femur. Projection of a pulsating femoral artery is shown by the *solid line*, a femoral vein projection by the *dotted line*. Entrance point of the wire tip is 2 cm from these vessels

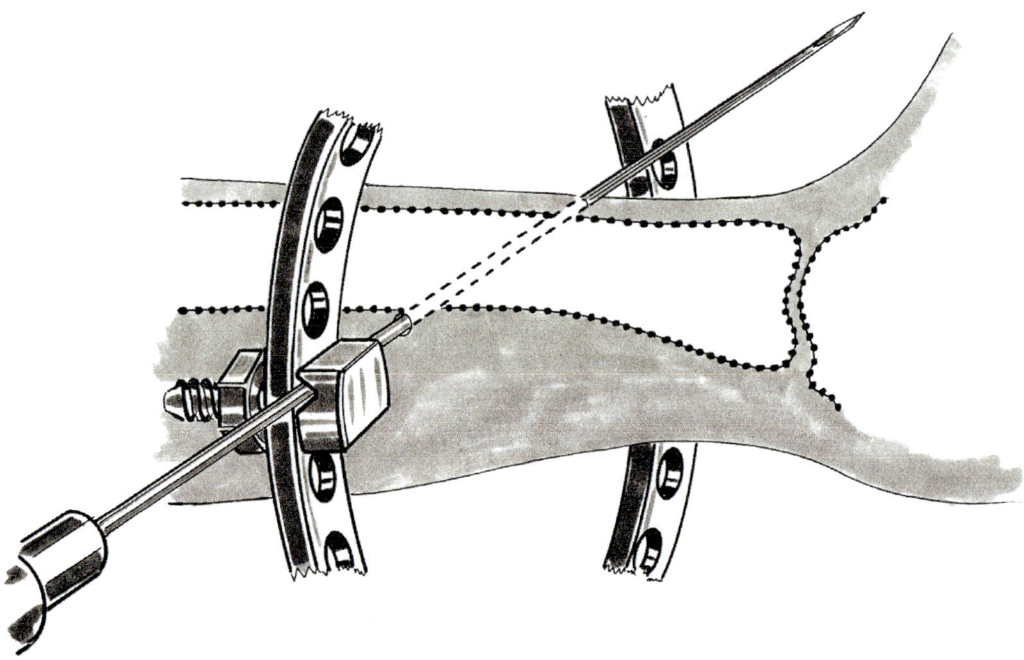

Figure 11.6: Simple guidance system to ensure correct K-wire introduction into the tibia. Section of a ring is shown with a loosely attached slotted fixation bolt at the entrance site. The wire is positioned on its groove, which prevents its deflection during introduction and drilling. The wire is shown being guided through the bone *(interrupted line)* and exiting at the side of the ring wall with the guiding bolt

4. The K-wire must be introduced slowly, pausing several times during the procedure to avoid burning of tissues, particularly bone and skin. It is recommended that a low-power drill with a speed of not more than 30 to 40 rpm be used. Low-speed wire introduction also permits moving aside such movable soft tissue structures as blood vessels and nerves, thereby avoiding serious complications (Fig. 11.7). Deep nerves and vessels situated along the tubular shafts of the bones are well protected with this slow penetration because they are surrounded by connective tissue and packed within the triangular or quadrangular sheaths formed by the intermuscular septums. These sheathed formations have a limited margin of movement (about 0.5 cm to 1.5 cm, depending on the extremity), and slow introduction of a K-wire also will push aside these structures, with minimal risk of wire tip penetration.
5. At the entrance and exit sites the skin must be supported by finger pressure to secure the exact point of wire penetration. The skin surface is manipulated according to the type of procedure being performed. In transfixation of an extremity with a nonmovable ring, the skin is held firmly and perpendicularly

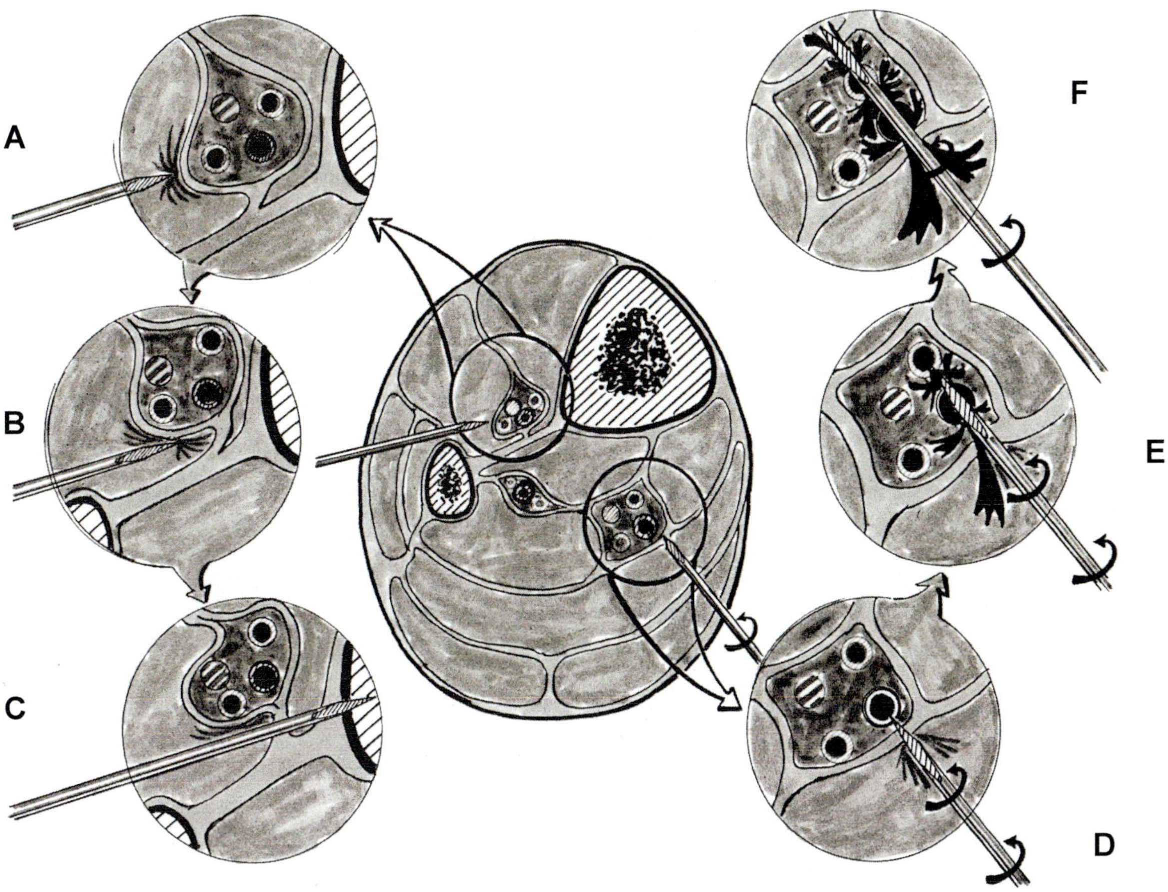

Figure 11.7: Cross section of the leg, with encircled nerve-vessel bundles. Effect of low-speed and high-speed K-wire tip introduction on the blood vessels and nerves. Tip of the wire, introduced slowly, makes contact with the bundle sheath (A), pushes it away without penetration (B), and continues into the bone (C). D-F, possible pitfalls of high-speed introduction of the wire include penetration of an artery (F)

against the underlying tissue. In a planned distraction the skin should be pushed toward the site of corticotomy (Fig. 11.8). In a planned compression the skin should be pushed away from the site of the compressed ends (Fig. 11.9). Shifting the skin in this manner prevents (or decreases) it from being cut by the wire during the course of distraction-compression and also prevents additional pain and unnecessary scar formation.

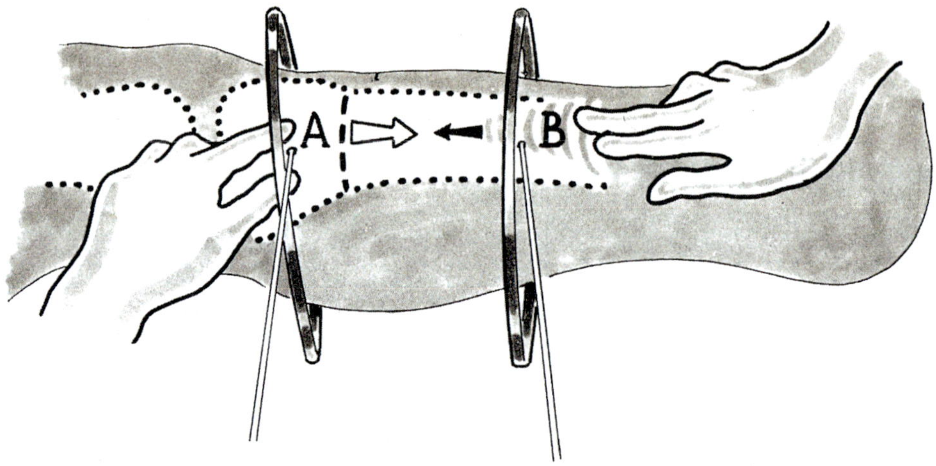

Figure 11.8: Skin support near various K-wire entrances into the tibia. A, point of entrance for the fixation of a nonmovable proximal supporting ring. *Interrupted line* shows site of tibial corticotomy. *White arrow* shows direction of distraction; *black arrow* shows direction in which skin is manipulated toward the site of corticotomy. B, point of entrance for the fixation of a movable middle ring

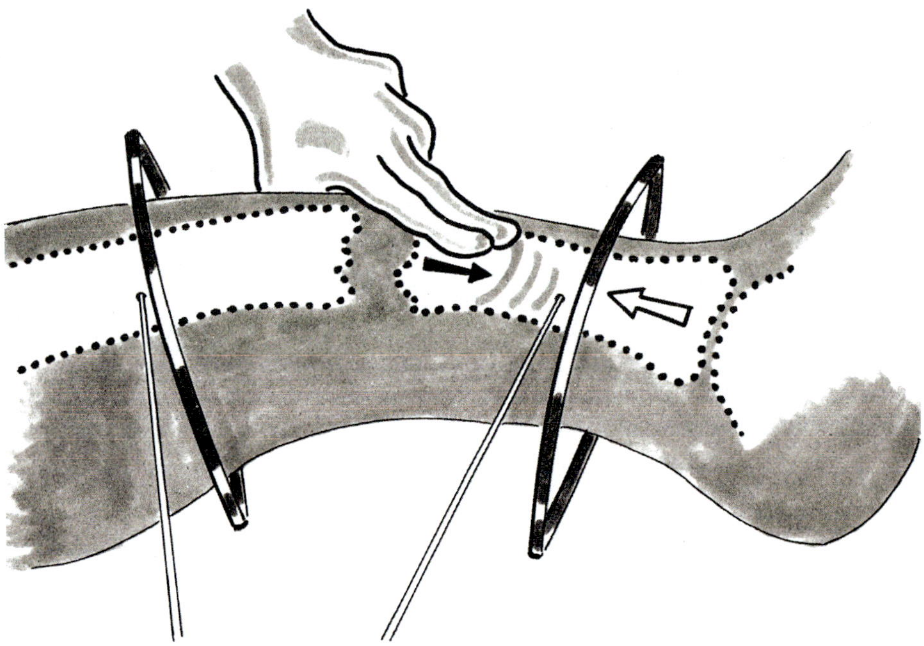

Figure 11.9: Skin support near the K-wire entrance site for the tibia with nonunion. *White arrow* shows direction of compression of the distal ring; *black arrow* shows direction in which the skin is manipulated at the site of the compressed bone fragment end

6. To prevent joint contracture, the muscles must be kept in a position of maximal functional length at the moment of wire penetration. The closer the wire insertion to the joint the more attention should be paid to this principle. With the distal tibia, the foot must be placed in plantar flexion during wire penetration of the muscles of the anterior compartments, and then must be put in a position of maximum dorsiflexion during insertion of the wire through the posterior compartment. It is also preferable to keep the knee flexed during this ankle wire introduction procedure (Fig. 11.10).

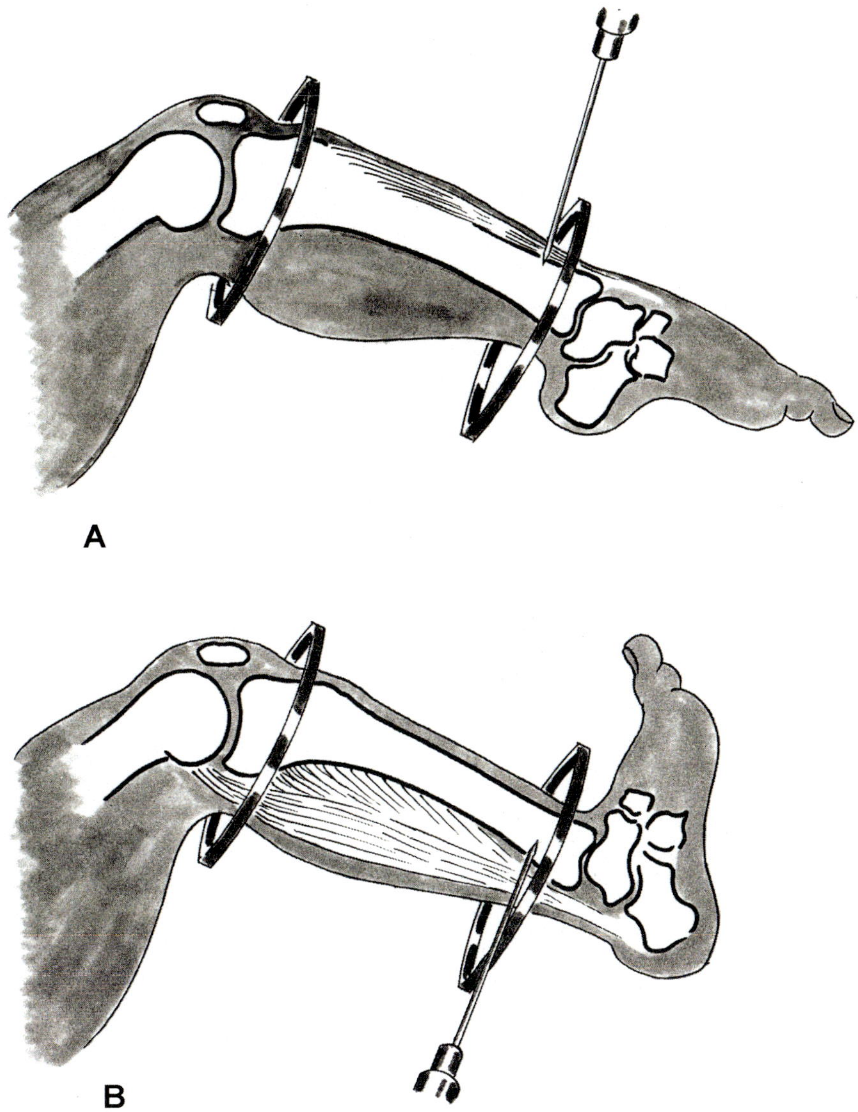

Figure 11.10: Prevention of ankle joint contracture. A, with introduction of a wire into the distal tibia, the foot is placed in plantar flexion during wire penetration of the muscles of the anterior compartment. B, with introduction of the wire through the posterior compartment, the foot is placed in a position of maximum dorsiflexion; the knee remains flexed

7. Each wire drilled through the bone must be introduced correctly at the first attempt. The rule is, one wire, one hole. Multiple holes resulting from incorrect wire positioning destroy compact bone through mechanical damage and through burning. The surgeon must consider that with multiple wire holes the subsequent loading from the distraction-compression movement at the same cortex location will further hasten bone destruction and resultant wire fixation weakening. Multiple drilling through bone marrow significantly destroys it and blood circulation, causing hematoma formation, delaying its ability for new cell development, and may even contribute to infection (Fig. 11.11).

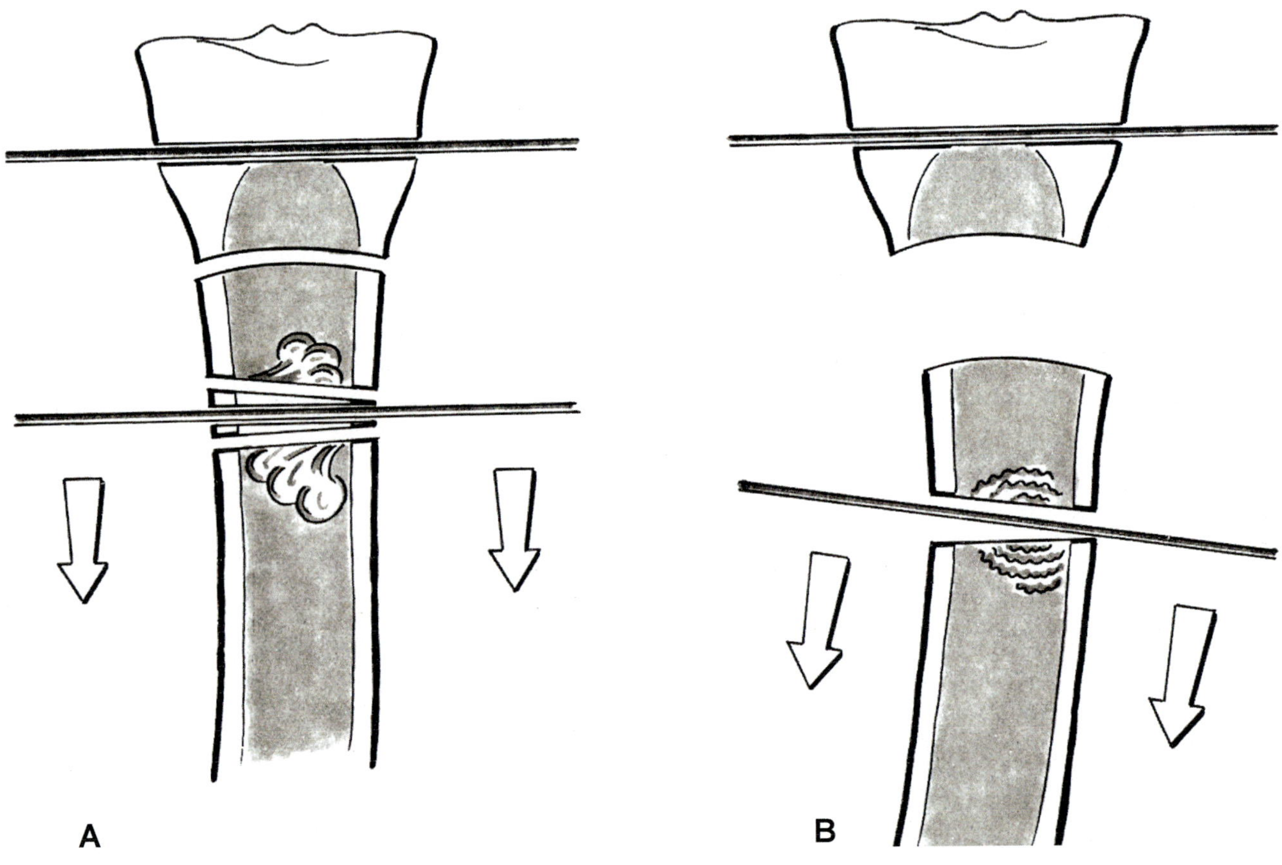

A B

Figure 11.11: Effect on bone cortex and marrow when multiple holes are drilled for one wire. **A,** schematic of a tibial segment with one wire introduced proximally through one hole and the second wire introduced distally, with three holes drilled, with the corticotomy site in between. *Arrows* show the direction of distraction. The *gray clouds* represent hematoma formation in bone marrow. **B,** same tibial segment after distraction. The proximal wire remains firmly fixed, but the distal wire now is loose because the cortex was mechanically weakened by multiple holes being drilled and by bone burning. The wire now is in a sideways position, and scar tissue replaces the hematoma

Surgical Technique

Bearing in mind these seven cardinal rules, the technique of K-wire introduction is as follows. The tip of the wire is introduced through the skin by simple puncture. Farther in, the tip is introduced through the fascia and muscles until it touches the cortical bone. All this is done by simple manual puncture, without drilling. As soon as a surgeon feels that the cortical bone has been reached, it is useful to slightly move the tip of wire up and down transversely to the bone surface, to ensure that the tip is not on the bone slope and will not slide down when drilling the wire through the cortex layer is begun. Once the wire is positioned correctly, low-speed drilling is commenced. To avoid bending of the wire and at the same time to maintain a straight trajectory, the wire should be gripped at the entry point with a wet sponge. It is important to be able to feel the passage of the wire tip through both sides of the cortex. When the second side of the cortex has been penetrated, drilling is terminated. Ideally, the wire is drilled through both sides of the cortex, passing through the bone canal and bone marrow. Transmedullary wire insertion rather than cortical insertion is important because it provides greater wire stability and helps prevent cortical osteomyelitis (Fig. 11.12).

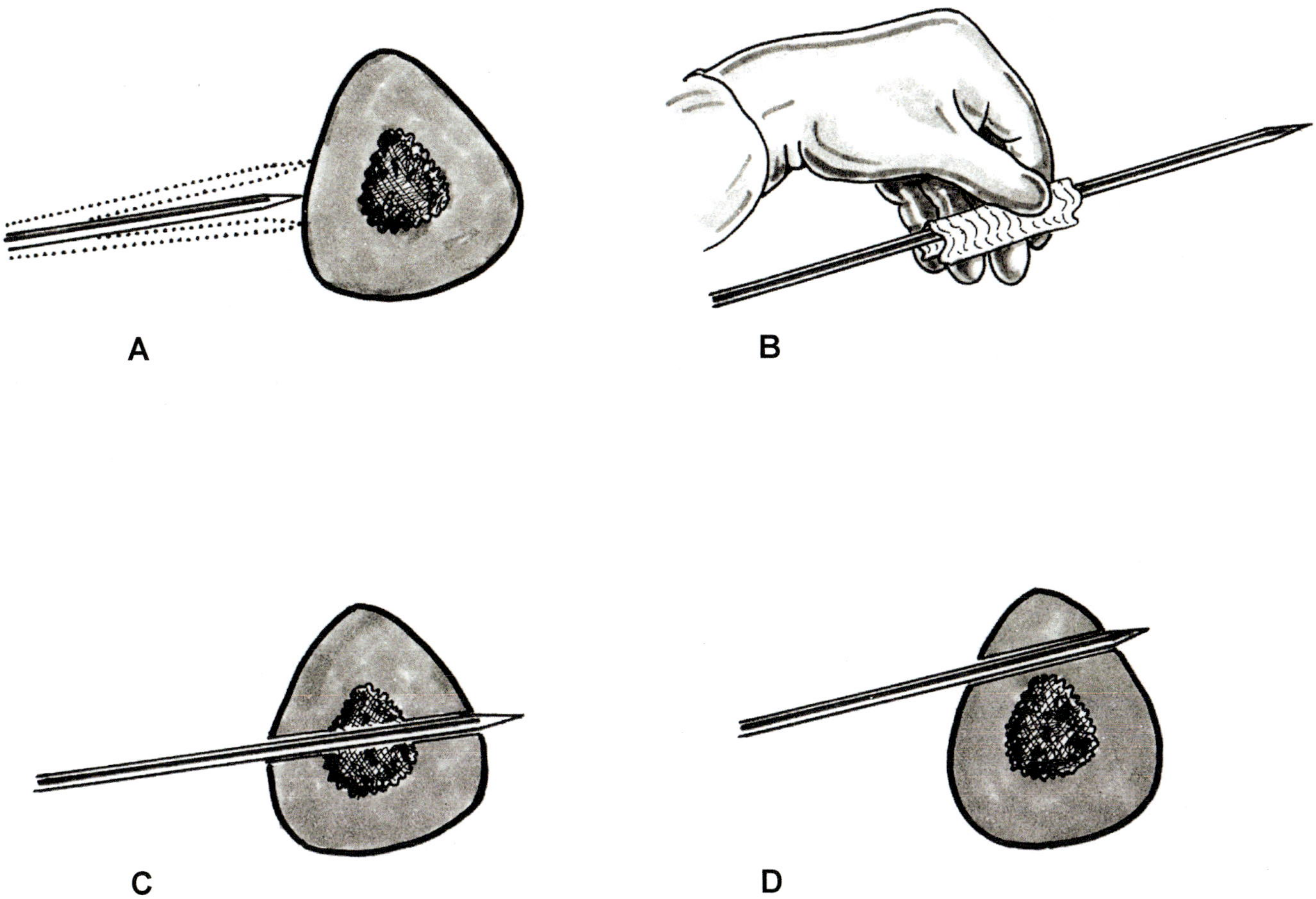

Figure 11.12: Technique of K-wire introduction into bone. A, wire tip is moved slightly vertically to make sure it is not on the bone slope and will not slide downward when drilling begins. B, wire is gripped with a wet sponge. C, wire is drilled through both sides of the cortex, passing through the bone canal and bone marrow transmedullary. D, wire is drilled incorrectly through the cortex, which can lead to the development of cortical osteomyelitis

At this moment the surgeon must try to pull the wire backward slightly. If it is firm and unmovable, the wire is in the correct position. If it pulls back easily the direction of drilling must be changed.

After passing the far side of the cortex the drill is disconnected, and wire insertion is completed by hammering with light taps to prevent perforation of major vessels and nerves, by pushing them from harm's way. As the wire progresses to the exit side, a practical and useful technical hint is to use the fingers to feel the tip as it emerges from the deep tissues. This palpation assures that the wire is proceeding in the correct direction. When the wire tip approaches the surface, the skin at the exit site must be manipulated in the same direction as at the entrance site (Fig. 11.13). Either the surgeon uses fingers or the skin-pulling device to align the entrance and exit sites.

Wire insertion is continued until the amount of wire protruding from either side of the extremity is approximately equal. Now the connection of the wire to the

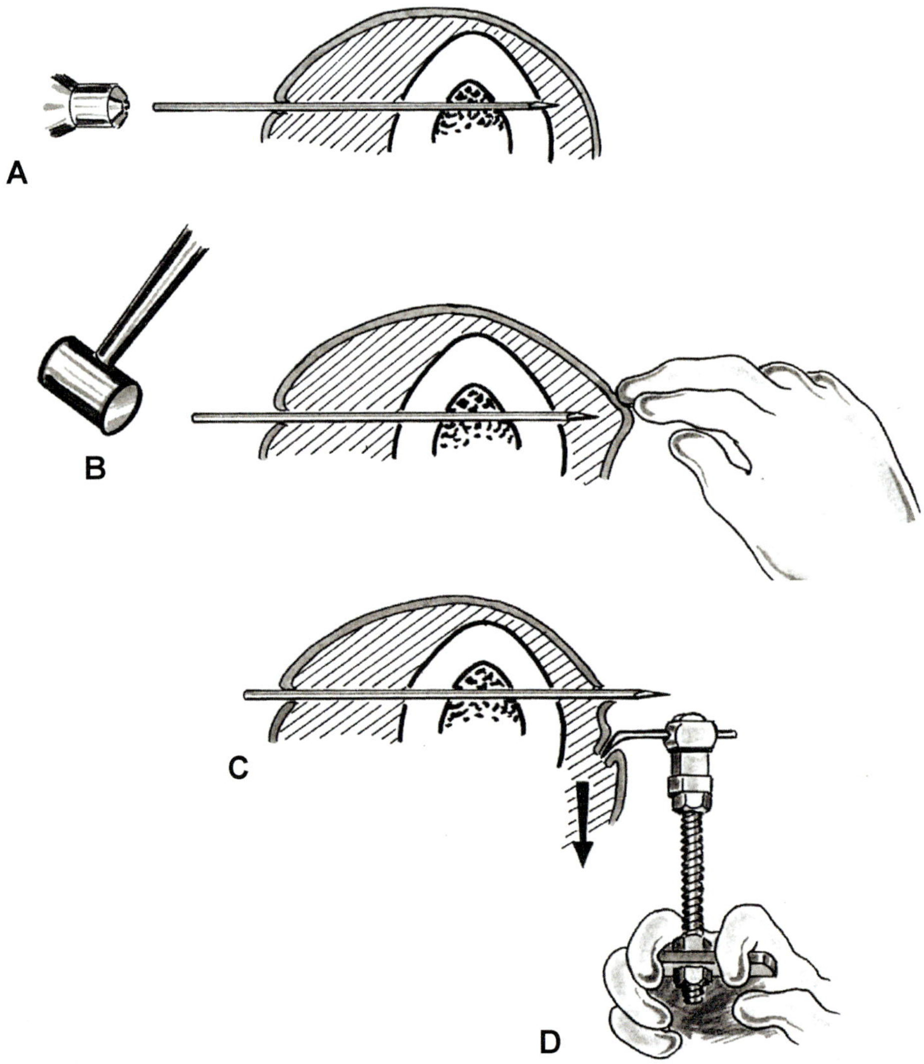

Figure 11.13: Wire introduction technique. Portion of an extremity cross section showing skin *(gray)*, muscles *(shaded)*, and bone *(white)*. A, after passing the far side of the cortex the drill is disconnected. B, continued wire insertion is completed by hammering with light taps. As wire insertion progresses, the emerging tip is felt by the fingers. C, wire tip emerges from the skin, and is manipulated by the fingers or, D, a special device consisting of the bent, sharp wire tip fixed to a short threaded rod, with a short plate as a base

ring begins. Another useful way of advancing only the olive wire is with pliers, grasping the exiting wire and pulling it through while an assistant holds the extremity firmly. Also, a 0.5-cm skin incision must be made at the portal of the olive stopper wire with a No. 11 blade.

WIRE POSITIONING ON THE SAME RING

Ring stability implies the prevention of side-to-side displacement and the absence of shearing movements. A well-stabilized ring has to be attached to the bone as if it were rooted to the ground. To achieve this level of stability, at least two wires criss-crossing at an angle as close as possible to 90 degrees and an additional offset wire are required. Because the neurovascular bundles are close to the bone, it is practically impossible to achieve a 90-degree angle between two wires at the same level. Nevertheless, in transfixing wires to each ring an attempt must be made to find a way to introduce two wires in the widest maximum angle. If the angle of introduction is 30 degrees or less, there is always a great possibility of side-to-side ring displacement. If the angle is between 30 and 45 degrees, there is a possibility of creating ring shearing movement (Fig. 11.14).

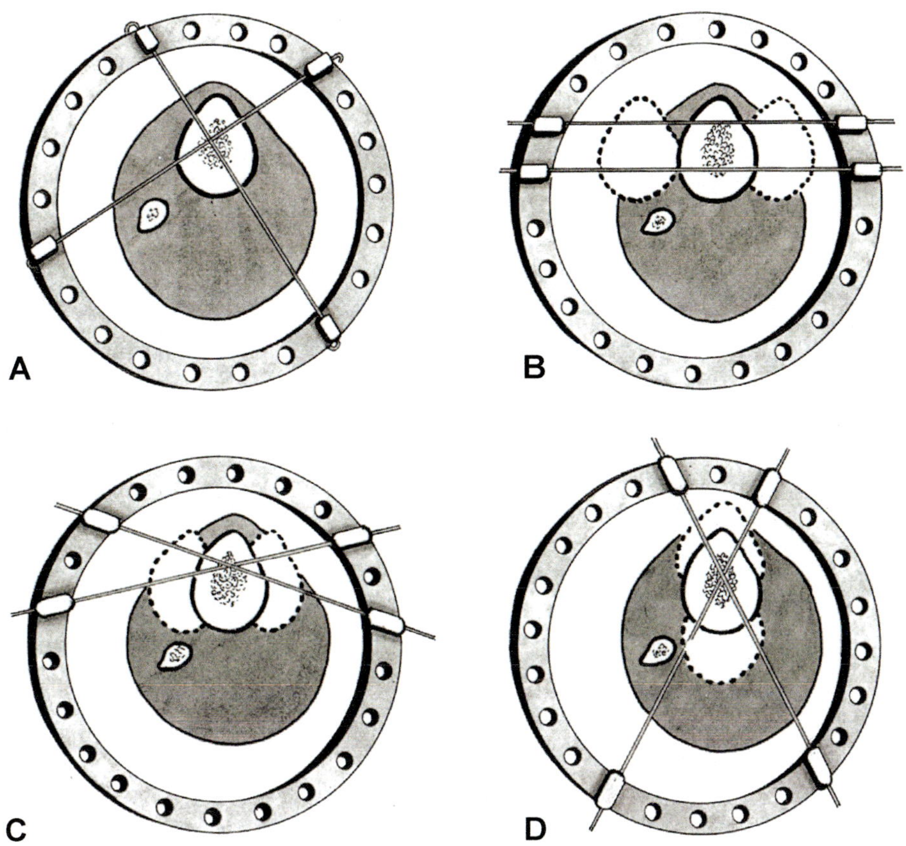

Figure 11.14: Wire positioning on the same ring. Leg cross section with two wires introduced through the tibia at different angles to each other. *Interrupted line* represents tibial displacement. A, wires are introduced at 90-degree angles, forming a very stable transfixion. B, wires are introduced parallel to each other. Such transfixion is unstable, and the tibia can be displaced all the way to either side. C, wires are introduced with 30-degree angulation in the frontal plane. This transfixion is not stable, and the tibia can be displaced slightly to either side. D, wires are introduced with 30-degree angulation in the sagittal plane. This transfixion is not stable, and the tibia can be displaced to either side

In addition to ensuring ring stability, wide angulation between the wires confers a second advantage: it brings about more even distribution of the loading forces on the bone cortex along the plane of the ring. This force distribution is an important consideration for bone fragment stability during the distraction-compression procedure (Fig. 11.15).

Side-to-side displacement can be prevented by using wires with the olive stoppers at both sides of the bone. To correct any shearing ring motion still present, wires introduced at different planes, with the so-called offset wires, will augment ring stability. This will also prevent wire contiguity in the bone marrow.

For greater ring stability it is useful in certain situations to leave a 3- to 5-mm gap between the ring wall and the introduced wire, then insert a washer (Fig. 11.16).

The rule is that *the wire should not be brought down to the ring; rather, the ring should be brought up to the wire*. This is done either by using washers or at times a post, support, or half-hinge. The choice depends on the size of a gap between the wire and ring. *Bending the wire down to the ring is strongly contraindicated because it will induce pain from the permanent pressure, and skin necrosis from the skin being squeezed between the ring and the bent wire* (Fig. 11.17).

In the relationship between two closely connected wires it is of practical importance to always maintain at least a 3-cm gap between their entrances or exits on one side. This gap prevents skin tightening, pain, and the spread of infection from one wire tract to another.

In some cases three wires can be transfixed to one ring. This is indicated for a ring when greater than

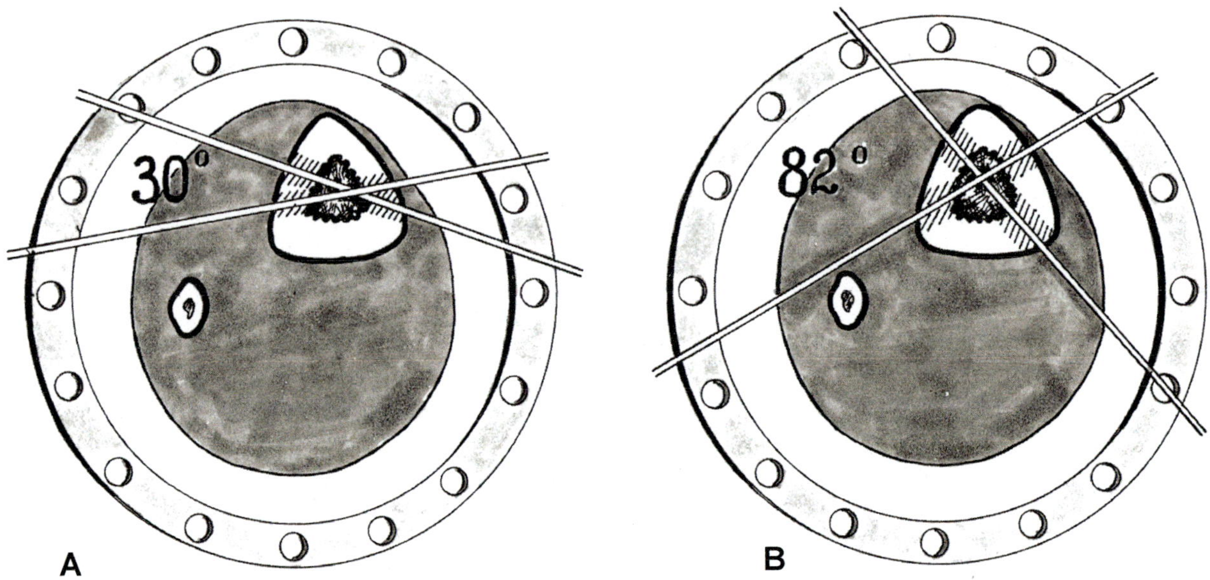

Figure 11.15: Distribution of loading forces on bone cortex. Schematic of a leg in cross section with the ring transfixed to the tibia by two wires at different angulations. *Diagonal lines* represent the distribution of loading forces. A, with the two wires introduced with 30-degree angulation, distribution of the loading forces is concentrated at a narrow part of the bone cortex. B, with the two wires introduced with 82-degree angulation, the loading forces are distributed evenly on the bone cortex

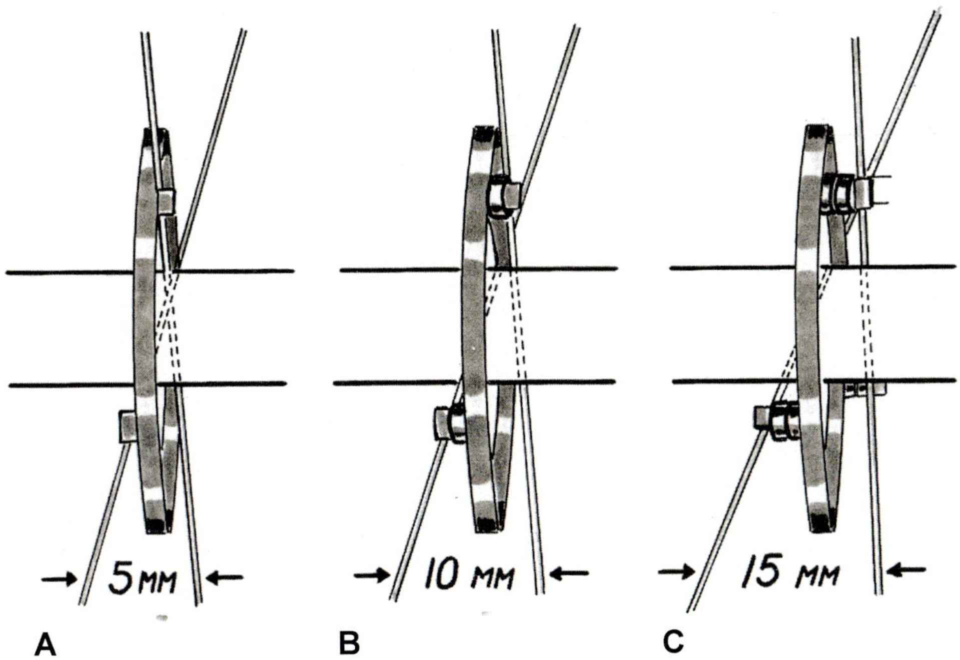

Figure 11.16: Ring stabilization with use of washers. A, wires are situated above and below the rings; therefore their planes are 5 mm from each other. B, wires are situated 3 mm off the rings, and single washers are used on each side. Thus the wires and their planes are 10 mm from each other and the ring position is more stable. C, wires are situated 5 to 6 mm from the rings, and double washers are used on each side. Thus the wires and their planes are 15 mm from each other and the ring position is very stable

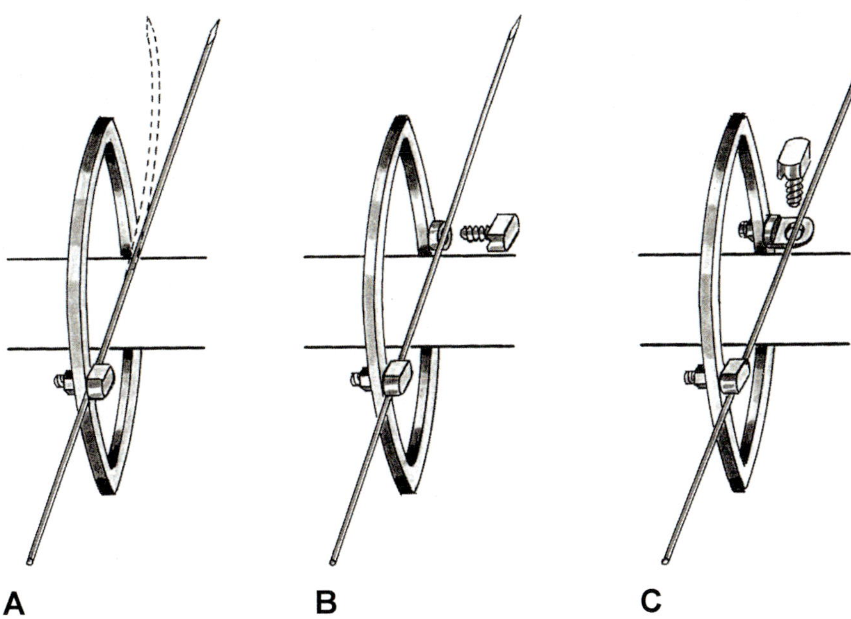

Figure 11.17: Wire-ring relationship when one side of the wire is some distance from the ring. A, wire never should be brought to the ring (shown by *interrupted line)*. B, ring is brought to the wire by using a washer. C, ring is brought to the wire by using a support

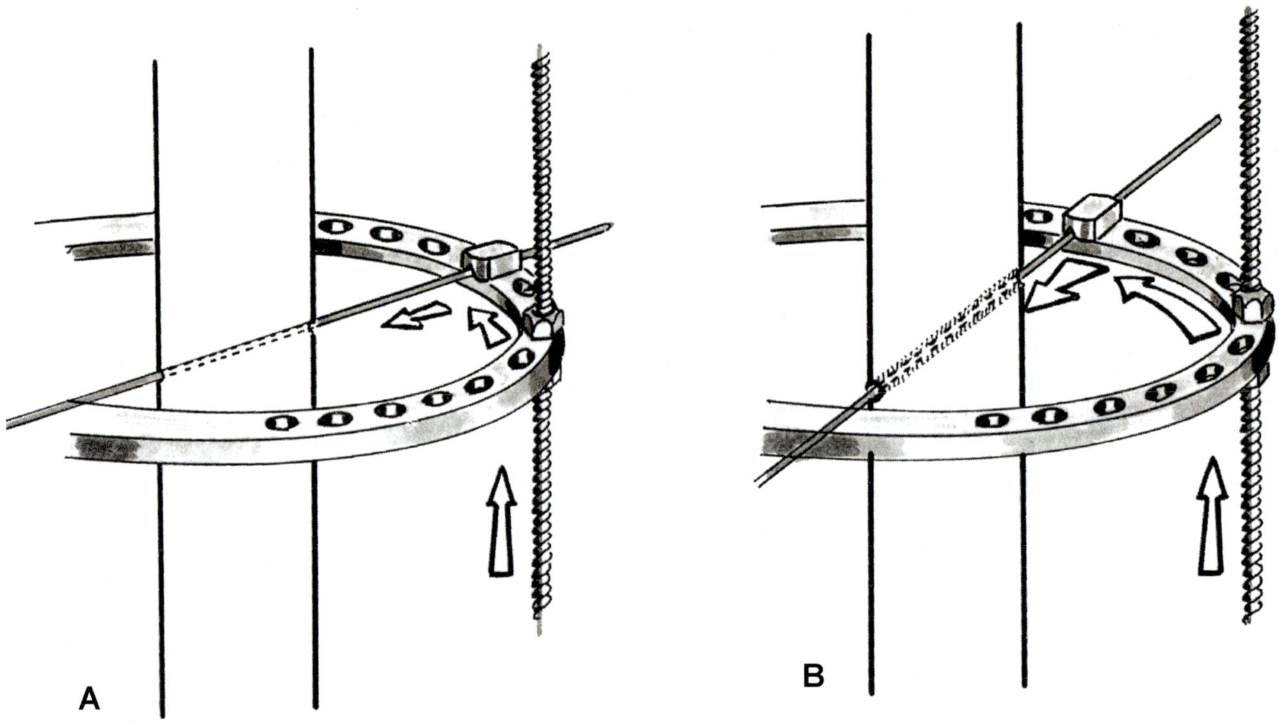

Figure 11.18: Relationship of the wire and ring connector. *Arrows* show distribution of axial loading. A, when the wire is close to the ring connector it bears smaller axial loads. B, when the wire is away from the ring connector it bears greater axial loads and therefore develops a larger diameter hole in the bone *(shaded lines)*

normal loading is involved, for example, for the main supporting ring at the proximal tibial metaepiphyses or for the pulling ring of a large bone fragment. The advantage of three-wire fixation is more even distribution of loading at the cross-section of the bone, at the level where the chief force is applied.

A wire should be fixed as close as possible to a ring connector (such as a threaded or telescopic rod) on a ring. Whether the wire is closer to or farther from the connector will affect loading characteristics. Distribution of axial loading is transmitted from ring' to ring through the ring connectors, and is passed on to the transfixing wires. The closer the wires are situated to the ring connectors the less axial loading they will bear. Thus it is important to try and fix the wires near the ring connectors. This prevents the formation of a large hole in the bone cortex, resulting from axial loading pressure, and also prevents wire breakage (Fig. 11.18).

OFFSET WIRE POSITIONING

Greater ring stability can be achieved through multi-planar wire introduction rather than through introducing multiple wires on one plane. If a wide criss-cross angle between two wires has not been attained, placing a third wire a short distance from the ring on another plane will increase its stability.

These additional wires on the ring are called offset, or drop, wires, and are fastened to a ring by two attached supports. The ring with offset wires represents a unit of

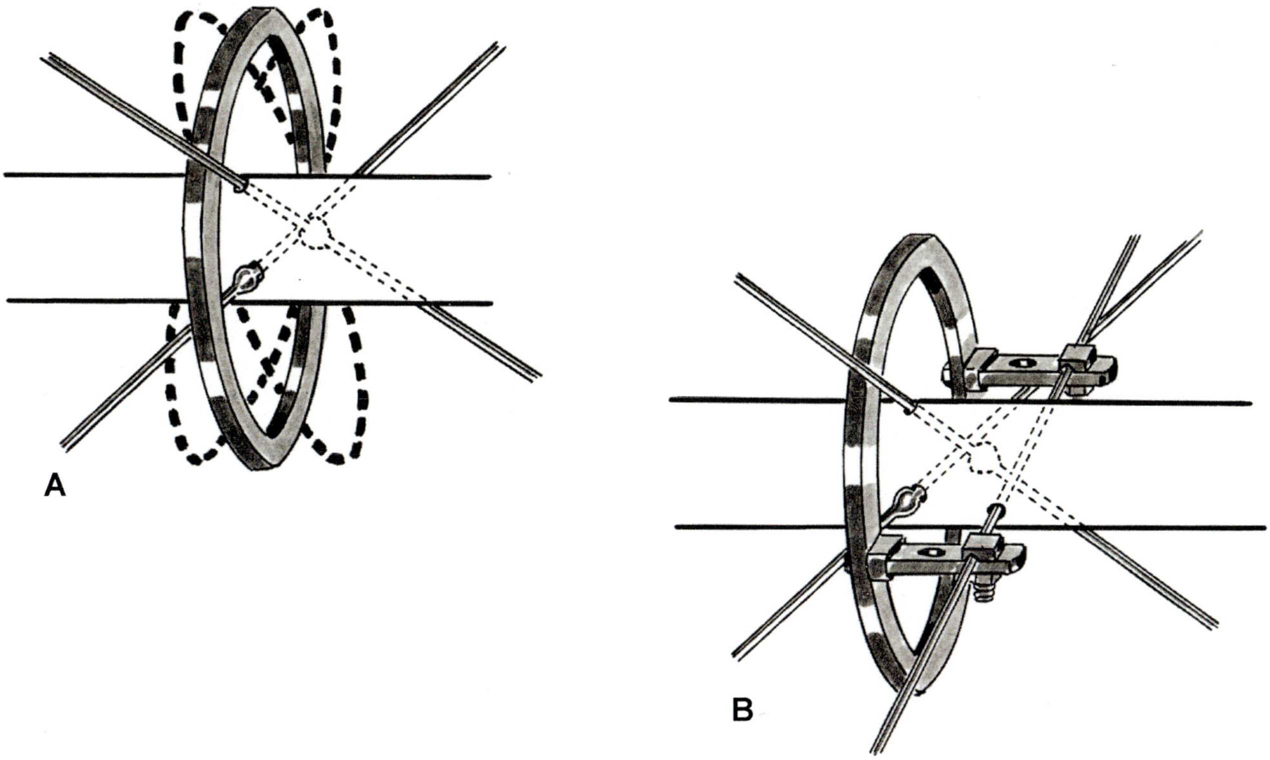

Figure 11.19: Ring stabilization through use of wires with stoppers and offset wire. A, ring is stabilized by introduction of two wires with olive-type stoppers on opposite sides of the bone. Shearing of the ring *(interrupted lines)* still is present. B, similar ring stability is augmented by the use of an offset wire, which is fastened to the ring by two supports

the frame. Another advantage of the offset wire is that, because it is away from the two main ring wires, it can be introduced in a direction different from that of the main ring wires. Thus the ring with offset wire becomes a multiplanar and multidirectional unit.

In some cases even two additional wires can be placed on both sides of the ring for stabilization. Spreading the wires vertically over a section of bone, rather than on one plane, makes the ring extremely stable (Fig. 11.19).

Dr. Ilizarov recommends the use of the offset wires rather than connected half-rings for additional support. In his practice, the more planes of fixation the rings have the fewer rings are required for the whole frame. The end result is that the entire frame construction is much lighter and thus easier for the patient to wear.

There is, however, one particular disadvantage to the adjacent or offset wire. Because it is connected to the ring by an extension part, it is not so stiff as it would be if connected directly to the ring; thus it cannot be tensioned as intensively as the wire connected directly to the ring. The offset wire is not recommended for use with the pulling-pushing movable ring. With the bone fragment movement, this wire can produce great pain and provoke wire tract infection.

PROPER DISTANCE OF WIRES FROM JOINTS, AND DIRECTION OF INTRODUCTION

When a ring is positioned near a joint the wires have to be introduced at a distance that allows the maximum joint range of motion. Three important anatomic and biomechanical conditions must be considered to assure proper distance and direction of the wires. First, the joint capsule is situated some distance from the joint gap, and this distance can be significant. For example, the top of the suprapatellar bursa of the knee joint can reach a distance of 4 to 5 cm from the upper patellar pole; the auxiliary recess of the shoulder joint reaches below the surgical neck level; the elbow articular capsule spreads above the coronoid and olecranon fossa; the ankle articular capsule spreads above the level of the tibia tendon grooves. All those joint specifications dictate careful planning and secure introduction of the wires near these joints to avoid penetration into the joint cavity and subsequent development of septic arthritis (Fig. 11.20).

Second, since anatomically there is a concentration of bone sulci at tendons near the joints, wire introduction must be directed so that it does not penetrate the tendons. This is especially important for the ankle and elbow joints. Penetration of the wire, and particularly the wire with an olive stopper, can produce tendon damage and decubitus ulcer with subsequent permanent joint contracture.

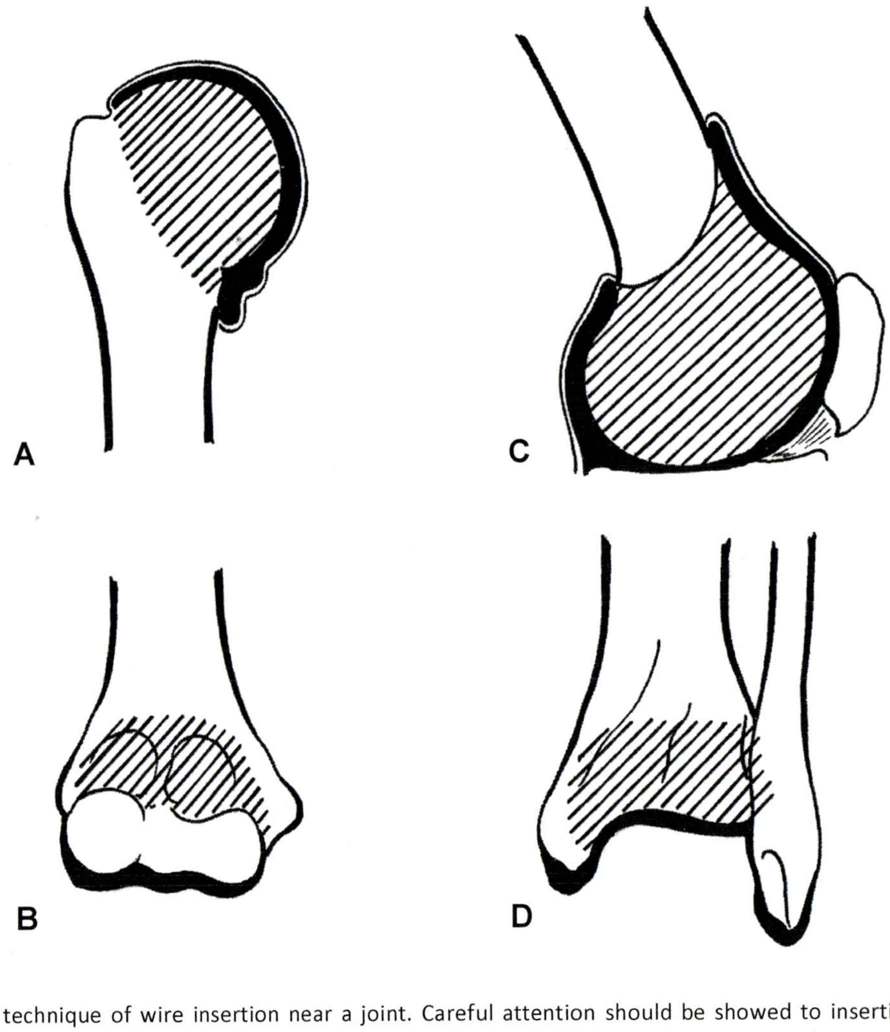

Figure 11.20: Proper technique of wire insertion near a joint. Careful attention should be showed to inserting the wire a proper distance from joint capsule to ensure as little restriction of range of motion as possible and proper direction of insertion to avoid penetration of tendons of the shoulder (A), elbow (B), knee (C), and ankle (D)

Third, the wires close to the joint should be introduced through muscle fibers that are stretched maximally. This precondition assures less pain and greater freedom of motion.

WIRES WITH STOPPERS

Originally Dr. Ilizarov manually bent a standard K-wire, creating a sort of Z-shaped stopper for firm bone fixation. But this Z-shaped end had the disadvantage of cutting through soft tissues and was not strong enough to withhold major loading. That problem stimulated Ilizarov to introduce the thicker wires (1.5 and 1.8 mm in diameter) with a soldered ball twice the wire diameter on it. This innovation, the olive wire, in turn increased the indications for its use (Fig. 11. 21). Now the olive-shaped stopper wire is turned out of a single piece of stainless steel, and is used for bone fixation, bone fragment displacement reduction, bone fragment deviation correction, technique of bone fragment pulling in an internal transport, interfragmentary compression, and in osteoporotic bone (sometimes with a washer).

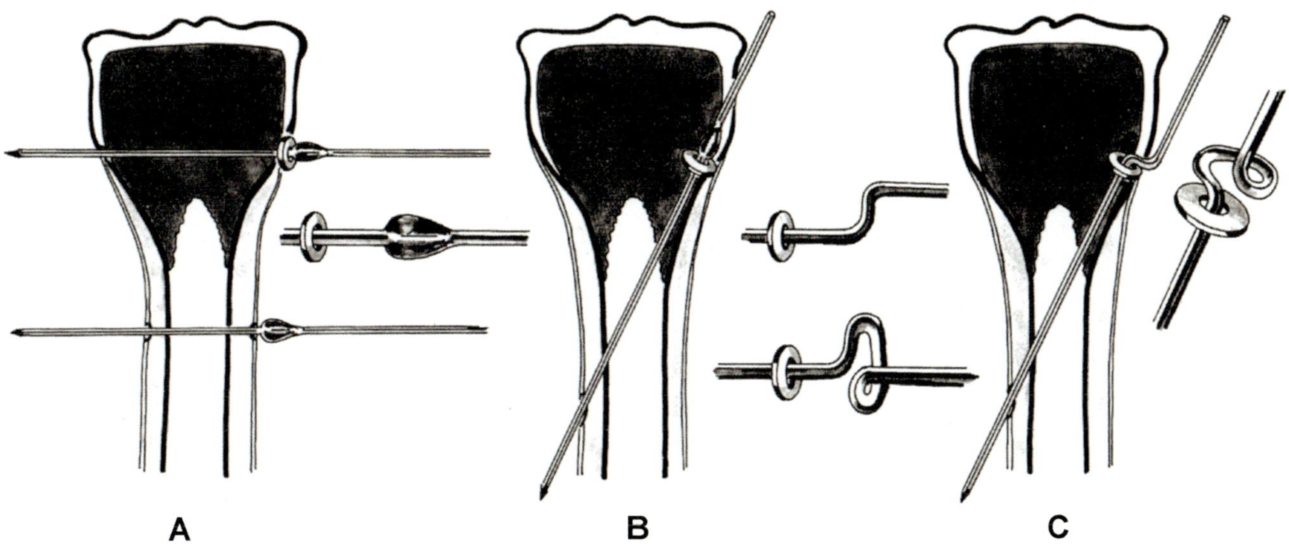

Figure 11.21: Wires with stoppers (olive wires) play an extremely versatile and important role in the Ilizarov technique. The olive wire (A) was developed by Ilizarov as an alternative to his early practice of bending and twisting the K-wire into Z-shapes (B and C). Note that washers are used in conjunction with stopper wires when they are introduced near a joint

WIRE TENSIONING

General Considerations

The obligatory rule is that each wire fixed to the ring must be properly tensioned. Only a tensioned wire can sustain the required loading forces and perform the task of stable frame support over the long course of treatment. *The quality of bone healing and/or bone regenerate development depends on the strength of wire tension* (Fig. 11.22).

Wire tensioning brings about a suitable balance in the stability and flexibility of the frame. Any motion between the protruded section of the wire and the skin tends to irritate the skin and create pain. The proper wire tension reduces pain and irritation, and prevents development of wire tract infection.

The exact strength of tensioning depends on (1) local frame construction (half-ring vs. full ring, offset vs. main ring wire); (2) local bone condition (osteoporosis vs. normal bone); (3) weight of the patient (small child vs. large adult); (4) functional wire loading (stabilization vs. distraction-compression).

The range of the wire tensioning strength is 50 to 130 kg. General recommendations for the suggested tensioning strengths are as follows:

1. Wire on half-ring: 50 to 70 kg
2. Offset (drop) wire, depending on size of the supporting posts: 50 to 80 kg
3. Single wire on a ring: up to 100 kg
4. Two to three wires on a ring in a young patient: 110 kg for each wire
5. Two to three wires on a ring in an adult patient: 120 to 130 kg for each wire
6. Wire with an olive stopper: 100 to 110 kg
7. Wires with olive stoppers used for interfragmentary compression, depending on bone condition; 50 kg.

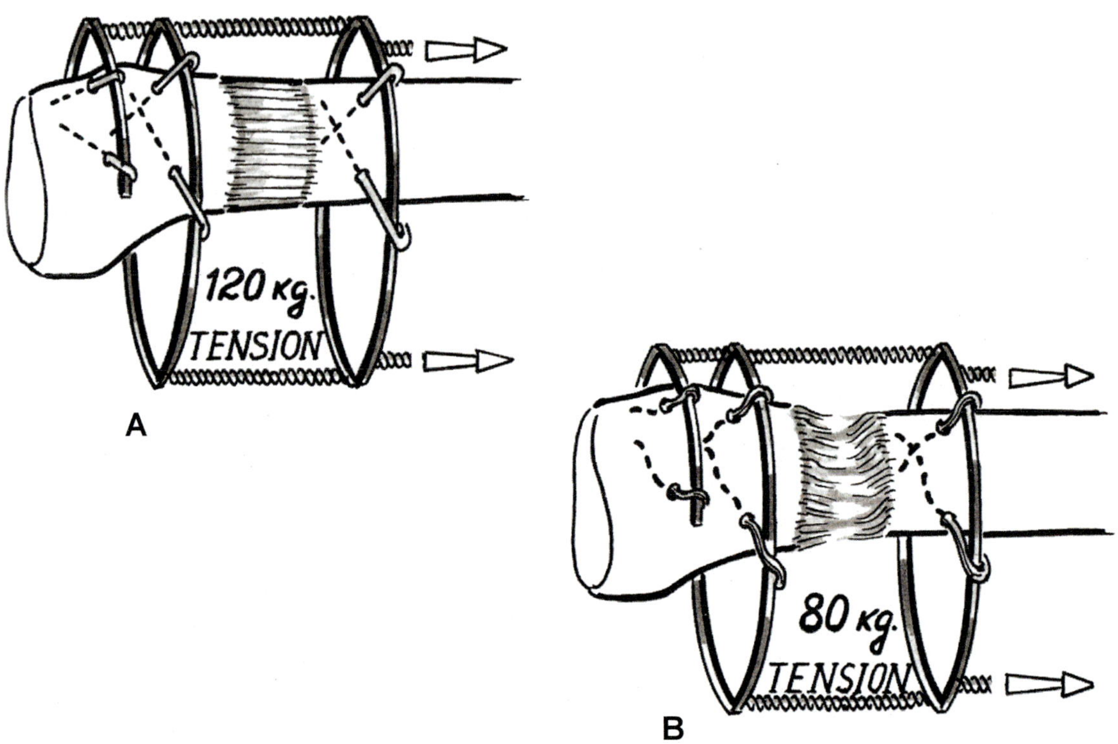

Figure 11.22: Schematic representation of distracted bone. Proper wire tension is paramount. Every wire fixed to bone and a ring must be correctly tensioned. A, correct wire tension greatly influences the quality of regenerate. B, inadequate tensioning adversely affects development of regenerate

The strength of tensioned wires is not constant during treatment, but can decrease or increase depending on the movement of frame parts due to distraction-compression, as a result of frame adjustments, or as a consequence of increase in the bone hole diameter produced by the permanent wire pressure.

The clinical signs of a decrease in tension strength are pain and skin irritation at the wire site. The radiographic signs of tension strength increase appear as concave wires bending with compression and convex wires bending with distraction of the bone fragments (Fig. 11.23).

Tensioning Technique

If properly tensioned, the thin K-wire develops stiffness almost equal to that of a thick pin. Correct wire tensioning ensures solidity and stability of fixation in the entire frame. In fact, wire tensioning is essential in enabling the wires to withstand enormous distraction and/or compression loading over the long course of treatment. There are several key guidelines for performing wire tensioning properly:

1. Tensioning of each wire must be done immediately after its introduction and fixation.
2. Tensioning must be performed with one end of the wire already firmly fastened to the ring; the tensioning is carried out on the end directly opposite this anchored end.
3. Tensioning of the wire with a stopper (olive wire) must be directed to the side opposite this stopper.

There are several different techniques of wire tensioning.

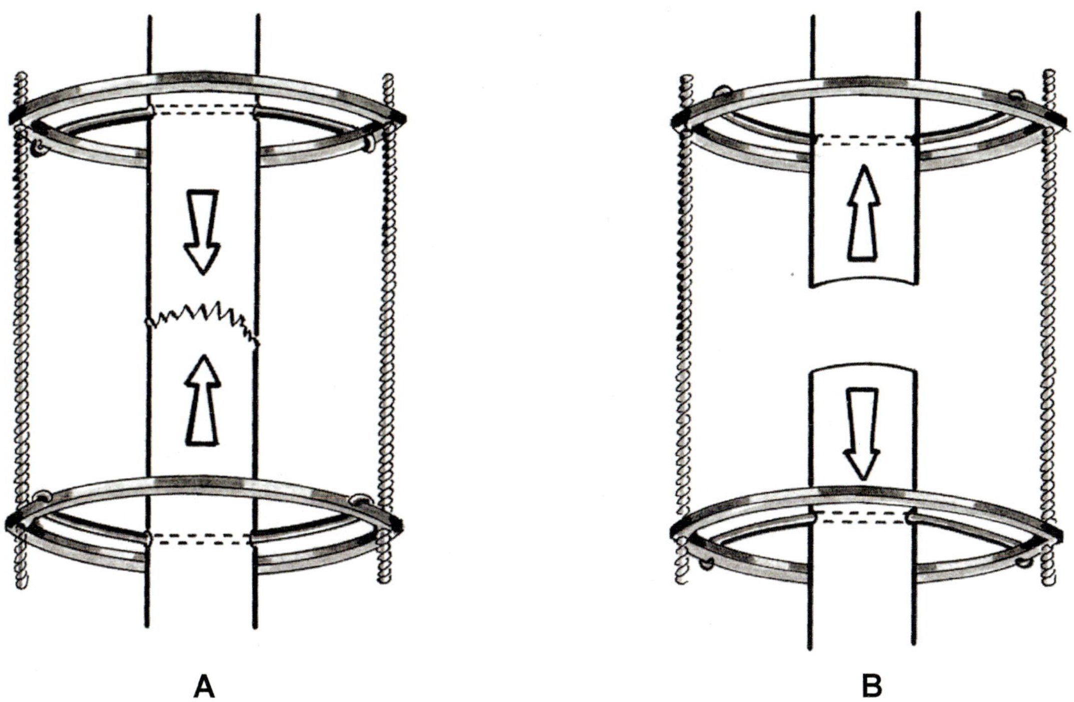

Figure 11.23: Schematic representation of radiographic signs of wire tensioning. A, wire becomes concave as it is bent with compressive forces. B, wire becomes convex as it is bent with distraction forces

The so-called Russian manual technique was introduced by Ilizarov at the time of initial development of the fixator, and it is still popular in Russia. This technique consists of firm wire tightening by turning the wire fixation bolt and the nut simultaneously for approximately half of a full turn (Fig. 11.24). This technique requires application of tremendous manual strength by the surgeon, and it has a disadvantage of not being quantitatively measurable in a definitive way. Frequently wire retensioning is necessary with this technique.

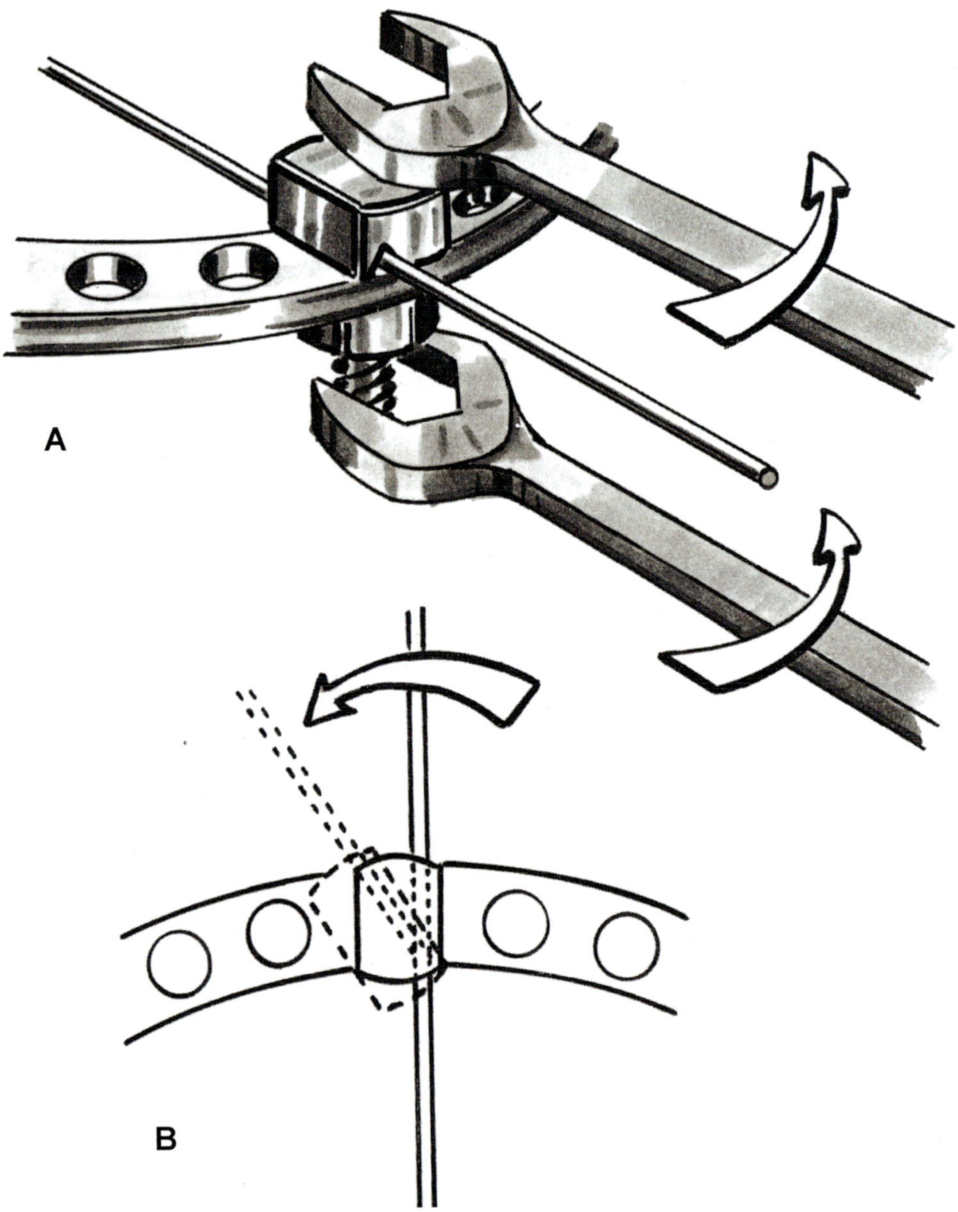

Figure 11.24: Russian "manual technique" of wire tensioning. A, firm wire tensioning is achieved by simultaneously turning a wire fixation bolt and nut with two wrenches approximately one-half turn. B, turning of the wire fixation bolt tightens the wire by bending it off the 90-degree axis with the ring, shown schematically above. This Russian technique has the double disadvantage of not being quantitatively measurable and of often requiring retensioning

The technique of tensioning with the original Ilizarov tensioner involves first fixing the wire to the ring with a bolt. The wire then is tensioned by clockwise turning of the handle (Fig. 11.25). This technique does not require great strength on the part of the surgeon, but is quantitatively nondefinitive.

The most recommended wire tensioning technique is use of a dynamometric wire tensioner (Fig. 11.26). At least three types of dynamometric tensioner have been introduced by Italian and French inventors since the Ilizarov surgical technique became popular in the West. Most wire tensioning now is performed with a dynamometric wire tensioner.

To tension the plain wire, one end first must be fastened firmly to the ring with the wire fixation bolt. The dynamometric tensioner then is connected to the opposite, unattached end of this wire (Fig. 11.27A). After proper tensioning is achieved, this end also is fastened to the ring. For balanced tensioning of two wires on one ring, two tensioners should be applied to the wires and tensioning should be performed simultaneously. If the jaws of the tensioner cannot be clamped directly onto the ring, the wire may be tightened by first inserting a hexagonal threaded socket, which acts as a spacer over it (Figs 11.27B and C).

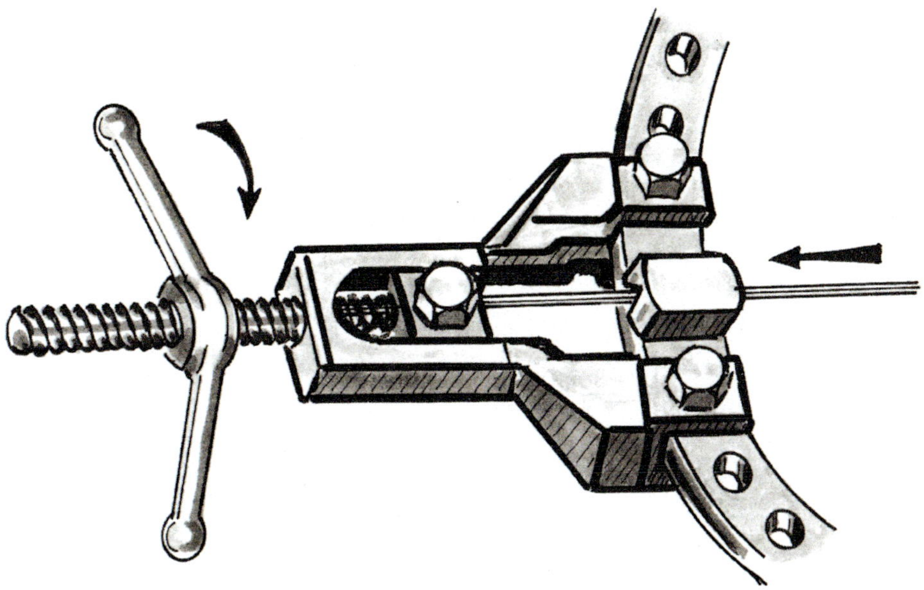

Figure 11.25: Original Ilizarov wire tensioner. Section of a ring is shown with the tensioner attached and the wire fixed by the bolt. *Curved arrow* shows turning of the handle; *straight arrow* shows direction of wire tensioning

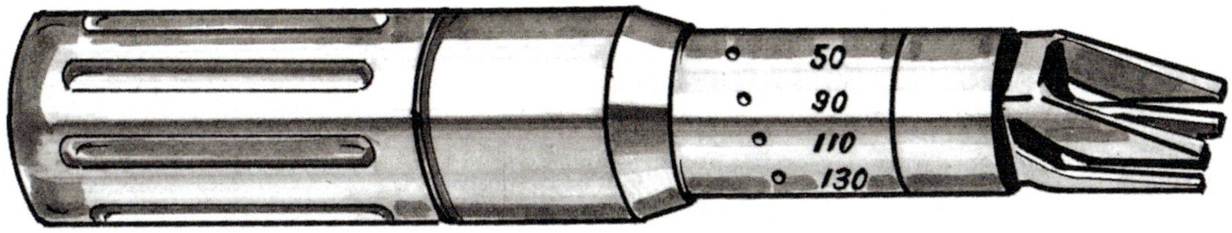

Figure 11.26: Dynamometric wire tensioner has both adjustable and fixed "jaws" *(right)*, which attach to the ring, and a central hole. Numbers represent the strength of tensioning, in kilograms

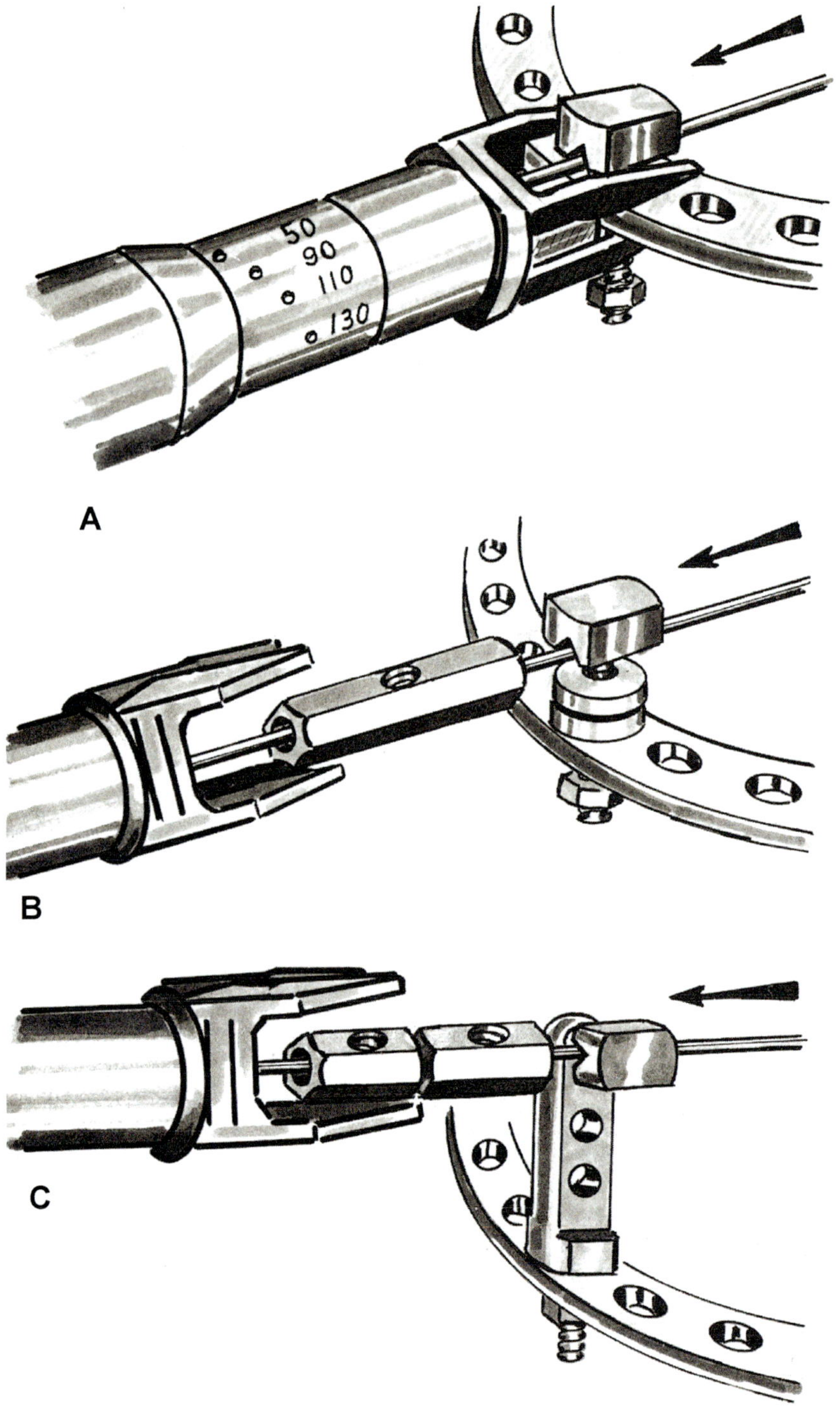

Figure 11.27: Technique of wire tensioning with the dynamometric tensioner, shown on a section of a ring. *Arrows* indicate the direction of tensioning. A, wire is on the same plane with the ring, and the jaw of the tensioner is attached to the ring edge. In this position the wire is easily introduced into the tensioner central hole. B, wire is raised above the ring with two washers. In this situation a hexagonal socket is introduced between the fixation bolt and tensioner, and the wire is introduced into the tensioner central hole. C, with the offset wire attached to the ring by a support, the two hexagonal sockets are used similarly as in B

AFFIXING WIRE TO RING

If correctly introduced into the extremity, both ends of a wire lie freely over the same side of the ring wall. Their exact position in relation to the ring holes determines the manner of their fixation. The three possible wire-ring hole positions are (1) wire over the middle of a hole; (2) wire near the edge of a hole; (3) wire between two holes (Figs 11.28A, C, and E).

The wire never should be manipulated from one position to another to suit its fixation to the ring; rather, it should be fixed to the ring in the exact position from which it emerges from the patient's skin (using a washer if there is a gap between the ring wall and the wire). The fixation or fastening of the wire to the ring is accomplished with either the cannulated or the slotted wire fixation bolt, or sometimes with the wire fixation buckle.

The choice of which part is used for fixating a wire is determined as follows:

1. If the wire is situated in the middle of the hole the cannulated bolt must be used.
2. If the wire is situated near the edge of the hole the slotted bolt must be used. The slot or groove must be opposite the side that is turned, for additional tension.
3. If the wire is situated between two holes the buckle must be used (Figs 11.28B, D, and F).

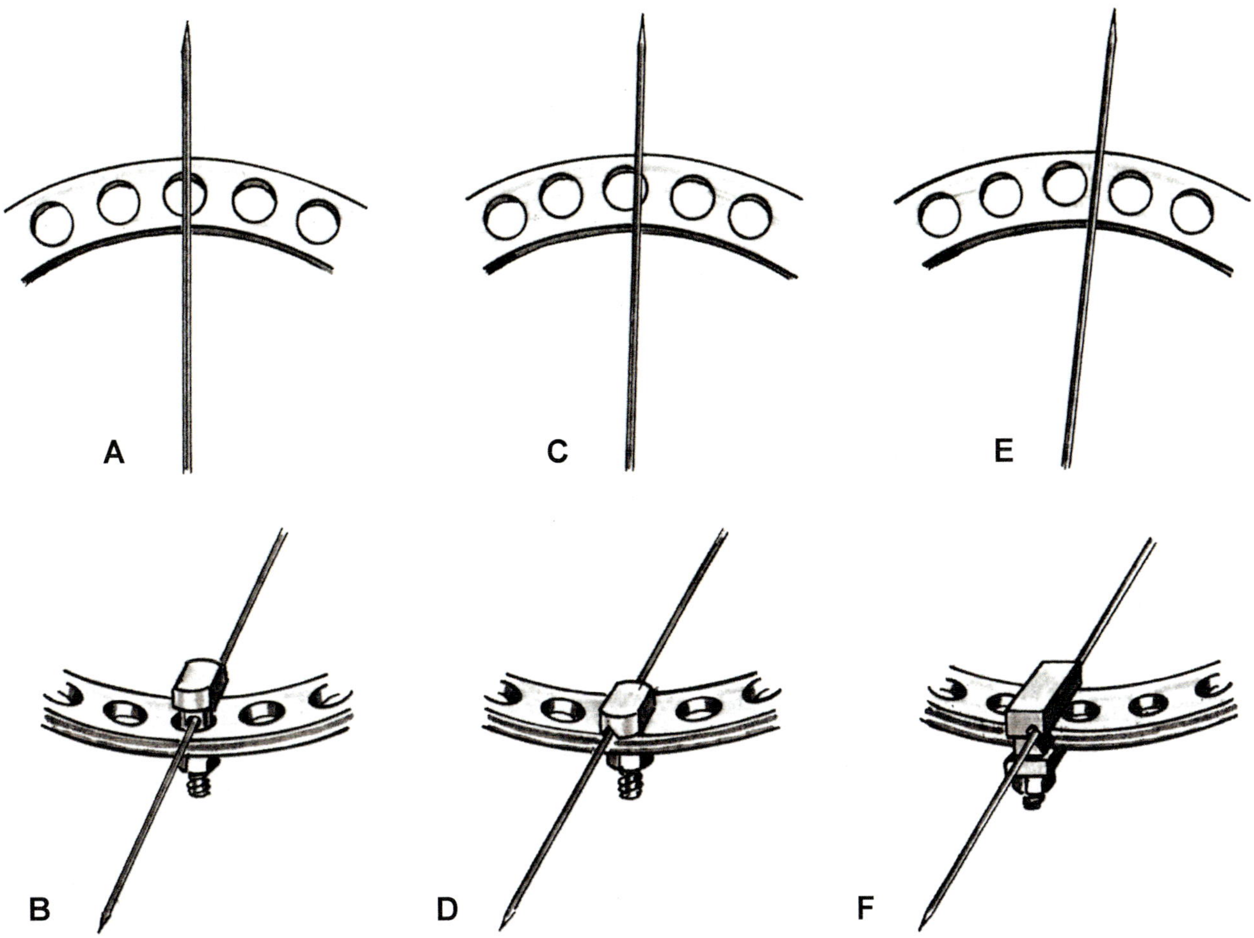

Figure 11.28: Position of wire in relation to ring holes, and types of fixation parts appropriate to each situation. A and B, wire is situated across the middle of the ring hole, and a cannulated bolt must be used for fastening. C and D, wire is situated near the edge of a ring hole, and a slotted bolt must be used for fastening. Note that the slot or groove must be opposite the side that is turned, for greater tension. E and F, wire is situated between two ring holes, and the slotted wire fixation buckle is used

The surgeon must avoid placing the wire close to the connection of two half-rings, but in certain situations this is the only choice. If so, the wire fixation buckle may be used for a dual purpose: to connect two half-rings and to fix the wire to the frame.

In some cases wire fixation must be performed away from the ring wall. In this situation a combination of supports is introduced into the nearest available hole and is brought to the wire, but not vice versa (Fig. 11.29).

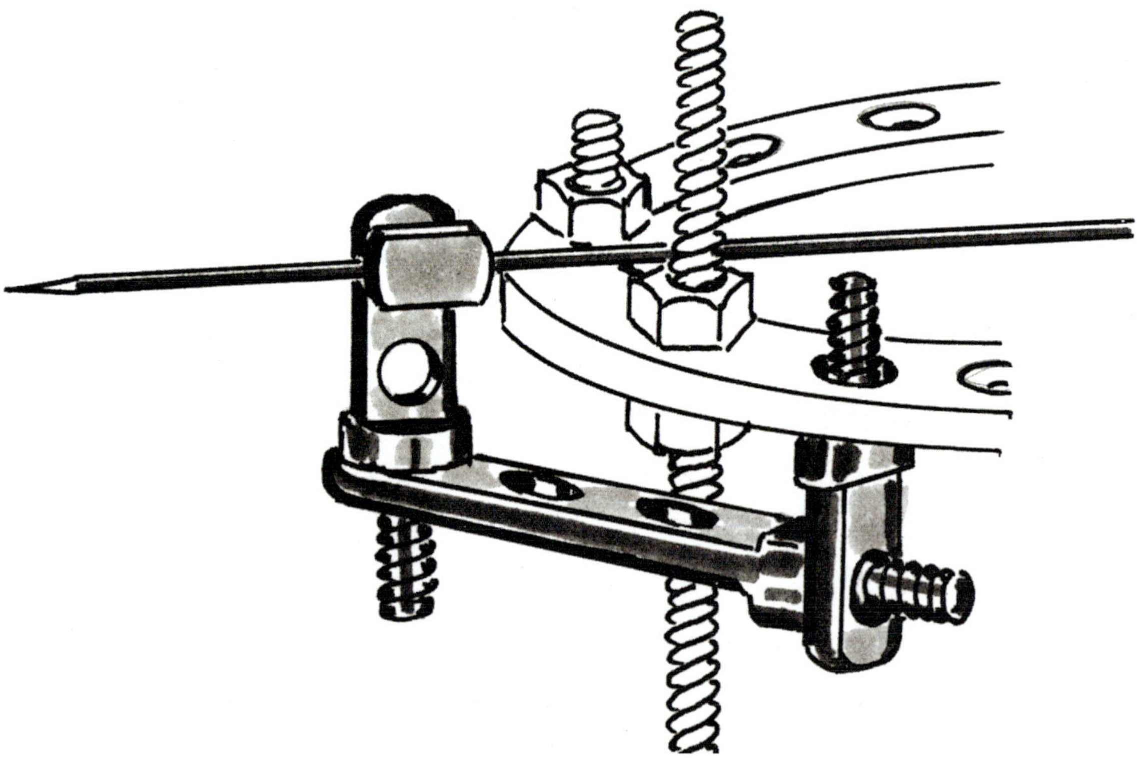

Figure 11.29: Sometimes a case requires the surgeon to perform wire fixation away from the ring. The combination of supports used to accomplish this task is shown. It is essential to restate that the wire is never brought to the ring, but vice versa

TECHNICAL HINT

WIRE TENSIONING

When tensioning wires with the Russian manual technique or with the tensioner without dynamometric scale, it is impossible to measure tension strength. In such cases there is a useful clinical tip that permits the surgeon to determine whether sufficient stiffness has been achieved. The surgeon listens to the tune of the tensioned wire when it is tapped lightly with an Ilizarov wrench. If the tone is high-pitched, the wire tension is stiff enough; if low-pitched, the wire must be tensioned further.

This practical clinical tip can be used not only after wire tensioning but also to verify the stiffness of tensioning over the long course of treatment, particularly for the wires of the movable rings.

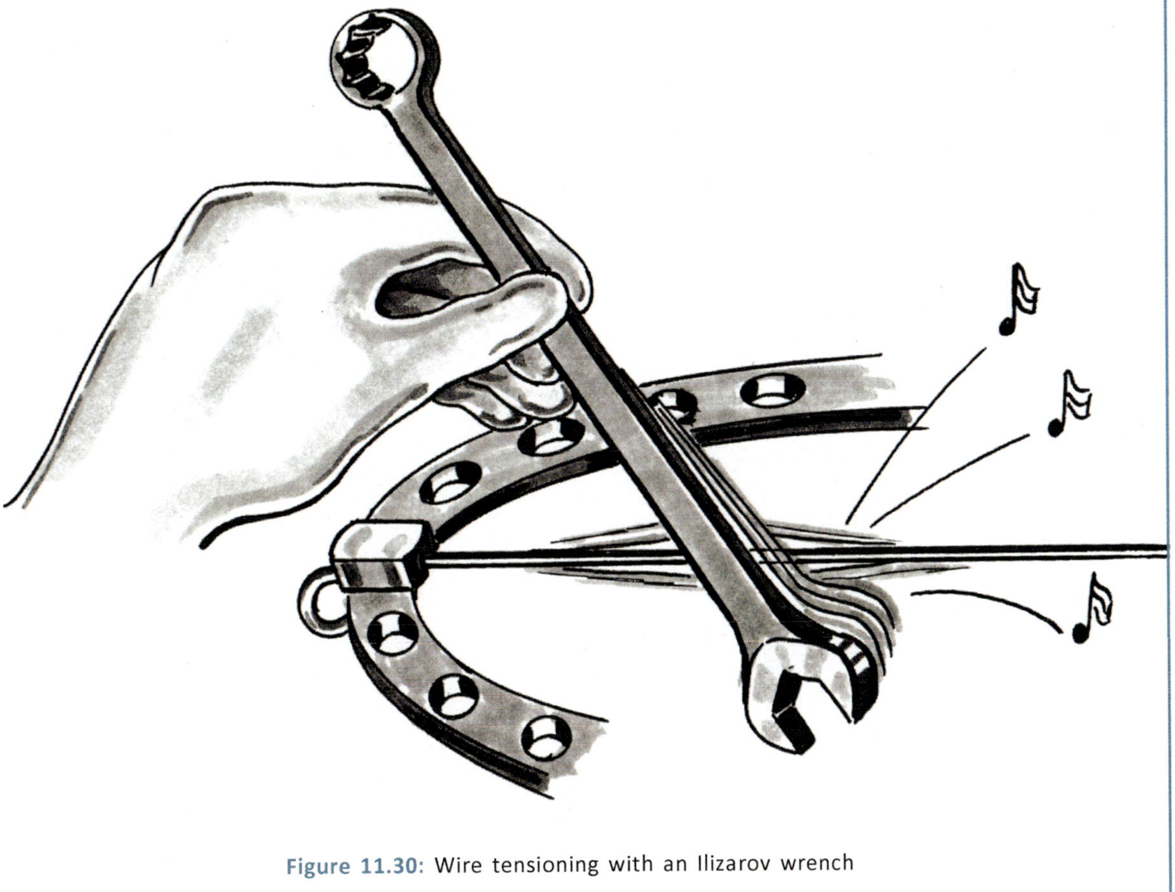

Figure 11.30: Wire tensioning with an Ilizarov wrench

REDUCING (CORRECTING) WIRE

The tensioning technique can be used not only to achieve the proper wire strength but also in some cases to reduce displacement of the bone fragments. In this way the tensioned wire becomes an instrument that corrects the malposition. Such a wire is called a reducing, or correcting wire. The principle of this reducing technique is based on the fact that the straight wire, introduced into a bone and then curved (or arched), is able to produce a shift of the bone toward the concave side of this arch (Fig. 11. 31).

There is a particular problem, however, in curving the straight wire inside the soft tissues: doing so can cause pain and even can produce necrosis if it is performed simply by changing the tensioning direction. Ilizarov uses one of his many practical tips for this problem. The wire is introduced all the way through the extremity at the site of minimum surrounding soft tissue. The free end that has emerged from the far side of the bone is bent toward the side of the desired bone shift, then is pulled back so that its point is even with the cortical bone. After this it must be hammered out again, because it is already bent and the tip would penetrate the skin at a different point

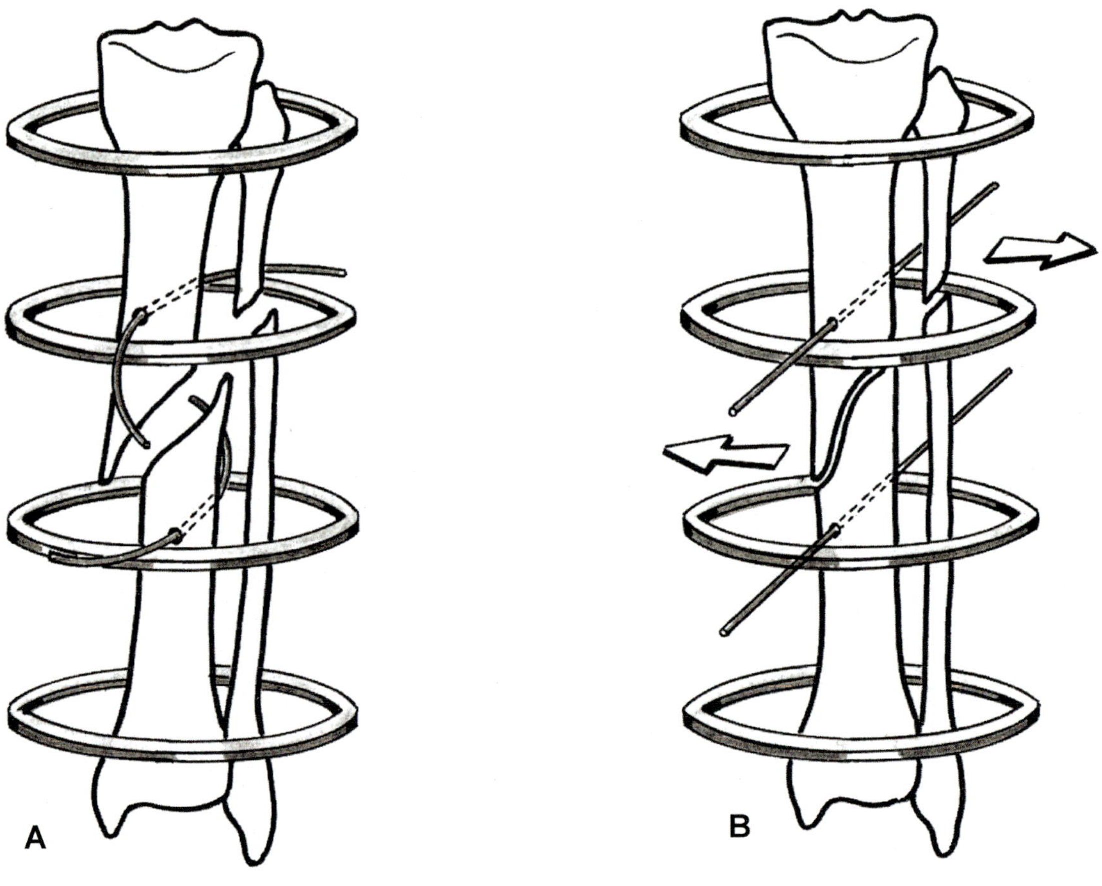

Figure 11.31: Technique of reducing bone malposition in which fragments are shifted by tensioning arched wires. A, two reducing wires are introduced into two displaced bone fragments and arched so that their concave sides face the site of displacement. B, same two wires after they have been straightened by tensioning and subsequently have brought the displaced fragments together

if reused. The same procedure is repeated with the second wire end, on the other side of the extremity. Finally, there will be an arched wire that when straightened via tensioning will shift the bone fragment (Fig. 11.32).

The reduction or correction of bone fragments also can be achieved with the linear translation technique. Two olive wires are introduced into the bone in opposite directions and then tensioned (Fig. 11.33). To perform bone shifting in this manner, it is advisable to use two tensioners simultaneously.

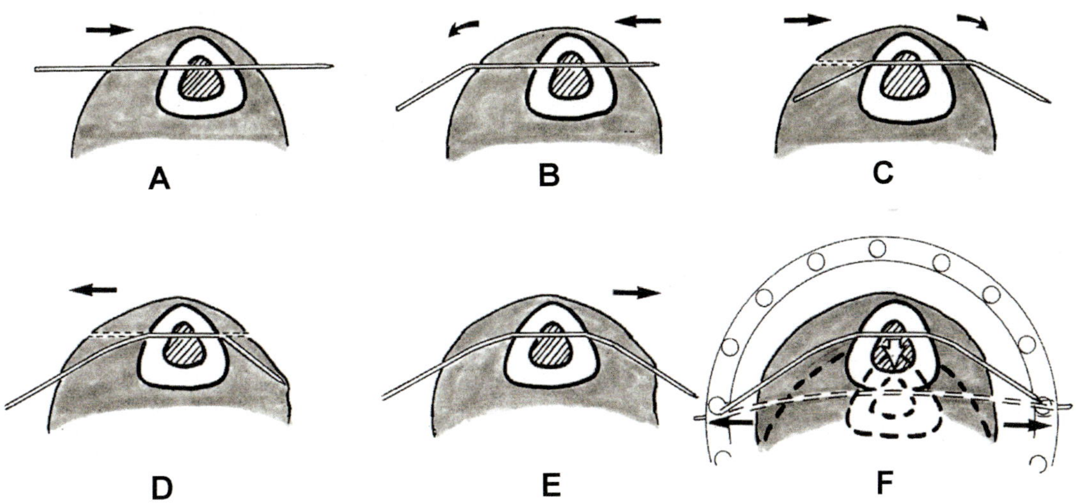

Figure 11.32: Technique of bending a wire for the application of corrective (reductive) forces. Partial view of an extremity cross section is shown, with the wire introduced through the bone and soft tissues. *Arrows* indicate direction of wire shifting and bending. A, wire is introduced completely through the bone. B, wire protruding end is bent approximately 30 degrees and pulled back up so that the tip reaches the far side of the bone. C, free end (portion on side of bone where introduction was made) of the wire is now bent approximately 30 degrees and is tapped back through the bone and soft tissues with a hammer. D, wire is pulled back up so that the second bent end plunges into the soft tissues. With this shifting, the first bent end emerges from the skin. E, position of the wire with continued reintroduction forward. Now the second end emerges from the skin. F, with the ring assembled and tension applied to both ends of the bent wire, it is straightened. This produces shifting of the bone and soft tissue to the concave side of the bent wire

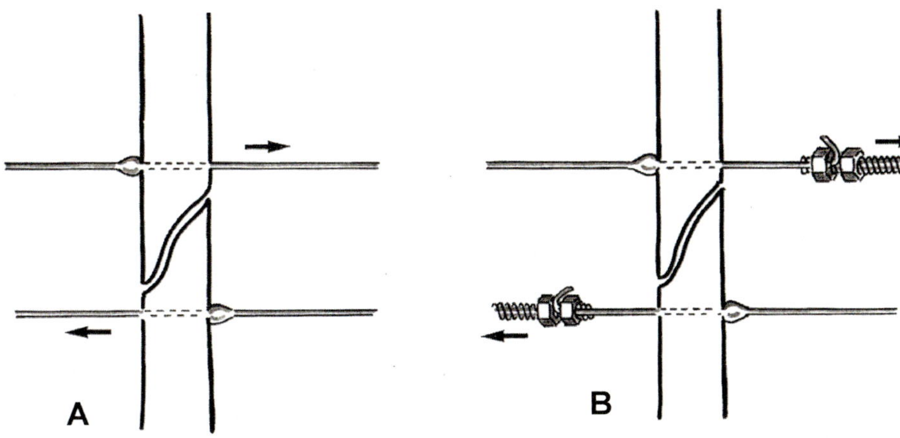

Figure 11.33: A, immediate intraoperative linear reduction technique. Two olive wires are introduced to the bone fragments in opposite directions then tensioned. *Arrows* indicate the direction of tensioning. B, postoperative linear reduction technique. If reduction cannot be performed on the operating table, olive wires may be attached to pulling devices and gradually reduced

If reduction (correction) cannot be performed immediately on the operating table, the olive wire(s) can be attached to the pulling device to produce gradual shifting.

WIRE RETENSIONING TECHNIQUE

Over the long course of treatment there is always a possibility that some of the wires will become slack as a result of metal fatigue and enlargement of the holes in the bone. This is especially true of wires connected to movable rings. When wires slacken they must be retensioned. As a rule, the slack wire produces pain, and sometimes inflammation, in the surrounding tissues. Production of a low-pitched tone when the wire is tapped confirms weakened tension and loss of stiffness. Retensioning is performed by applying two wrenches simultaneously to the head of a fixation bolt and a nut and slowly turning both of them a quarter-turn or half-turn. The wire pitch tone should be rechecked after this retensioning. Wire retensioning can be painful, and in many patients requires some kind of local anesthesia (e.g. numbing spray and/or 1% lidocaine injection). If there is need to retension several wires, it is advisable to sedate the patient or administer general anesthesia. If there is need for significant wire retensioning, it is performed with reapplication of a wire tensioner (dynamometric or simple) on one end of the wire, which is loosened, then refastened with a bolt.

On rare occasions wire retensioning cannot be performed because there is complete lack of wrench access to the wire fixation bolt and nut (i.e. all nearby ring holes are occupied). This situation dictates wire replacement, which is in fact a full-fledged adjustment procedure.

WIRE CUTTING AND BENDING

Wire cutting and bending may seem insignificant, but in fact are essential. The way in which free wire ends are cut and bent can have significant impact on the patient's health, and sometimes the physician's. The sharp ends of wires that protrude and are unprotected will scratch and can penetrate the physician's hand or skin. In the current climate of widespread hepatitis and human immunodeficiency virus infection, grave complications may result. Therefore wire cutting and bending can be considered a very significant part of the entire procedure and should be performed according to the following rules:

1. To protect the physician from skin penetration or scratches each wire's sharp end must be cut immediately after wire introduction and before tensioning and fixation to the ring.
2. Both ends of the wire, approximately 5 to 6 cm, must be left free. This is important so that the wire can be gripped by the tensioner should the need for wire retensioning arise in the future.
3. Both ends of the wire are bent into loops wrapped around the ring wall, with their tips tucked below the ring (Fig. 11.34).

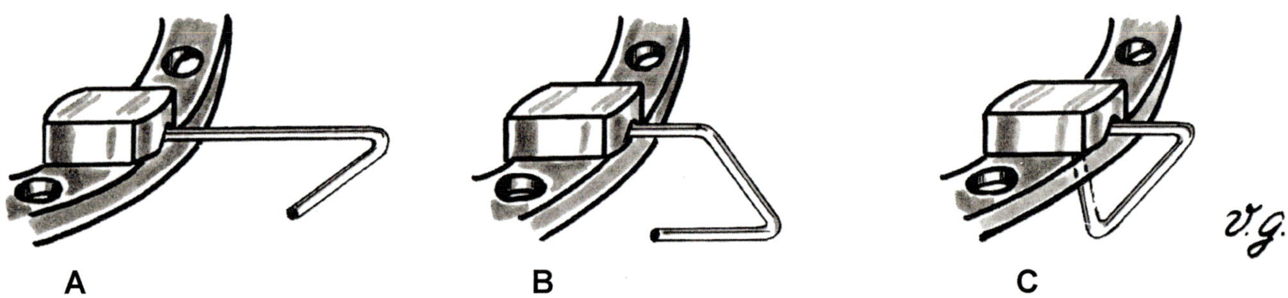

Figure 11.34: Technique of wire bending. Section of the ring is shown with the wire fixed to a fixation bolt and cut 5 to 6 cm out of it. A, distal part of the wire end is bent at a sharp angle. B, proximal part of the wire end is bent near the bolt to the side of the ring. C, loop made by the two sharp angles by bending and turning the wire around the ring's wall. The end of the wire thereby is secured under the ring wall and cannot scratch or puncture the patient's or physician's skin

GUIDEWIRE

In the technique of bone fragment distraction there is always a possibility of fragment deviation. This is especially true for cases requiring two levels of distraction and for those with large bone loss replacement by the bone transport technique. To prevent such deviation, in the 1960s Ilizarov introduced a technique of guiding (or directing) insertion of the wire lengthwise into a bone medullary cavity (Fig. 11.35).

The use of the guidewire is only for axial stabilization of the moving fragment. As such, its proximal end must be above and its distal end below the fragment level. One of its ends (usually proximal) is buried in the bone canal, and the opposite end attached to a nonmovable ring frame.

The choice of site for guidewire insertion depends on the direction of distraction. In this respect, it is more secure to introduce it distally to the site of corticotomy. A small skin incision, 0.5 to 1.0 cm, is made over one of the most prominent bone parts (e.g. condyle, epicondyle, or malleolus). The smooth wire is introduced into the bone medullary cavity by drilling it through the cortex strictly in a tangent direction. It is important to consider the bone architecture at this level, because the trabecular portions continue some distance from the condyles. The best way to control introduction of the guidewire is with the assistance of an image intensifier. As soon as the wire tip penetrates the trabecular part of the bone and emerges into the medullary (marrow) cavity, the drilling must be stopped.

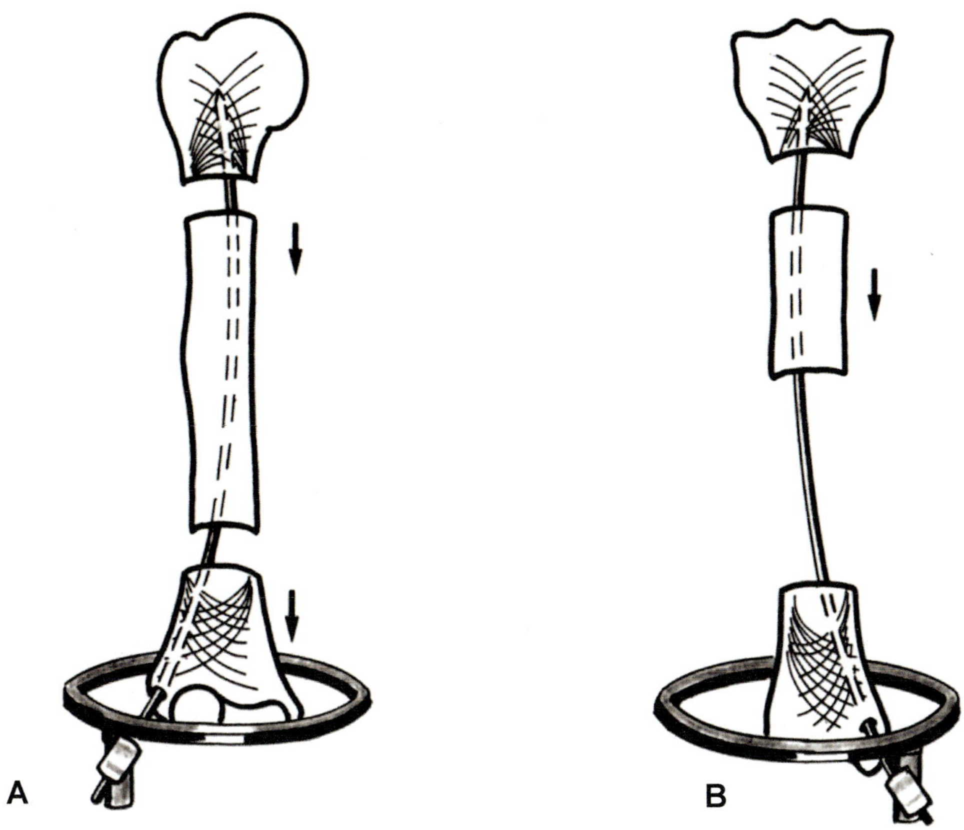

Figure 11.35: Technique of guiding (directing) wire insertion to prevent bone fragment deviation with distraction. *Arrows* show the direction of distraction; *curved lines* at bone ends represent the level of the trabecular portions. For the purpose of simplicity, only nonmovable distal rings are shown, to which the guidewires are attached with posts. A, humerus with two levels of corticotomy. Guidewire is introduced through the lateral epicondyles. B, tibia with resected middle part and a proximal corticotomy. Guidewire is introduced through the medial malleolus

The guidewire must not be drilled along the bone marrow, it may become arched (or curved) and can destroy the internal organization of the marrow.

Further wire introduction is performed with gentle hammering. If the wire is positioned centrally or near the internal bone wall, the injury to the marrow structure with its abundant blood vessel nets can be minimal and will not cause permanent damage (In many cases of malunion, nonunion, or infection the bone marrow already may have some degree of destruction). Conversely, possible bone fragment deviation and its subsequent correction can provoke far worse complications. In any case, the indications and contraindications for use of the guidewire always must be balanced.

In a procedure in the lower leg with a stiff or fused ankle the guidewire can be introduced from the heel, proximally (Fig. 11.36). It is drilled through calcaneus, talus, and the trabecular part of the distal tibia, starting laterally to the sustentaculum tali. Further introduction is achieved by hammering. If there is an incision and a bone medullary canal is opened, the wire can be introduced into it and hammered distally through the tibia, talus, and calcaneus from outside the heel. As soon as the proximal end of the wire is levelled with the wedge of the tibial distal fragment the wire is introduced retrograde into the proximal fragment.

Removal of the guidewire is accomplished by simply pulling it out of the bone. This is not always easy to do,

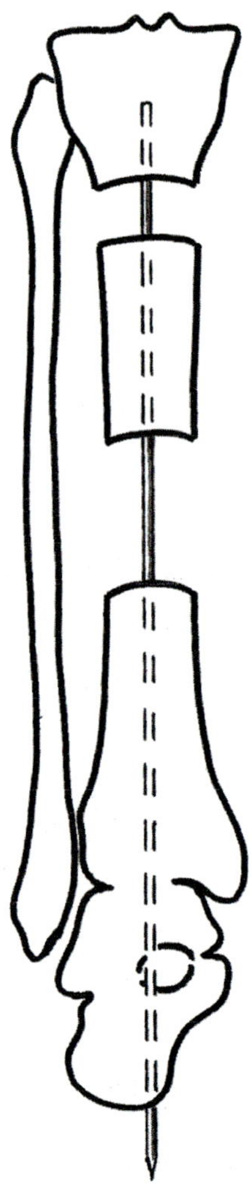

Figure 11.36: Technique of introducing the guidewire through a fused (stiff) ankle and subtalar joint. Tibia with the middle part resected and proximal corticotomy are shown. Guidewire can be introduced from the heel proximally or through the bony defect distally

because the wire can be arched and its tip may be deep in the trabecular part of the opposite side of the bone. In some cases this wire has to be left in the bone, and its protruding end cut.

PULLING OR TRACTION WIRE

In the technique of internal bone transport Ilizarov introduced yet another practical use for the K-wire: as a connecting device between the movable bone fragment and the traction mechanism. Balancing the tractional forces requires two wires. If one pulling wire is used, the guidewire must be used to prevent fragment deviation.

There are three types of pulling wires. Their common feature is the existence of some type of stopper on the proximal end, which is attached to the bone. There are wires with the olive stopper, with the Z-shaped wire twist, and with the hooked end. Each of these wires has its own indications and method of introduction (Fig. 11.37).

The stoppers must be situated distal to the level of the bone osteotomy (corticotomy) and at the bone fragment proximal level. Introduction of the pulling wires must be performed before the corticotomy, to prevent excessive bone fragment shearing and bone marrow damage. Thus the level of wire insertion must be planned and marked in advance.

There are three ways to introduce the pulling wire:

1. Drilling it obliquely through both bone cortices.
2. Drilling it obliquely through one cortical wall and introducing it further by hammering it into the medullary cavity, with exit from the skin below the bone fragment distal end (this requires control with an image intensifier).
3. Drilling it through one cortical wall at the level of the subsequent corticotomy, with further introduction by hammering and then bending the proximal end to make a hook, which is caught on a bone fragment edge.

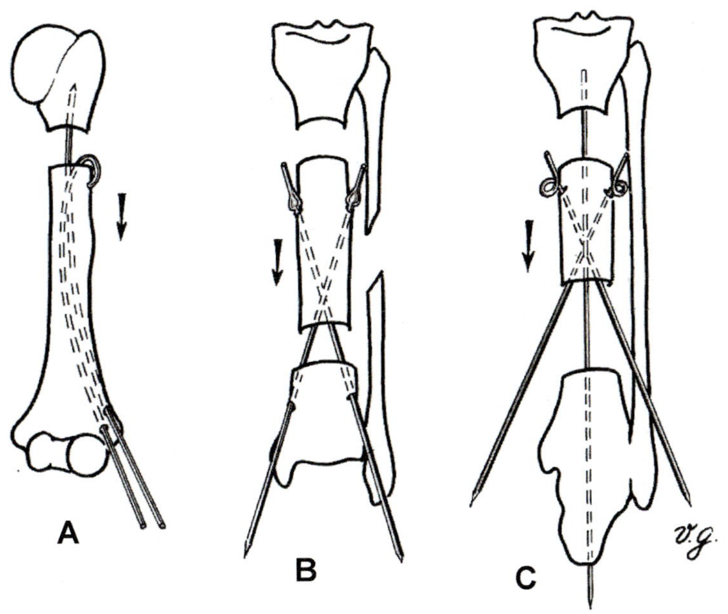

Figure 11.37: Technique of introducing three types of pulling (traction) wires. *Arrows* indicate direction of pull. A, smooth wire is introduced into the humerus through the lateral epicondyle, and extracted at the site of corticotomy. It then is hooked with a needle-nose pliers and is fixed to the bone edge. To prevent distal fragment deviation the guidewire is advanced into the proximal fragment. B, two olive wires are shown introduced obliquely into the tibia just below the proximal corticotomy site and drilled down into the distal fragment through a second corticotomy. They are cut near the olives to prevent soft tissue injury during distraction. Their exit sites are located above the malleolus. Because these two pulling wires produce well-balanced traction, there is no need for a guidewire. C, in a case similar to that in B, the two smooth wires are introduced obliquely into the middle fragment with a Z-shaped bend to create stoppers. They exit at the site of the bone resection. To prevent middle fragment deviation the guidewire is introduced through the heel and drilled up to the proximal fragment

The distal end of any of the three types of pulling wire is connected to the traction device. Removal of the pulling wire can be performed only retrograde to the direction of traction.

BONE FIXATION WITH HALF-PINS

The half-pins measuring 4 and 5 mm in diameter were introduced by the Italian surgeons Catagni and Cattaneo for use in a special device for proximal femur fixation (Fig. 11. 38). Although it contradicts the Ilizarov doctrine of the importance of the stiffness and elasticity achieved through small-diameter tensioned wires, use of half-pin bone fixation occasionally is preferable to use of K-wires. If half-pins are used for nonmovable supporting ring fixation, they do not interfere significantly with the tissue regenerating resources. If they are used in addition to the wire fixation with movable rings their interference with tissue regeneration is even less significant.

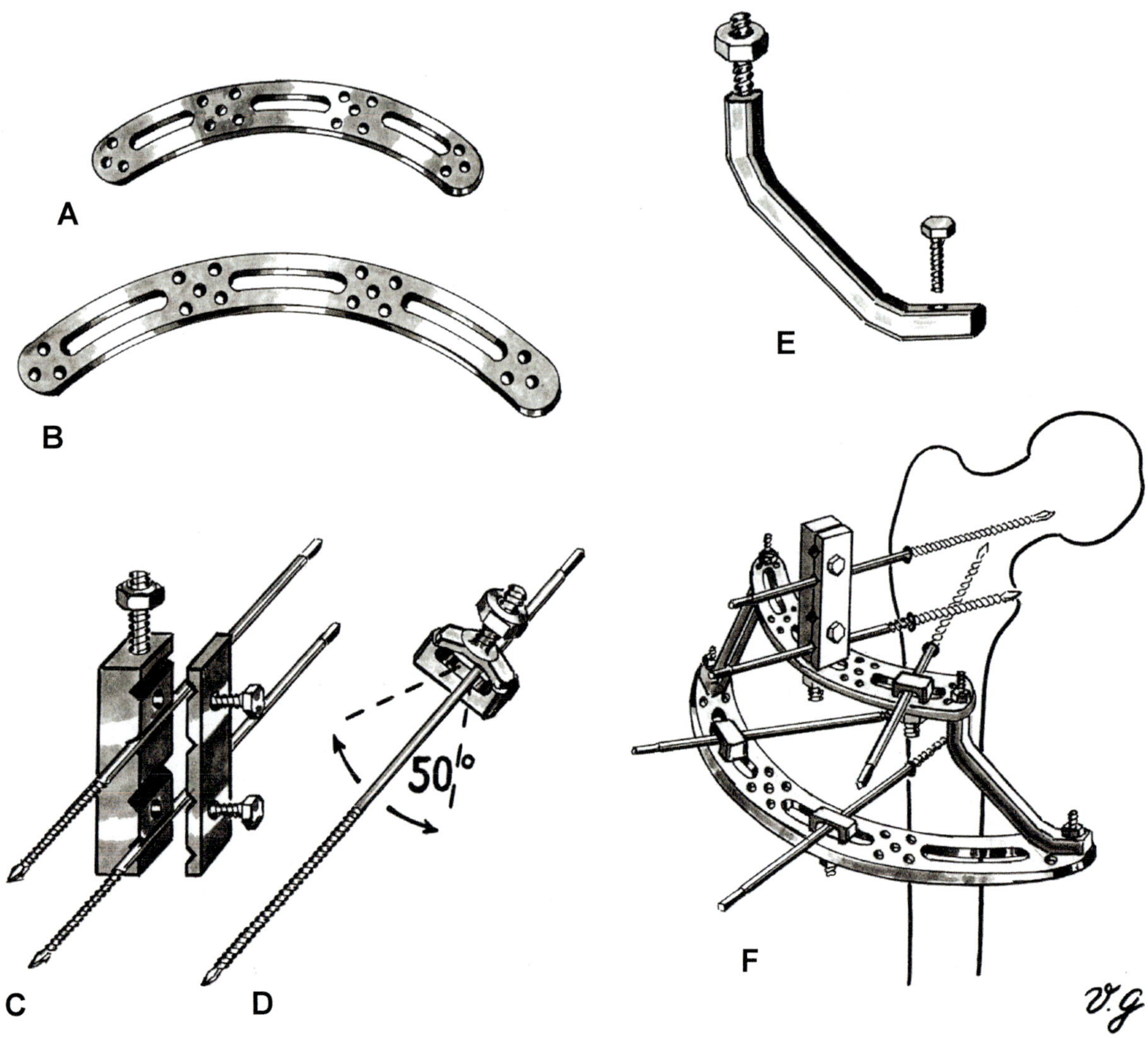

Figure 11.38: Set of parts provided for half-pin introduction, and assembled special device for proximal femur fixation. A and B, 90-degree and 120-degree arches, C, multiple pin fixation bolt assembled with two half-pins before being tightened. D, single pin fixation bolt with a half-pin. The 50-degree permissible pin direction angle is shown. E, oblique support connector. F, proximal femur device assembled and fixed to the bone with five half-pins

The chief indications for use of half-pins are:

1. Anatomic considerations at the limb level, where neurovascular structures may be compromised easily.
2. When the application of a ring is impractical and has to be replaced by the arch.
3. When necessary additional support is required, after wire fixation already has been applied.

The two types of half-pins are those with the interrupted threaded end and those with the continuous conical threaded end.

Half-pins are available in three sizes: 120, 150, and 180 mm long. The tip of the threaded end is bayonet shaped, and can be drilled easily into bone cortex. It is recommended that the bone be predrilled with the 3.2-mm diameter drill bit (or with the 4.4-mm diameter bit when introducing the 5-mm pin). In the case of severe osteoporosis the pin can be introduced without predrilling. It is of prime importance to place the half-pin so that both threaded sections of the pin are in full contact with the bone cortices (Fig. 11.39). The pin with a continuous conical threaded end is used primarily for

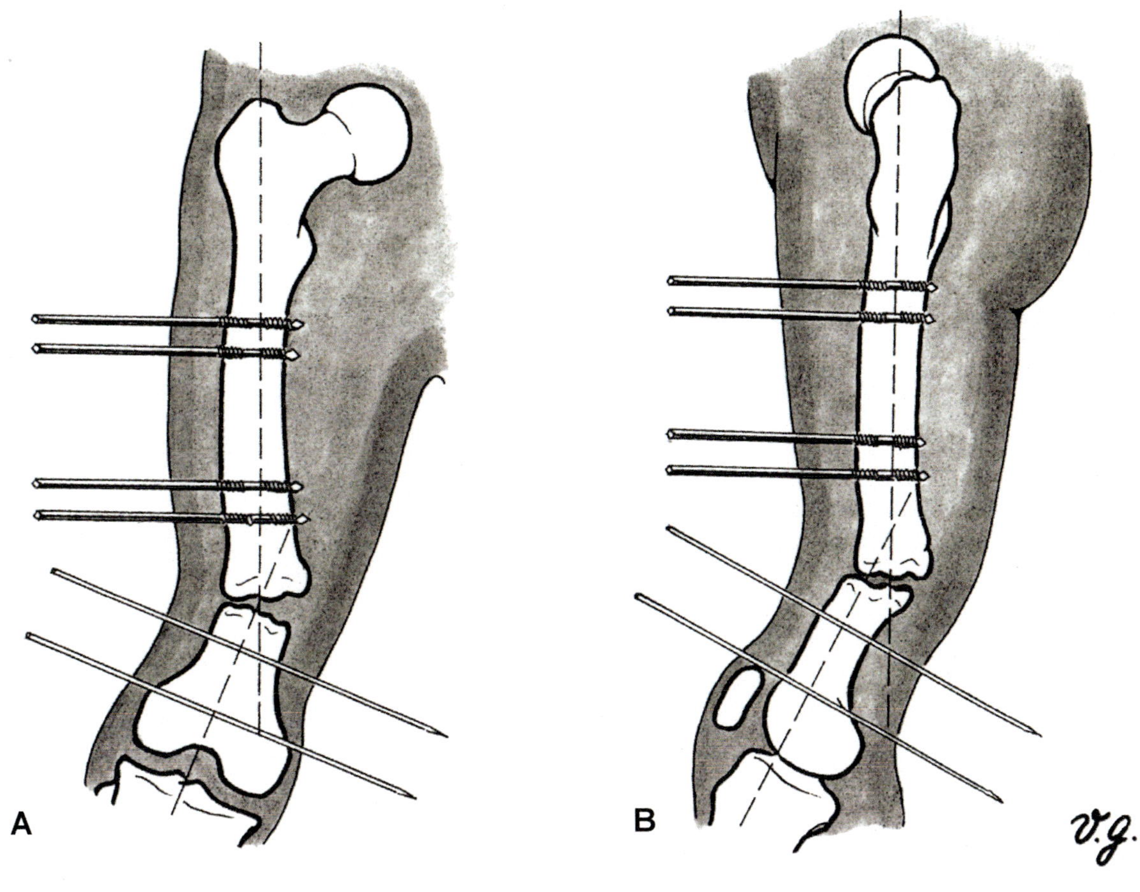

Figure 11.39: Combined introduction of half-pins and K-wires to the femur with distal nonunion and valgus and recurvation deformities. A, anteroposterior view. B, lateral view. In both views the half-pins with threaded ends are introduced so that both threaded portions are immersed in the bone cortex. All four pins are introduced into the proximal nonmovable bone fragment, and the K-wires are introduced into the distal movable fragment. In this manner fixation stability and elasticity are secured

the proximal humerus (Fig. 11.40) and for the femur (Fig. 11.41).

The half-pin must be tightened to the femoral arch or ring without bending. If it is bent before tightening, there is the risk that it will break near the attachment to the bone. The half-pin is fixed to the femoral arch by the single pin—fixation bolt.

To connect the half-pin to the ring the threaded socket or bushing may be used. It is worth noting that if the half-pin is used in addition to wire fixation on the same ring, tightening is conducted only after the wires are tensioned. This prevents pin bending. Frequently after tightening the long free end of the half-pin protrudes above the femoral arch, and must be cut with the large bolt cutter while the patient is under anesthesia. This is a very painful procedure that cannot be performed postoperatively.

Fixation with the half-pin on the movable ring has the disadvantage of leaving a large scar. Moreover, it may irritate the skin and deep soft tissues, cause significant

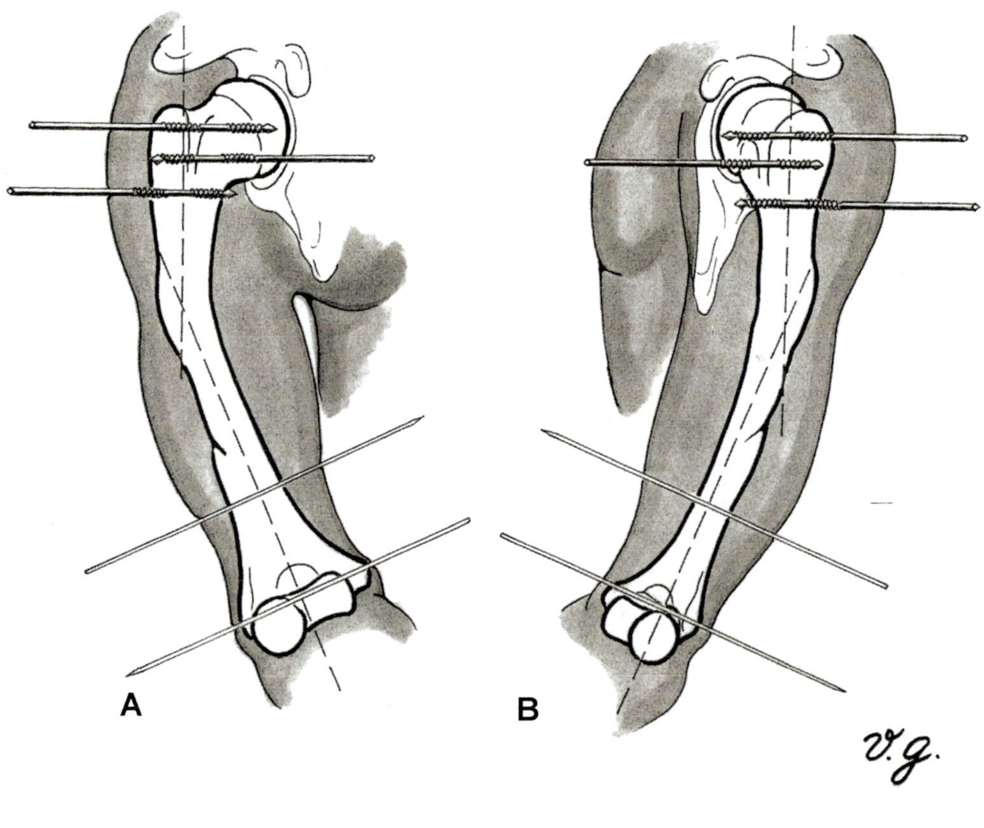

Figure 11.40: Combined introduction of half-pins and K-wires to the humerus with shortness and deformity. A, anteroposterior view. B, lateral view. In both views the threaded portions of the pin ends are immersed in the bone cortex

pain, and provoke pin tract infection more often than does fixation with the wire. Thus we recommend using as few half-pins as possible for the movable rings.

Removal of the half-pin is achieved with the reverse motion of the hand-drill attachment. Because the possibility (although it is infrequent) of a weak point existing close to the threaded portion of the half-pin, possibly due to metal fatigue, hand drill unscrewing always must be performed carefully, without sudden or great application of force.

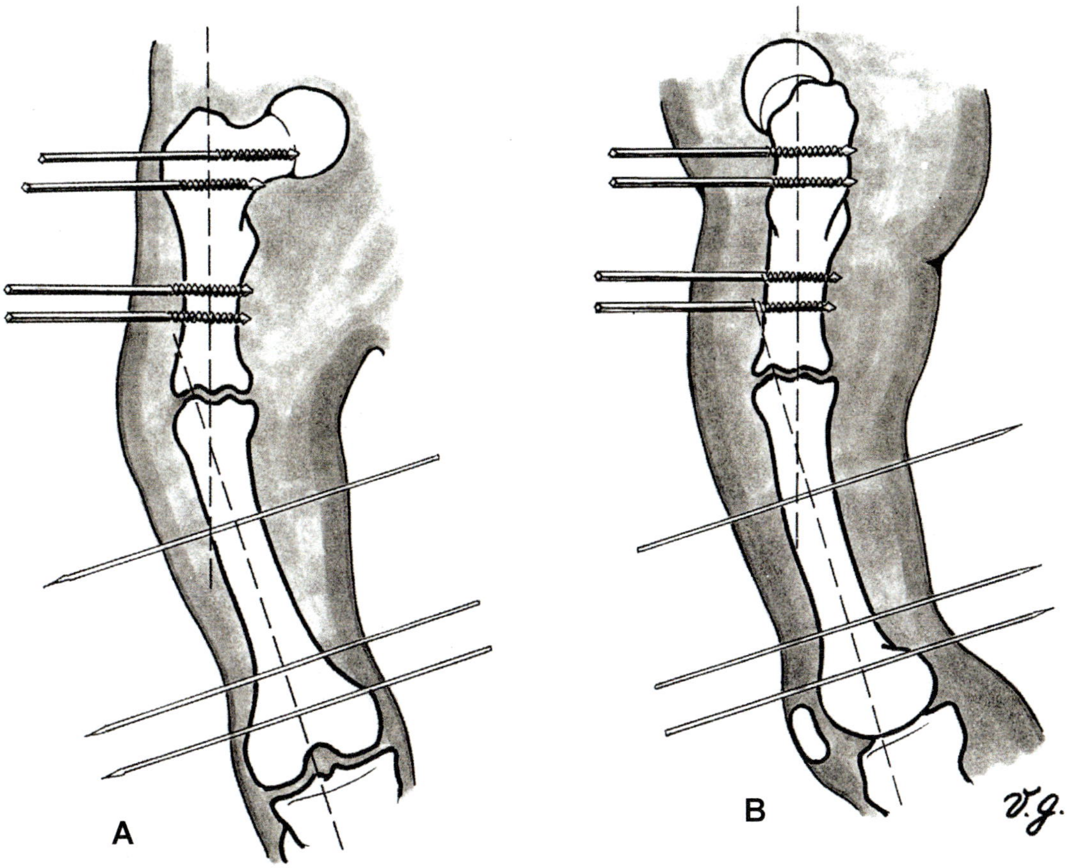

Figure 11.41: Combined introduction of half-pins and K-wires in a femur with nonunion in the lower third and varus and antecurvation deformity. A, anteroposterior view. B, lateral view. In this case the deformities may be corrected by distal fragment realignment using the compression-distraction technique. Movable distal fragment is shown transfixed by the K-wires on two levels. Proximal fragment is used to bear the supporting nonmovable arch and ring, and is shown fixed by half-pins on two levels (two threaded half-pins for each supporting frame component). The surgeon should pay particular attention that all half-pins and K-wires are introduced perpendicular to the long axis of the bone fragments. In both views the half-pins with the continuous conical threaded end are introduced so that the threaded areas are immersed in bone cortex. All four pins are introduced into the proximal nonmovable bone fragment, and the K-wires are introduced into the distal movable fragment, securing stability and elasticity of fixation

PART THREE

Clinical Techniques

12 Chapter
Ilizarov Corticotomy (Compactotomy) Technique

After the fixator frame is assembled properly and transfixed securely to the bone, the next stage of the Ilizarov procedure is to perform bone transection for distraction and correction. The generally accepted osteotomy technique was modified by Ilizarov in the 1960s. Clinical observations led him to believe that only a well-preserved vascular net at the site of the bone transection would contribute to full-blooded regeneration. The minimal surgical trauma to the bone and surrounding soft tissues, with the preservation of their bone-forming segments, optimizes the biologic conditions necessary for new bone development.

The Ilizarov osteotomy technique consists of cutting through compact bone only, with preservation of the periosteum and bone marrow. Ilizarov's discovery of the corticotomy technique is an interesting historical anecdote. For years he tried many bone cut variations. In one case, to lengthen a short leg stump with a very poor blood supply he left all the surrounding tissues and bone marrow intact. The surgery was successful beyond anyone's expectations. This observation brought about the development of a new technique, the corticotomy or compactotomy.

ANATOMIC AND PHYSIOLOGIC CONSIDERATIONS

It is well established that the periosteal bone surface is responsible for growth in bone width and that the endosteum carries out the phases of bone formation alternating with phases of bone resorption. In the process of bone healing, new lamellae of the haversian system are deposited in new concentric layers. Cortical bone is remodeled, after it is cut, by bone cells deposited on the periosteal, endosteal, and haversian canal surfaces. With gradual dilatory lengthening through the bone cut, billions of new cells develop. Ilizarov's observations confirmed Wolff's (1892) law of bone transformation, that is, form follows function. For development of the bone collagen columns, that is, of the lengthening, deposited along lines of the mechanical stress, the first and most important condition is preservation of local blood circulation. Normally two-third of the cortical bone blood supply comes from the nutrient artery located in the bone marrow. It gives rise to the abundant net of the peripheral arteriolar branches and capillaries that enter Volkmann's and haversian canals. The periosteal arterioles provide one-third of the blood supply. In the case of bone destruction,

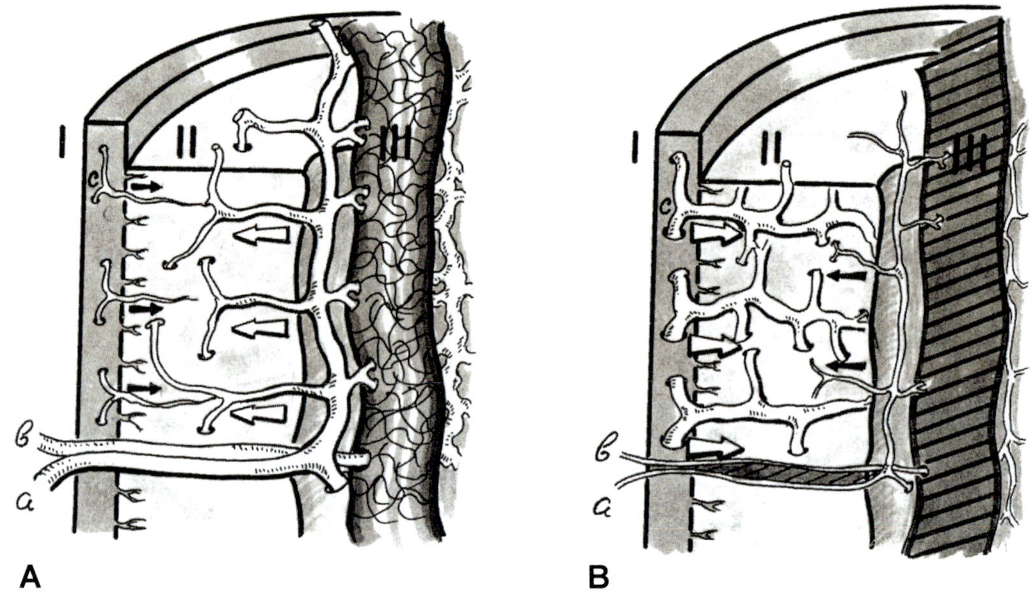

Figure 12.1: Schematic representation of a bone segment transected longitudinally and transversely. I = periosteum, II = compact bone, III = bone marrow, a = nutrient artery, b = commissary vein, c = periosteal arterioles. *White arrows* show direction of the main blood supply; *black arrows* show the direction of the additional blood supply. A, under normal circumstances, up to two-third of the blood supply for the compact bone comes from the nutrient artery with a well-developed net of haversian system collateral vessels, and the remainder of the blood supply comes from the periosteal arterioles. B, with the obliteration of the nutrient artery and bone marrow *(shaded area)* the main compact bone blood supply comes from the periosteal arterioles (direction now reversed), and only a small portion comes from the marrow side

such as after a cut, with bone marrow interruption or obliteration, there is complete or partial nutrient artery dysfunction. The periosteal arterioles begin to increase and extend their function as the main source of the cortex blood supply (Fig. 12.1). This suggests that to optimize the anatomic and physiologic conditions for new bone formation after division and distraction, the preservation of both endosteal and periosteal blood supply is of great importance.

In the Ilizarov procedure the bone cut serves three main purposes:

1. To create mechanical conditions (a gap) necessary for the development of distraction
2. To store the new bone-forming cells that were developed during lengthening and deposited along the lines parallel to the mechanical stress
3. To develop the area with increased blood circulation necessary for increased metabolic transformation of local tissues.

These preconditions are the basis of the Ilizarov osteotomy modification. To perform this, Ilizarov developed an intricate and elegant surgical technique performed through a very small skin incision, the corticotomy or compactotomy.

CORTICOTOMY TECHNIQUE

Transection of the cortex around a bone without cutting the bone marrow and periosteum is a delicate procedure, and must be performed extremely carefully and patiently. The best way to describe it is in stages.

1. The length of the skin and soft tissue incision is only 0.5 to 1.0 cm (Fig. 12.2).

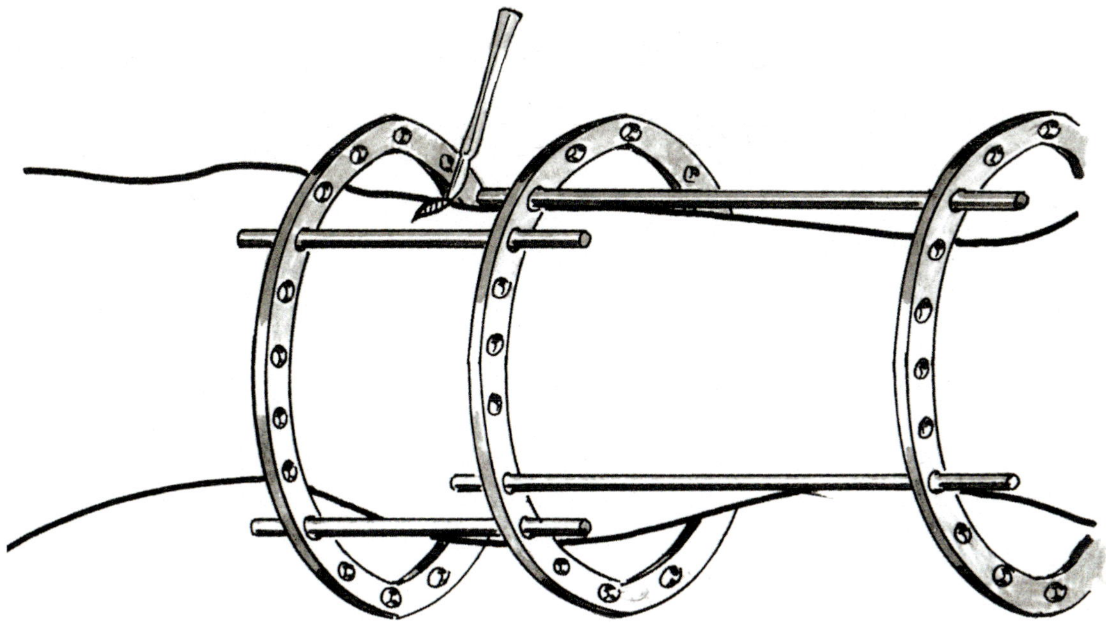

Figure 12.2: Three-ring frame applied to the leg. Transverse, small skin incision is made at the proximal metaepiphyseal site

2. Location of the incision must be at the site where the bone is situated close to the skin. This helps control the direction of transection more precisely (Fig. 12.3).
3. The cortex transection must be performed with a small osteotome, preferably 0.5 cm wide. This guarantees that its edge does not slip too deeply into the periosteum or bone marrow sides (Fig. 12.4).

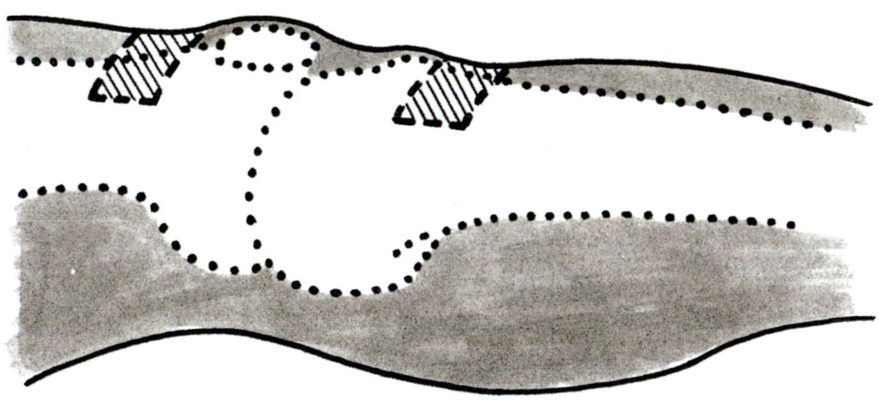

Figure 12.3: Lower femur and upper tibia with the bones outlined on the skin. *Shaded squares* designate location of incisions for corticotomy

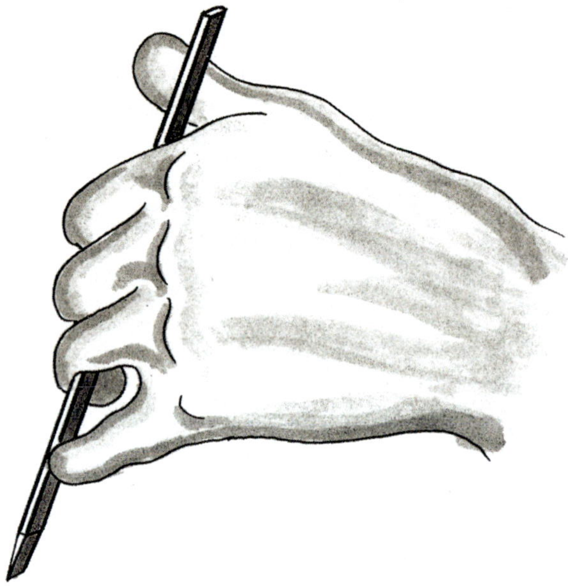

Figure 12.4: Osteotome 0.5 cm wide is recommended for corticotomy

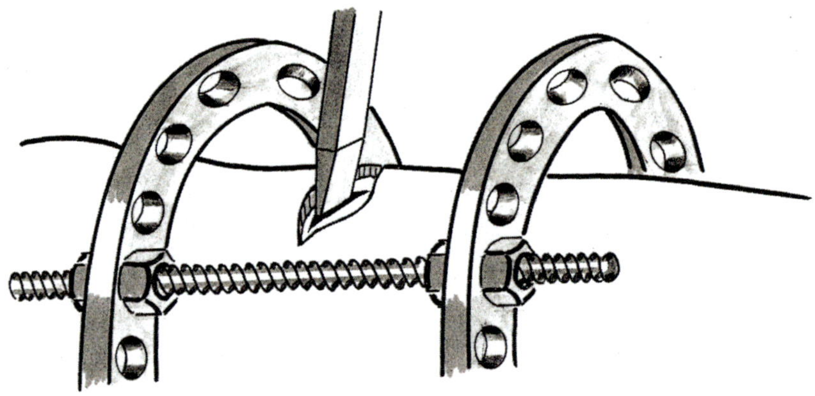

Figure 12.5: Corticotomy site between two rings. Note direct transverse cut through the periosteum, without separation and cleavage, at the site of the incision

4. Periosteum separation and cleavage at the site of the initial bone cut must be avoided. A direct transverse cut through the adjoining periosteum made by tapping the osteotome is recommended. This protects the periosteal arterioles from destruction and prevents hypoplastic bone regeneration at the section of the initial cut (Fig. 12.5).
5. After the periosteum is cut, the cortex transection is begun by further hammering. Because the hammering is done with the narrow osteotome, it must be done in a fan-shaped manner, directing the osteotome tip laterally and medially without extracting it (Fig. 12.6).
6. During these stages of the procedure there usually is almost no bleeding from the wound. As soon as the osteotome tip penetrates the endosteum layer it penetrates some vascular structures. Appearance of dark blood with fatty inclusions is a sign of penetration into bone marrow (Fig. 12.7).
7. At this stage the surgeon stops tapping in a straight (vertical) direction and continues by spreading the transection laterally and medially. It is important that the surgeon be able to feel the cortex resistance and listen to the sound of the tapping. It is also important that the tip direction be changed to divert the adjoined cortex segment proportionally

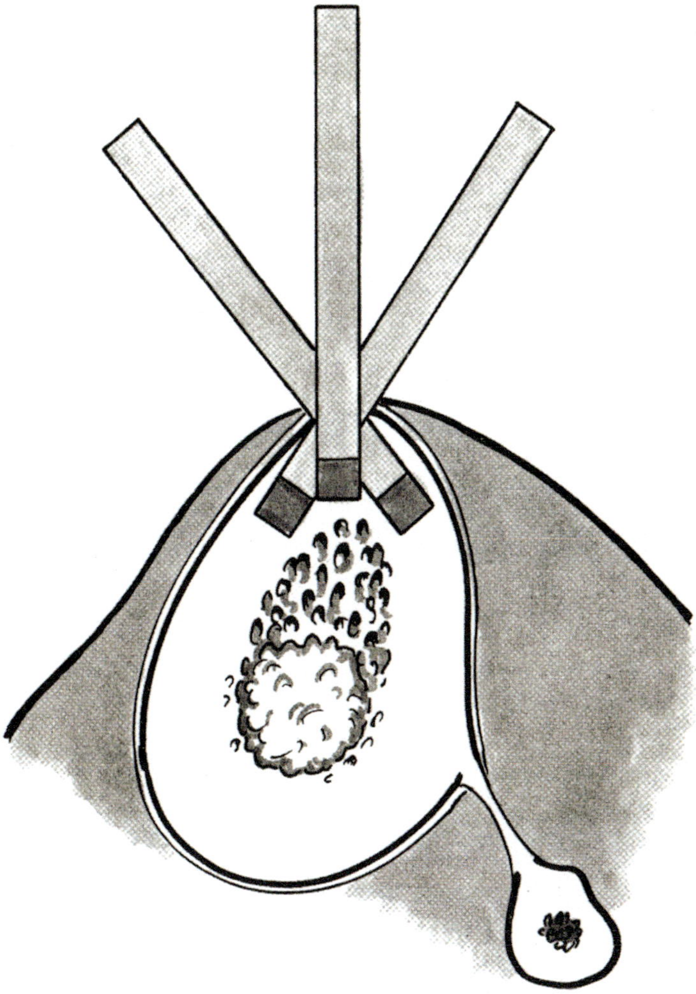

Figure 12.6: Partial cross-section through the upper part of the leg shows the tibia and fibula. Anterior cortex of the tibia is being transected by the osteotome. Transection is done in a fan-shaped pattern

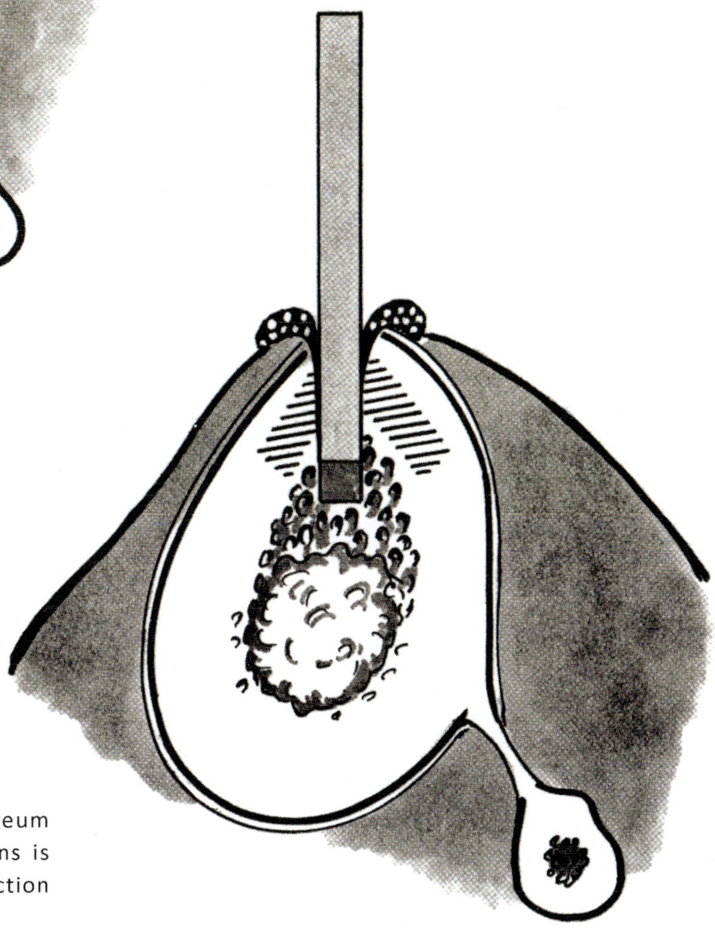

Figure 12.7: Osteotome tip penetrates the endosteum layer. Appearance of dark blood with fatty inclusions is a sign of penetration and the signal to stop introduction of the osteotome

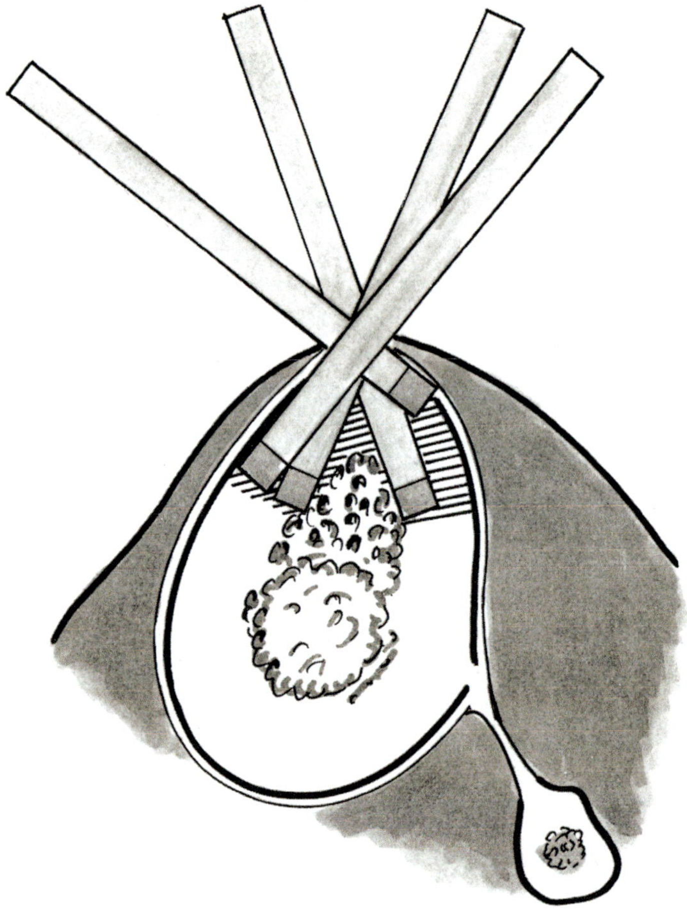

Figure 12.8: Tapping of the bone is continued by spreading the transection laterally and medially

(Fig. 12.8). The high-pitched sound is a sign of compact bone splintering. As soon as the sound changes to a low pitch and the feeling of bone resistance is lessened, the fan-shaped hammering must be stopped. These are signs that the osteotome tip has penetrated the periosteum.

8. After the adjoining cortex wall is transected, the continued direction of the osteotome must be changed (preferably without its extraction). Depending on the shape of the bone cross section, transection is directed alternately along the medial and lateral cortex walls (Fig. 12.9). Again, this must be performed while monitoring cortex resistance and high-pitched sound. If the osteotome tip slips into the periosteum or endosteum, its direction must be corrected. Moreover, an assistant can control the tip position by feeling it with his or her fingers (if the bone is situated close to skin).
9. When the transection of the bone walls is complete there will be signs of penetration outside of the cortex in two side points located opposite the initial cut. A triangular transection is developed (Fig. 12.10).
10. At this point the tapping is ceased and the osteotome handle turned alternately with pliers, with its position at the farthest medial and lateral

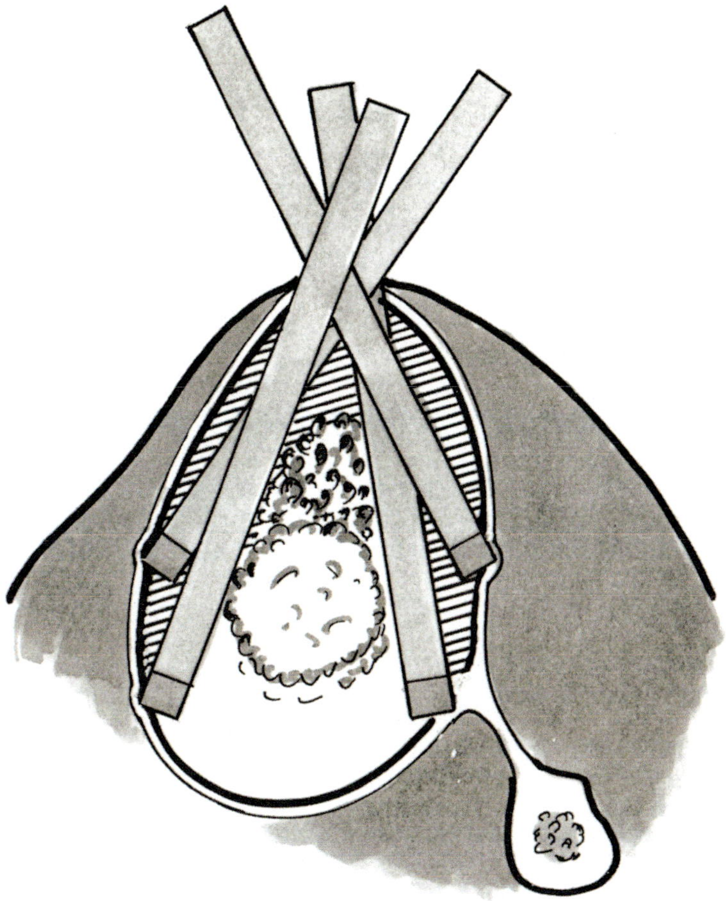

Figure 12.9: Tapping of the bone now is directed along the medial and lateral walls alternately

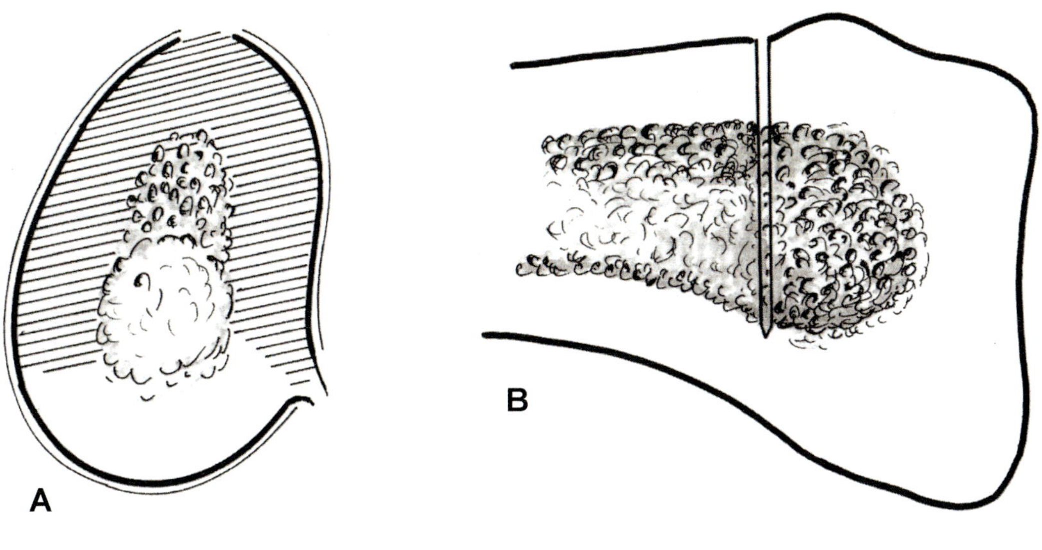

Figure 12.10: Transectional (A) and lateral (B) views at the corticotomy site of the proximal tibia. *Shaded area* indicates already transected part of compact bone

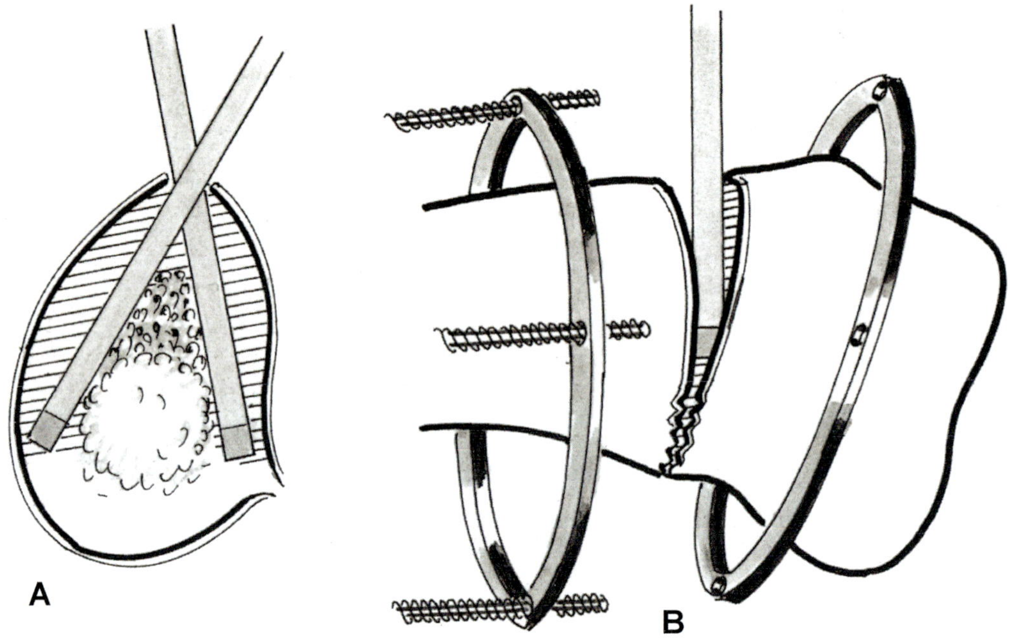

Figure 12.11: A, *shaded segment* represents the cut through the bone to the posterior wall. B, same compound bone cut shown in lateral view, with the osteotome handle turned with pliers

transection corners (Fig. 12.11). Usually, there already is a microcleft in the bottom wall cortex, and the cracking sound of its divergence should be the sign of the completed corticotomy.

11. To facilitate corticotomy, we (V.G.) introduced the T-shaped osteotome in two versions: straight and curved. The sharp cutting leg of the osteotome is covered by the narrow crossbar with smooth edges. This instrument is called a corticotome (Figs 12.12A and B). We recommend starting with the straight corticotome. By tapping it, the sharp-pointed vertical leg of the T-shaped tip is introduced through the periosteum into the compact bone. Then the smooth, rounded crossbar is placed under the periosteum. With further transection the periosteum is protected from its cut, and penetration into the bone marrow canal also is prevented. Because the crossbar is thin and narrow, it does not separate the periosteum significantly. As soon as transection of medial and lateral bone walls is accomplished, the straight corticotome must be replaced with the curved osteotome. Further tapping cuts the bone almost completely.

The advantage of the corticotome is that its crossbar is placed between the periosteum and the compact layer. This prevents the periosteum from being cut and ripped. At the same time the crossbar preserves penetration of the cutting leg into endosteum.

The corticotomy technique with the use of the corticotome is essentially the same as with the regular osteotome. The only difference is that the straight corticotome must be replaced by the curved one at the moment when the farthest medial and lateral bone wall corners have been reached. The tapping of the curved corticotome farther on allows further cutting of compact bone, up to the posterior wall (Figs 12.12C and D). The corticotomy then is completed by the rotatory movements described above.

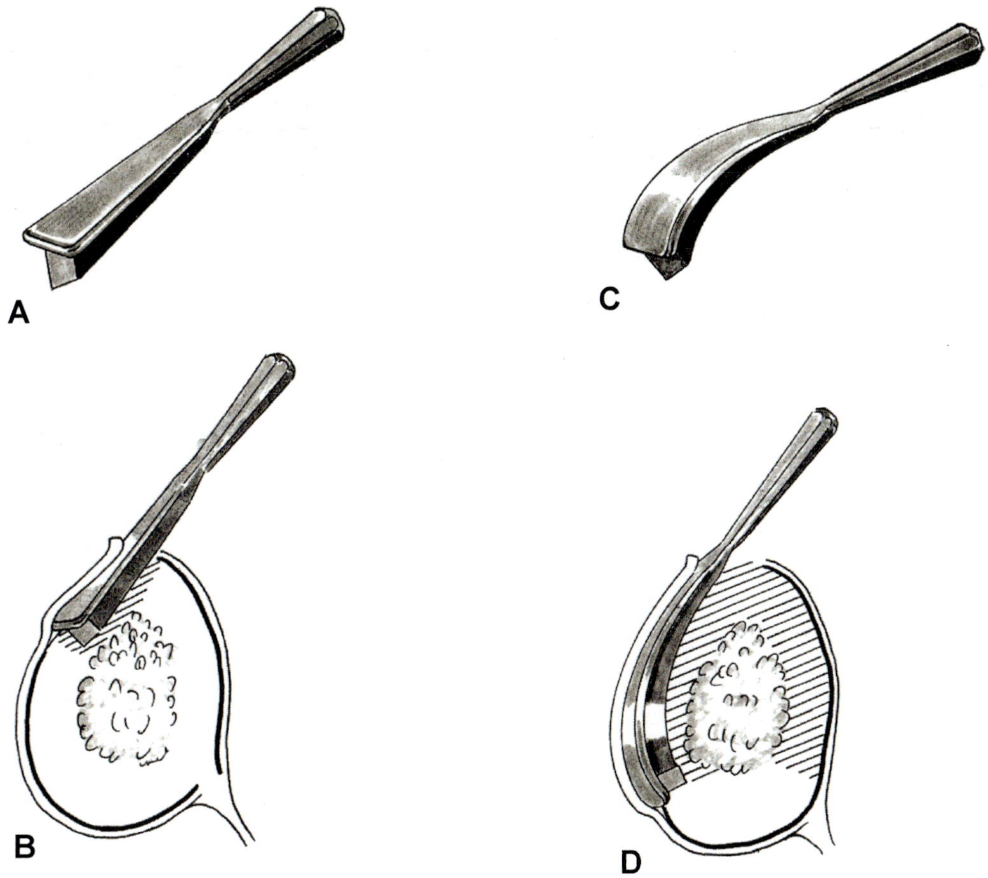

Figure 12.12: Use of the osteotome (corticotome) for corticotomy. A, straight corticotome with T-shaped blade. B, cross-section of tibial bone. Introduced into the bone cleave, the straight corticotome cuts the compact bone wall, thereby preventing periosteum damage and securing penetration into the bone marrow canal. C, curved corticotome with a T-shaped blade. D, cross-section of tibial bone. Introduced deep into the bone cleave, the curved corticotome cuts the corner at the posterior bone wall, preventing periosteum damage and securing penetration into the bone marrow canal

12. The osteotome is removed, and careful rotational movement must be performed by distal ring rotation (after fibular osteotomy, in the case of the leg). If there is a risk of nearby nerve damage, the rotation is performed toward the opposite side. For example, with the corticotomy at the proximal tibia the peroneal nerve can be damaged with internal rotation; thus only external rotation has to be performed (Fig. 12.13).
13. With the disconnection of the two rings and rotational movement, it is easy to displace the bone fragment alignment at the site of corticotomy. Any displacement at this level can produce damage to the bone marrow with its vessels and periosteal arterioles. This will be reflected in bone regeneration, bringing about its delay or hypoplastic formation. To prevent this the surgeon must hold these rings firmly with two hands at the moment of their disconnection (Fig. 12.14), and continue to hold them up to the moment when they are reconnected at a minimum of two or three points. Attention also must be paid to the ring levels and the correspondence of the holes.

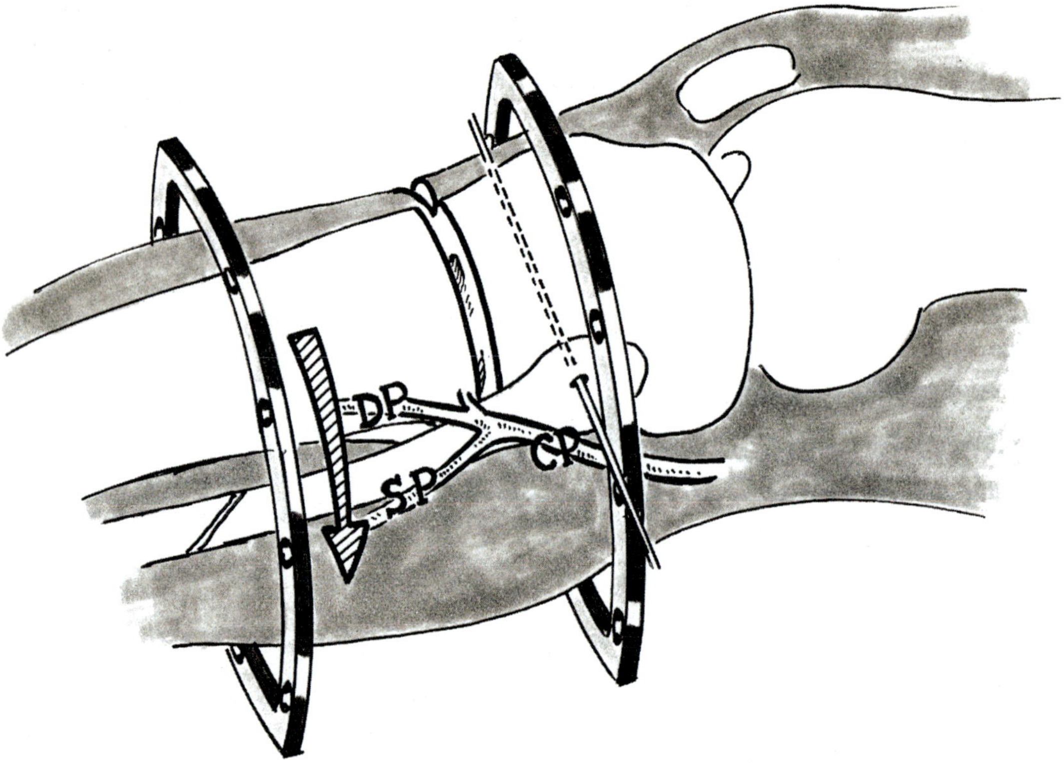

Figure 12.13: Partial view of the proximal tibia after corticotomy. CP = common peroneal nerve, DP = deep peroneal nerve, SP = superficial peroneal nerve. *Arrow* shows direction of external rotation of a distal ring. At the proximal ring the wire transfixes the head of the fibular and tibial metaepiphyses

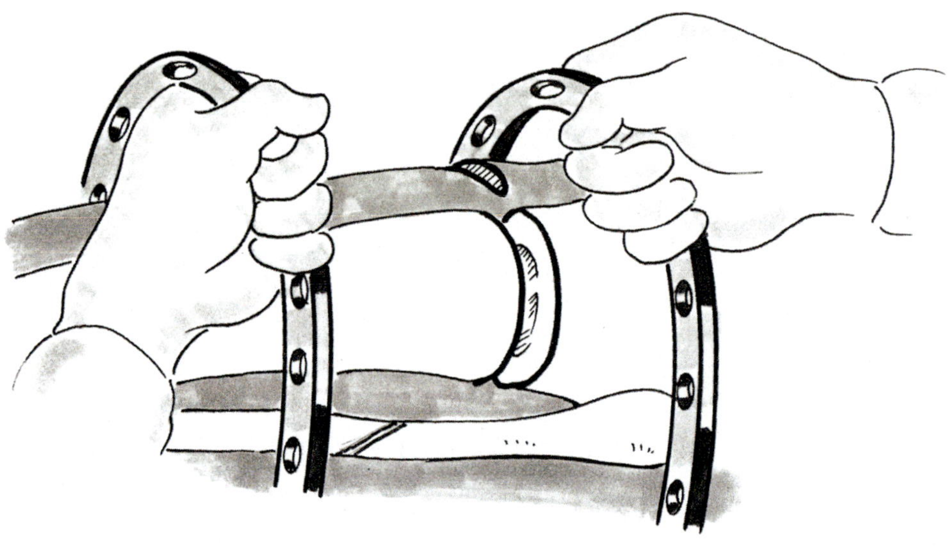

Figure 12.14: Partial view at the corticotomy site. To prevent corticotomized bone displacement, the rings above and below the corticotomy must be held firmly in place until the rings are reconnected completely

14. Because it still is easy to overlook some displacement, it is recommended that bone alignment be examined by introducing a fingertip into the skin incision. As the surgeon continues to hold the rings, the assistant feels the fragment correlation and suggests how to correct it. It is also useful to check the alignment correction by introducing a threaded rod in the corresponding holes of the rings. Proper alignment of the rod helps to orient the bone fragments (Fig. 12.15).

15. Regardless of confirmation of completion of the corticotomy, there always is the chance that it is not complete. This is because it is difficult to succeed in achieving a transverse cut of the posterior bone wall. In some cases a wedge-shaped crack occurs. It allows some movement at the site of corticotomy, and this can confuse the surgeon (Fig. 12.16). Thus radiographic imaging on the operating table is necessary before the wound is closed. Two views should be

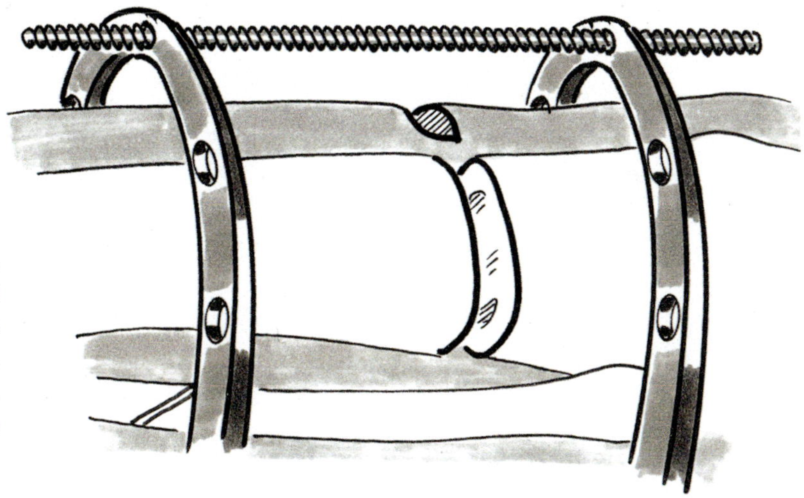

Figure 12.15: Partial view at the corticotomy site. To confirm correct alignment of the corticotomized bone, a threaded rod is introduced in the corresponding holes of the rings above and below. If the rod lines up with corresponding ring holes, the alignment is correct and will help to orient the bone fragments

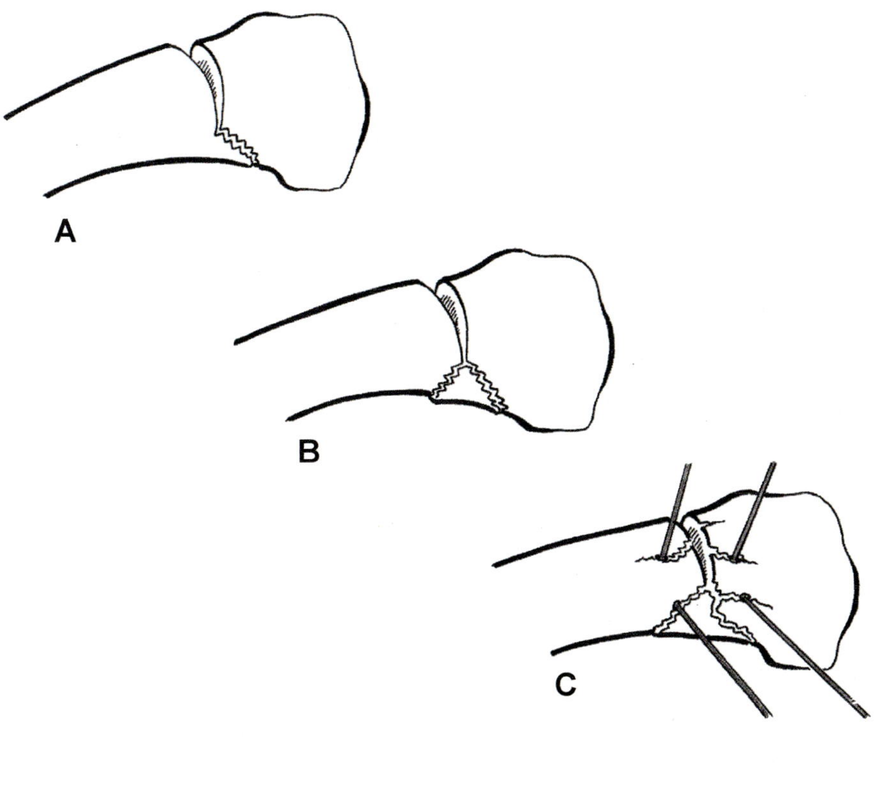

Figure 12.16: Three identical views of the proximal tibia after incomplete corticotomy, which can prevent distraction. A, oblique fracture of the posterior upper tibia at the site of thick soleal line. B, butterfly-type fracture of the posterior upper tibia. C, comminuted fracture, which extends to the sites of wires introduced too closely

obtained: anteroposterior and lateral. To view the corticotomy gap better, it is recommended that approximately 5-mm distraction be produced before the radiograph is obtained.

16. The wound is closed only after the surgeon is convinced that the cut through the compact bone is complete. Usually two or three 3-0 nylon sutures are adequate for closure. Some skin laceration may result while the direction and angulation of the osteotome are changed. Such laceration must be avoided by retracting the wound edges with the rakes.
17. Minimal distraction must be maintained for several days before further distraction is started. This gap of 2 to 3 mm cannot damage the vascular net. On the contrary, it contributes to the initiation of local tissue rebuilding. It stays filled with a hematoma, necessary for early development of microblood lacunae. These lacunae are the blood pools and precursors of the new vessels, appearing as early as the third to fifth day. This is exactly the time to start distraction, which brings about tension forces on the walls of the newly formed vessels. And from this regeneration begins.

LEVEL OF CORTICOTOMY

In choosing the corticotomy level, anatomic, biomechanical, and physiologic factors must be considered.

Anatomically, it is important not to cut the nutrient vessels. The entrance canal usually is located in a middle part of a tubular bone. Avoidance of the bone transection in its center is a wise precaution.

The anatomic texture of the bone segment chosen for corticotomy is also important. The most suitable segment is the relatively thin compact layer, situated at the level of the transition of the medullary cavity into trabecular bone. There is much less probability of the bone vascular net cutoff there.

Biomechanically, it is important to consider the proximity of the bone cut to a joint. In no case can the corticotomy interfere with its motion. Because the bone segment must be large enough to accommodate a supporting ring or two rings situated between the joint and bone transection, the estimated distance must be at least 6 to 7 cm.

Physiologically, it is important to evaluate the condition of the local tissues at the segment of planned corticotomy. Scars from previous injuries, infection, or surgery will interfere with osteogenesis. Bone structure changes (e.g. zones of sclerosis, porosis, or cyst formation) also can delay or prevent bone regeneration. Therefore the surgeon must evaluate carefully preoperative roentgenograms and sometimes must request preoperative angiograms, bone scans, and computed tomography, if necessary.

The metaepiphyseal segments of the bone are the most suitable levels for corticotomy (Fig. 12.17).

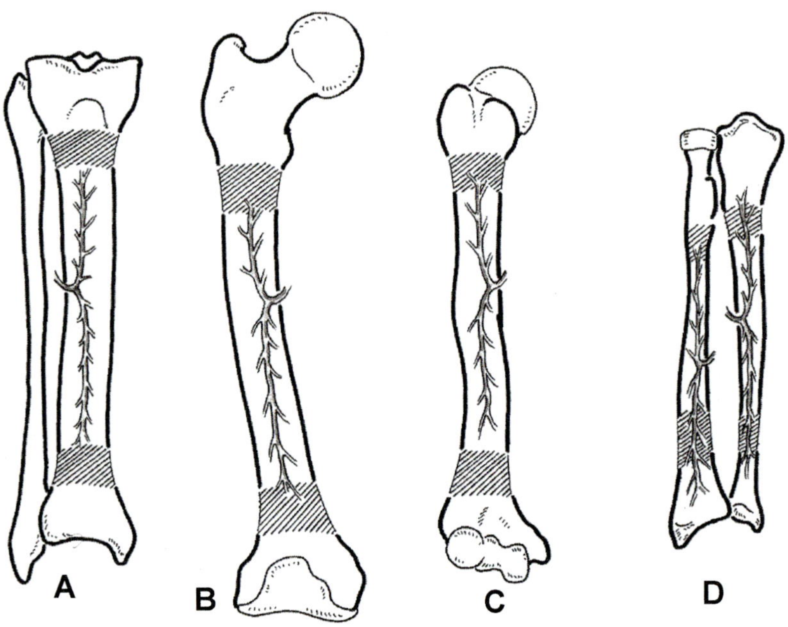

Figure 12.17: Metaepiphyseal zones *(shaded)* of the long tubular bones, which are the most suitable levels for corticotomy. Projection of the nutrient vessels is shown. **A,** proximal and distal tibia. **B,** proximal and distal femur. **C,** proximal and distal humerus. **D,** proximal and distal ulna and radius

MONOFOCAL AND BIFOCAL CORTICOTOMY

Depending on the goal of treatment in a particular patient, the corticotomy can be performed at one level (monofocal) or two levels (bifocal) on the same bone. Simultaneously cutting and lengthening a bone at two levels substantially reduces the duration of treatment.

In general, the monofocal corticotomy is indicated for (1) lengthening up to 5 cm; (2) bone fragment transportation up to 5 to 7 cm; (3) stimulation of local blood circulation in the limb without significant lengthening but generation of osteogenesis (e.g. in pseudoarthrosis or nonunion); (4) gradual correction of bone deformity.

The bifocal corticotomy is indicated for: (1) lengthening up to 10 to 12 cm; (2) bone fragment transportation up to 10 to 16 cm by shifting them toward each other; (3) simultaneous lengthening at one level and correction of deformity at another level; (4) stimulation of osteogenesis in metabolic disorders (e.g. Paget disease, osteogenesis imperfecta, Ollier disease).

RADIAL BONE CUT AND FIBULA RESECTION

If corticotomy is to be performed on one of the two bones in a limb (e.g. forearm or lower leg), a second bone cut is necessary for lengthening and correction. For the forearm this second bone in most of the cases is the radius. Ulnar ray defects frequently are associated with malformation of the radial ray, as for example in congenital radial pseudoarthrosis, radial deviation of the hand, and Madelung deformity. The level of the second bone cut must be chosen with consideration of the segment of interosseous membrane between the two cuts: the bigger it is the more force has to be applied to control bone alignment during lengthening or correction (Fig. 12.18).

In most cases the Ilizarov procedure is performed on the lower leg. The fibular osteotomy must precede tibial corticotomy, because otherwise it would be impossible to test tibial rotation.

Three anatomic areas are important to avoid in choosing the level of fibular cut: the tibiofibular joint, with the closely situated common peroneal nerve; the

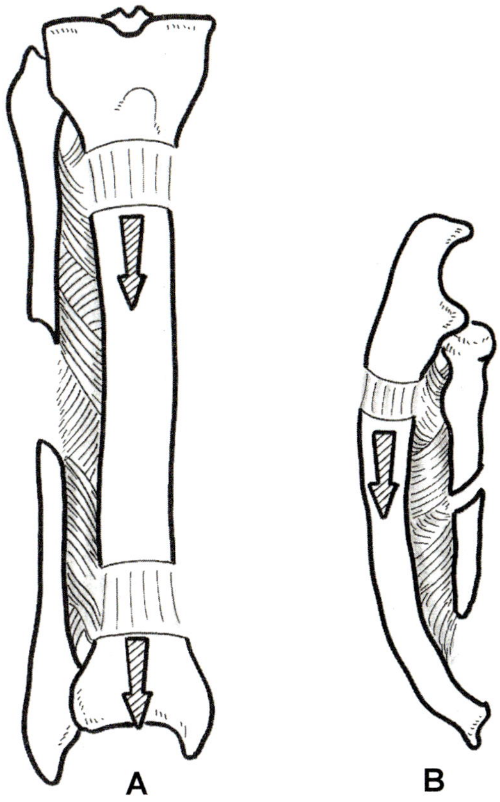

Figure 12.18: Level of the second bone cut in corticotomy of the tibia and ulna. *Arrows* indicate direction of distraction. A, 1- to l.5-cm resection is recommended at the middle part of the fibula. B, osteotomy of the middle part of the radius

tibiofibular syndesmosis; and the interosseous membrane. This cut should never be made too close to the bone ends, because it can interfere with joint function.

The leg interosseous membrane is a strong structure to which the anterior and posterior tibialis muscles are partially attached. It keeps both bones parallel to each other, which is important during lengthening. The fibula can be considered a natural splint for the tibia. This has practical meaning in tibial lengthening. Regardless of the level of monofocal or bifocal corticotomy, the fibula must be cut at a different level than the tibia to prevent tibial deviation. The recommended level for osteotomy of the fibula is in the middle part of its slender body (see Fig. 12.18A).

It is always expedient to perform fibular segmental resection rather than simple osteotomy. A cut of 0.5 to 1 cm guarantees necessary shifting of the fibula. It also prevents the possibility of premature fibular healing.

CORTICOTOMY OR OSTEOTOMY FOR PARTIAL BONE DEFECT REPLACEMENT

To overcome partial segmental bone loss combined with nonunion, Ilizarov introduced the technique of forming a split-off fragment that is shifted gradually to cover the defect. This is supposed to induce local osteogenesis and fill up the defect and nonunion itself. The compact bone is cut in the oblique rather than the transverse direction, through just one cortex. In this case, preservation of only the periosteal arterioles is possible. The chipped-off fragment must be large enough to make a ceiling-like covering.

Before making the periosteal incision, one or two olive wires are introduced in the oblique direction. Careful planning must precede their introduction so that the chipped-off fragment may be brought down to the desired site.

The compact bone cut is performed with the narrow osteotome in an angled position. It is preferable to try to do it subperiosteally (Fig. 12.19).

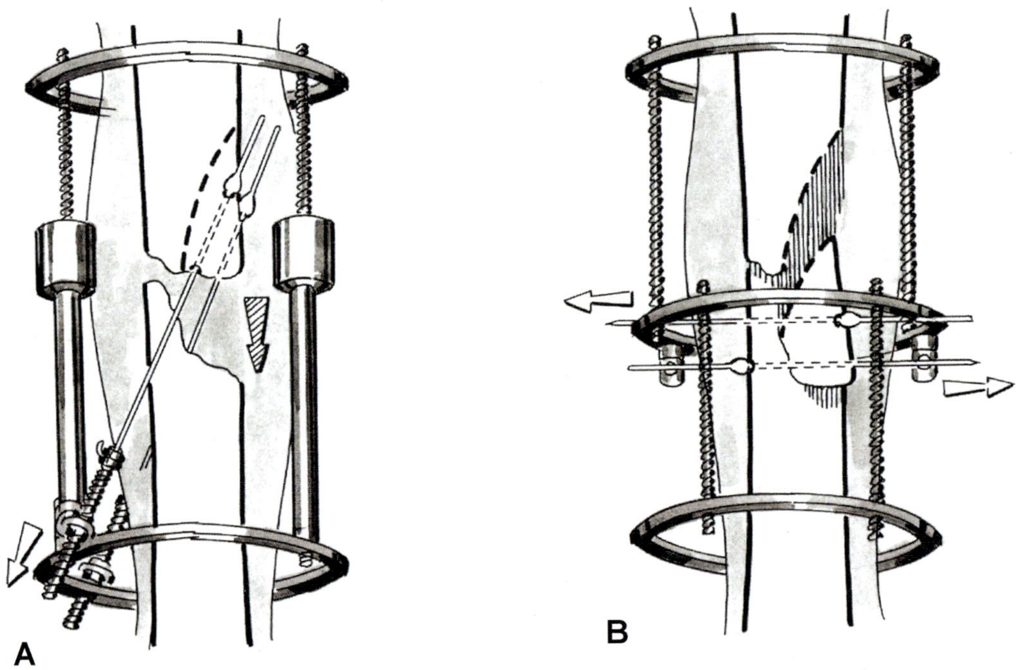

Figure 12.19: Split-off osteotomy technique for correction of a partial segmental defect. **A,** two oblique pulling wires with olive stoppers are introduced into the proximal fragment. Osteotomy is shown by the *interrupted line. Shaded arrow* indicates shifting of the osteotomized segment; *white arrow* indicates direction of forces that transport the free fragments. **B,** same split-off segment after gradual shifting is transfixed to the distal fragment by transverse wires with two stoppers. *Shaded segments* represent bone defect filled with regenerated tissue and zones of nonunion healing. *Arrows* show direction of bone fragment transport via the olive wires

S-SHAPED OSTEOTOMY FOR PURULENT OSTEOMYELITIC CAVITIES

To eliminate purulent osteomyelitic cavities at any site of bone, Ilizarov developed a technique of transectional osteotomy through the cavitary region. Because there usually are many connected and isolated cavities, the osteotome must be directed so as to open all of them. To achieve this, the cut usually is made in the shape of an S (Fig. 12.20).

This transection does not require careful preservation of local blood vessels because there are none. What it predisposes to is a dramatic change in the local metabolic environment. The use of apparatus to generate tension at the site of the S-shaped osteotomy brings about development of new vessels and stimulates osteogenesis.

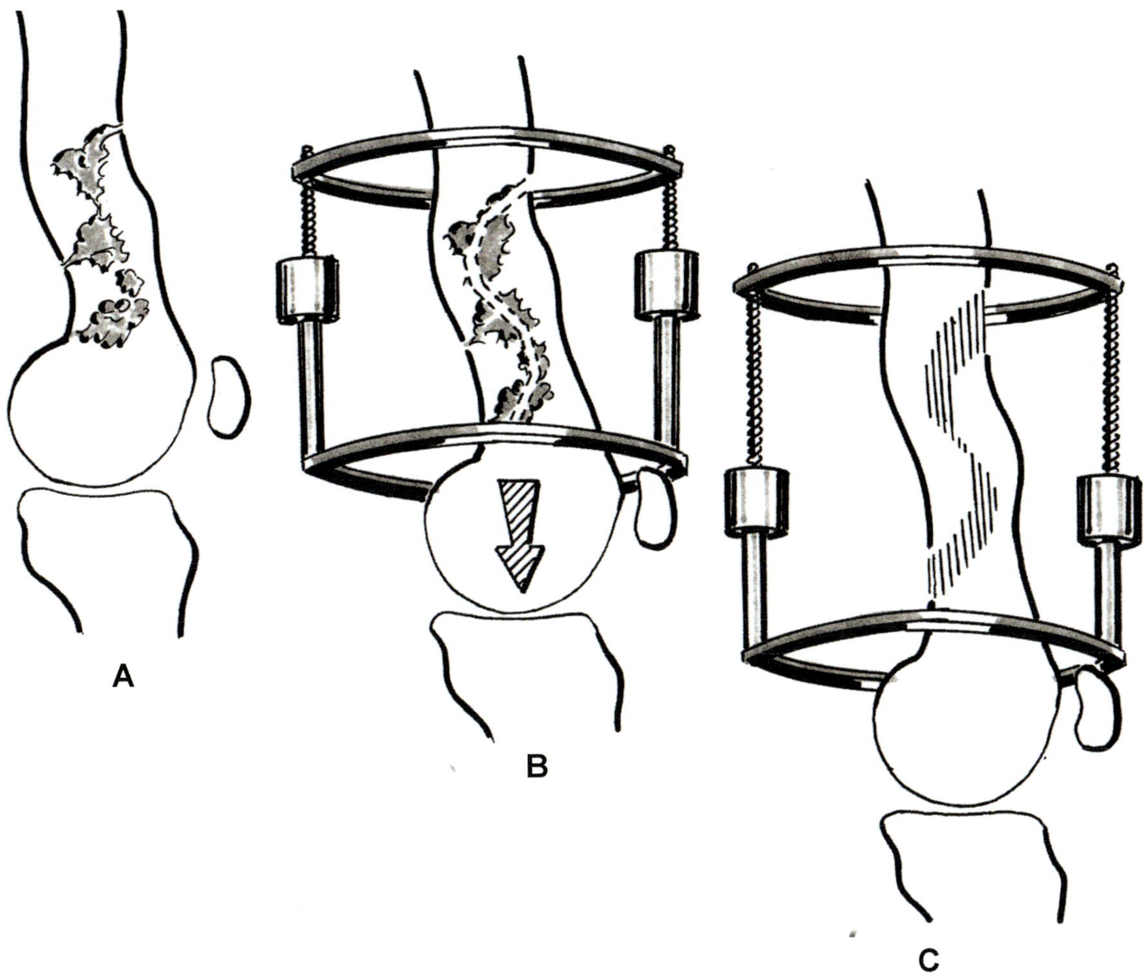

Figure 12.20: Distal femoral segment with osteomyelitic cavities, and frame applied. A, note purulent cavities. B, *interrupted line* represents S-shaped osteotomy. *Shaded arrow* shows direction of distraction. C, healed cavities (shaded area)

CORTICOTOMY FOR TRANSVERSE SHIFTING AND BONE WIDENING

If transverse tension is applied to the intraosseous membrane between the tibia and fibula with its longitudinal splitting and subsequent medial traction, it can stimulate osteogenesis and neovascularization. With this technique it is possible to reinforce and thicken the tibia or to repair a defect (Fig. 12.21).

The longitudinal splitting of the lateral side of the tibia with distraction can be used for thin limb widening (reshaping). This is also indicated for revascularization in circulatory limb disorders (e.g. endarteritis obliterans, Buerger disease) and for closure of trophic ulcers of any cause.

The technique of longitudinal bone splitting is as follows (Fig. 12.22):

1. Three or four small (1 cm) periosteal incisions are placed on the posterolateral fibular surface, all in a straight line.
2. A corresponding number of wires with olive stoppers are drilled transversely through these incisions in the direction of planned traction. The stoppers are set against bone, and the wires cut off just behind them.
3. Several drill holes are introduced into the bone, arranged in a straight line below the level of the wires.
4. Transverse cuts of the anteromedial half of bone cross-section are made with an osteotome, above and below, forming the proximal and distal ends of the fragment.

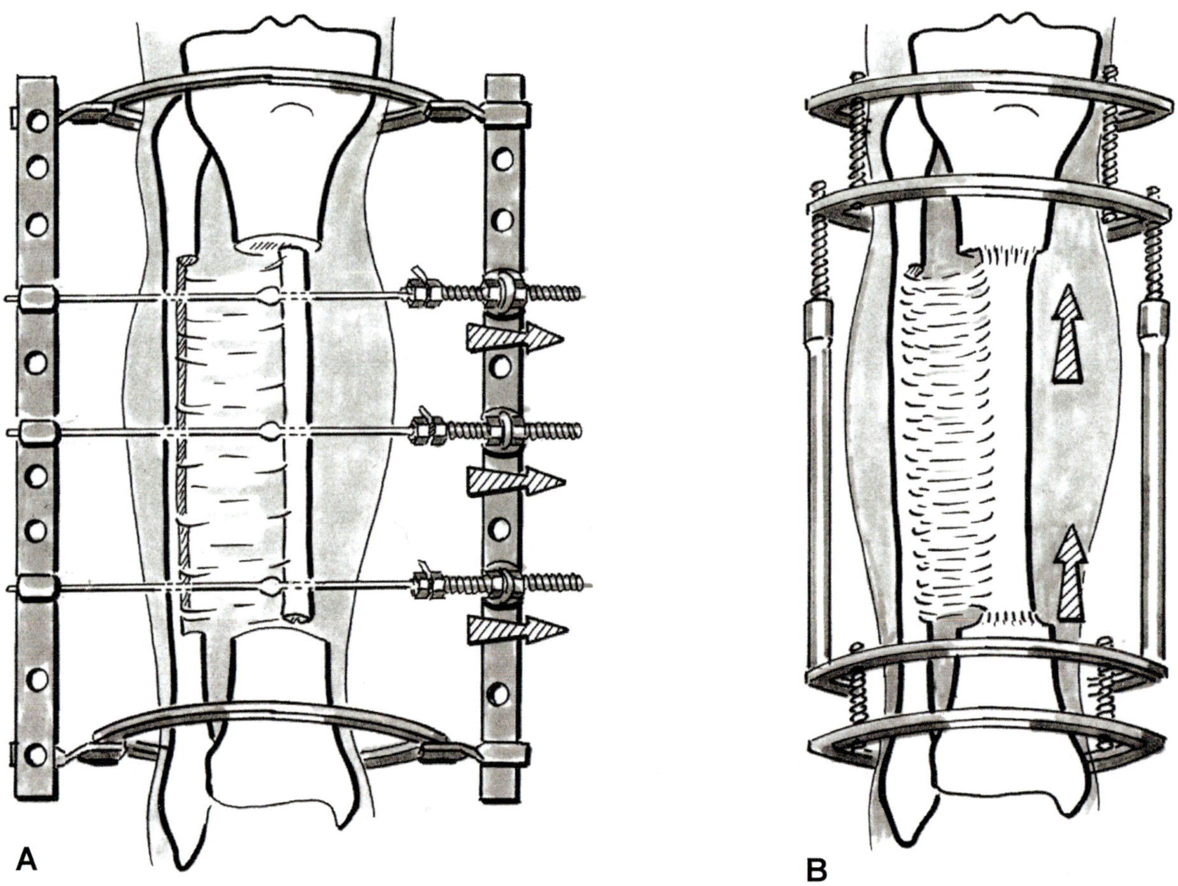

Figure 12.21: Osteotomy technique for transverse bone shifting in a tibial diaphyseal defect. A, tibial defect is being replaced by the transverse shifting of longitudinally split fibular segment. *Arrows* show direction of shift. Two-ring frame is reinforced with two long connecting plates. B, transverse shifting is accomplished. Frame is reinforced by two additional rings replacing the plates. Compression direction is shown by *arrows*

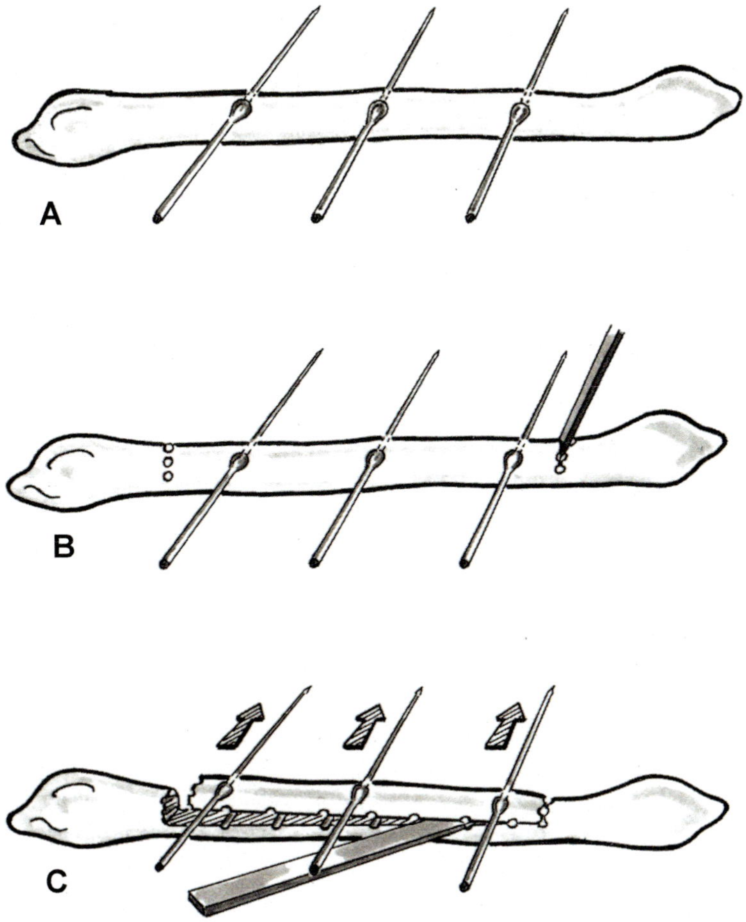

Figure 12.22: Technique of longitudinal fibular splitting for transverse shifting. A, three wires with olive stoppers are introduced into the fibula. B, two transverse cross sectional cuts are made above and below the wires. C, with longitudinal osteotomy performed between the drilled holes, the split-off fibular fragment is prepared for transverse shifting. *Arrows* indicate direction of transverse distraction

5. Several drill holes are made longitudinally. Careful bone cutting is done in a longitudinal direction, moving the narrow osteotome from one drill hole to another.
6. After completing this cut under direct visualization, the split-off fragment is prepared for gradual distraction in the transverse direction.

Typical mistakes that occur with the corticotomy technique include:

1. Skin incision too large.
2. Periosteal separation at the site of initial bone cut and around the bone.
3. Use of an oversized osteotome.
4. Poor choice of level of corticotomy.
5. Destructive hammering of the compact bone.
6. Direct cut through bone marrow canal.
7. Induction of the bone cut into the nearby wire tract.
8. Injury of the nearby magistral vessels and nerves.
9. Performance of the twisting osteotome maneuver before cuts are completed through medial and lateral bone walls.
10. Loss of fragment alignment.

Any of these mistakes can complicate bone regeneration.

13 Chapter

Hinges

The Ilizarov fixator is a very versatile device; unlike other fixators it can be used to treat virtually any type of deformity. This is achieved through the use of hinges between the rings, which secure and establish angulation essential for correction of the deformity. Subsequently, the hinges are used as pivotal (rotation) point components for the necessary straightening.

The positioning, orientation, and number of hinges are critical factors for deformity correction. Used in combination with distraction-compression devices (graduated telescopic rods), the hinges make it possible gradually to correct deformities, with simultaneous transformation of the bone and soft tissues. For example, hinges can promote straightening of an angulated nonunion with concurrent compression. The hinges also can help to achieve skin stretching, neovascularization, and softening of a scarred area, thus influencing the local tissue orientation as a result of the tensionstress during correction of the deformity.

The advantages of using hinges are as follows:

1. They constrain motion in a specific plane or planes.
2. They provide a specific fulcrum for calculation of and control of specific correction of angulation or displacement.
3. They provide biologic adaptation of tissues to new desired positioning.

For the hinges to be effective there must be sufficient gap created at the level of bone distraction, and wires with olive stoppers (or any kind of stopper) should be used to control and stabilize the bone(s). In rare cases, such as in children and in patients with bone diseases (e.g. osteoporosis, Paget's disease, osteogenesis imperfecta), bone straightening can be achieved even without creation of a distractional gap. If plain wires without stoppers are used as fulcrums, they must cross the bone perpendicularly at 90 degrees to prevent displacement.

There are several different ways to configure Ilizarov hinges, which are assembled easily from standard parts (Fig. 13.1):

1. Two female half-hinges connected to the threaded rods.
2. One male half-hinge and one female (the male half-hinge must be attached to the ring or connecting plate).
3. Two supports connected to each other.
4. Two posts connected to each other.
5. One support and one post connected to each other.
6. Two plates connected to each other.
7. The plate with the support or the post connection.
8. The combined two-axis hinge.

These hinges are described in chapters 8, 9, and 10. The common feature of all the hinge configurations is that they have a connecting bolt as the axis of rotation.

The bolt is fixed by the lock nut with the nylon insert or with two thin half-nuts tightened to each other. These nuts must secure the connected parts but not be so tight as to prevent their free rotation or motion.

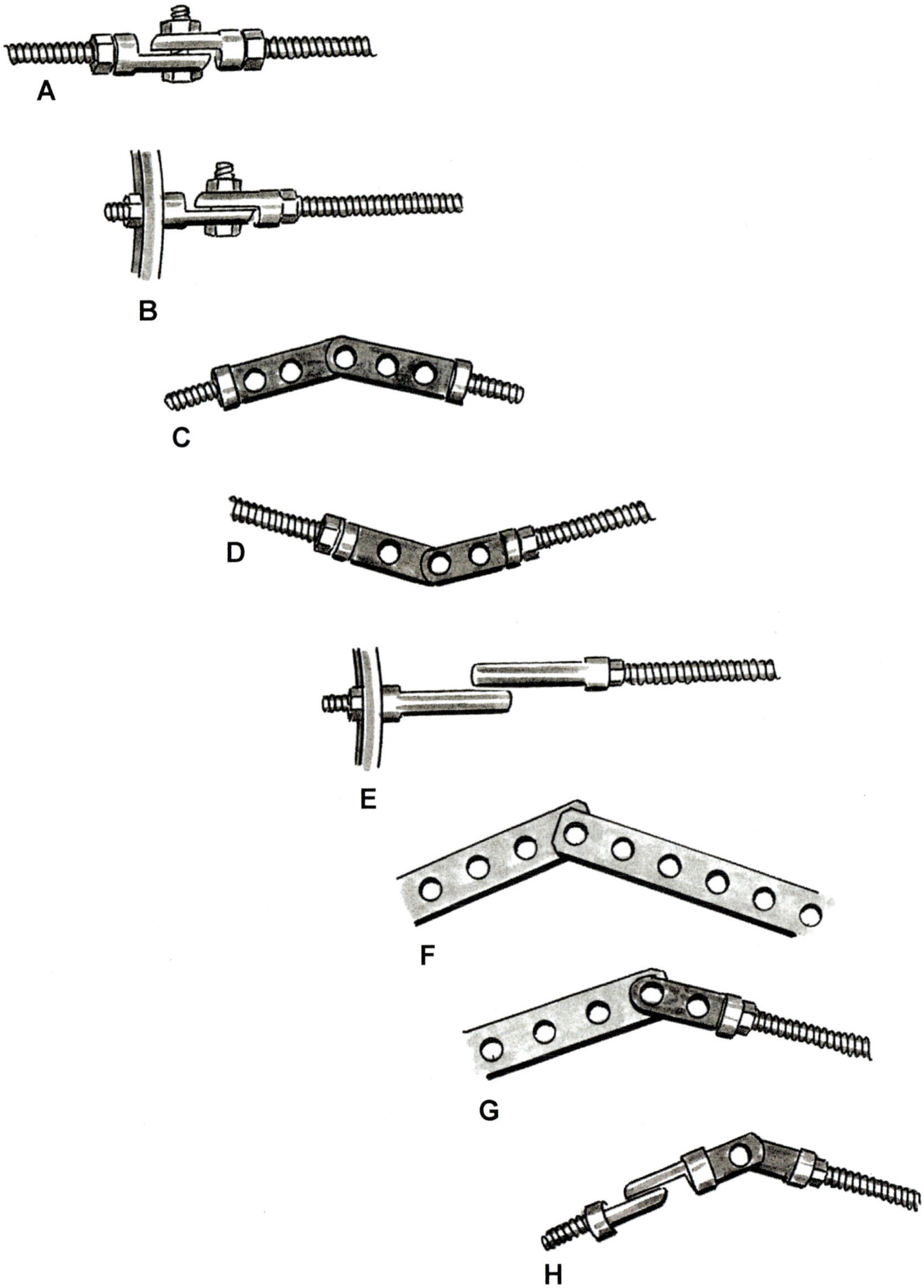

Figure 13.1: Various hinges. A, two female half-hinges. B, one male half-hinge and one female half-hinge. C, two supports. D, two posts. E, one support with one post. F, two plates. G, one plate with one support or post. H, combined two-axis hinge with two half-hinges

The location of distraction-compression devices in relation to the hinges depends on the planned straightening; they can be placed at the concave or convex side of deformity. It is advisable to use two devices, thereby distributing the forces evenly.

POSITIONING OF HINGES

In planning to use the hinges with the frame, their exact position has to be calculated. The best way to do this is to transfer the bone positions (from the roentgenogram) to paper and draw in the location of the hinges. This must be done in two planes: frontal (anteroposterior) and sagittal (lateromedial).

Depending on the type of deformity, the dominant plane for correction of recurvation and antecurvation deformities is the sagittal plane; for valgus and varus deformities the frontal plane; for combined deformities the plane with the most evident and functionally important curvature (Fig. 13.2).

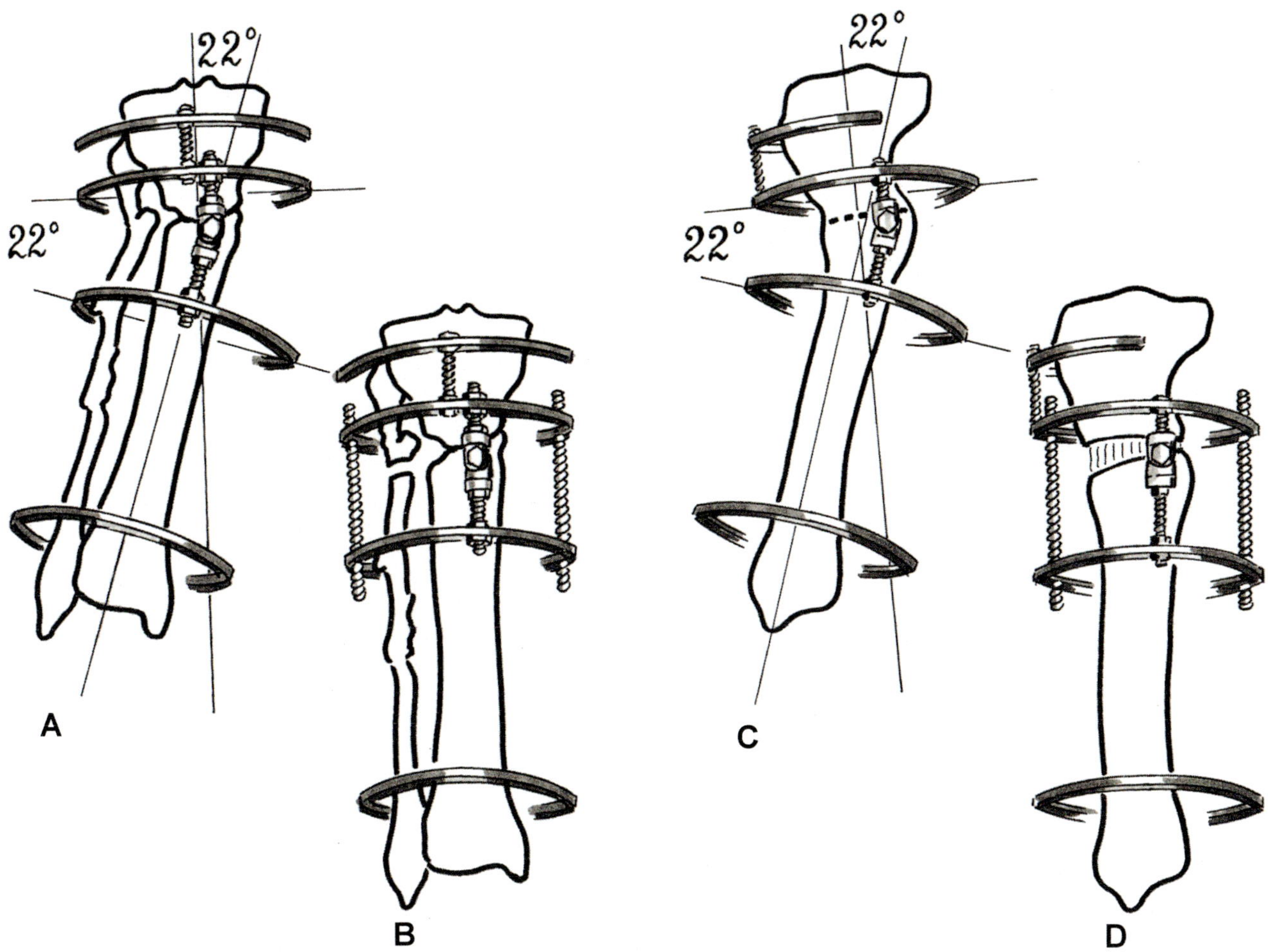

Figure 13.2: Positioning of the rings with the attached hinges. A, in tibial valgus deformity of 22 degrees with nonunion, the rings near the curve are positioned perpendicular to the axes of the proximal and distal fragments and at the angle of 22 degrees to each other. The hinge angle is equal to the deformity angulation. B, after hinge straightening the rings are parallel to each other. This position is the most suitable for introducing the ring connectors, and is very stable. C, in tibial recurvation deformity of 22 degrees the rings near the curve are positioned perpendicular to the axes of the proximal and distal fragments and at an angle of 22 degrees to each other. The hinge angle is equal to the deformity angulation. *Interrupted line* represents corticotomy level. D, after hinge straightening the rings are parallel to each other. This position is the most suitable for introducing ring connectors, and is very secure

Several important parameters must be considered in hinge positioning:

1. Two rings to which hinges are attached must be strictly perpendicular to their bone fragments; they must either start perpendicularly and end angulated, or vice versa. This predetermines further straightening and secures the corrected fragments (Fig. 13.2).
2. Two hinges located at the opposite sides of deformity usually are required for stability (Fig. 13.3).
3. The hinge rotation axis must be situated on the horizontal level of the deformity apex. If two hinges are used, both must be on that level (Fig. 13.4).
4. It is critically important that hinges of the same plane are oriented along the same plane as the deformity (Fig. 13.5).

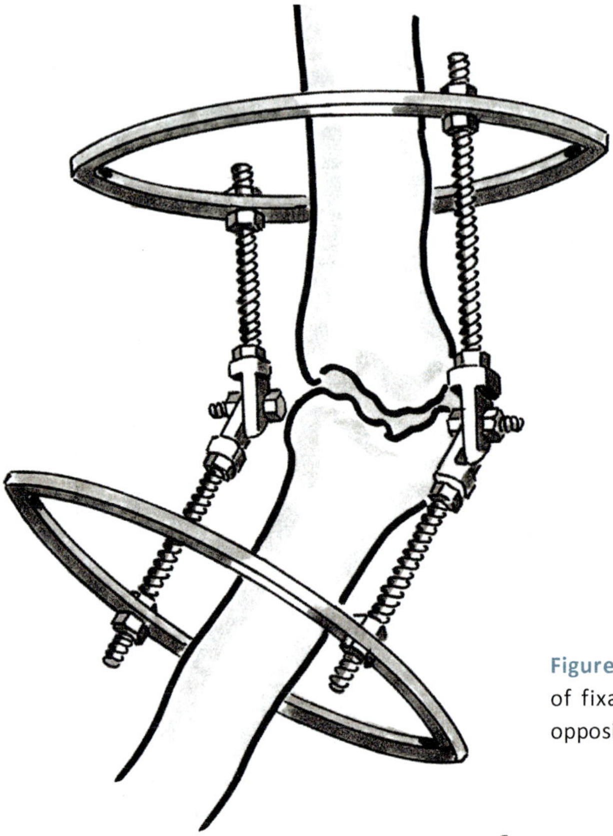

Figure 13.3: Hypertrophic pseudoarthrosis with angulation. For stability of fixation during gradual straightening, two hinges are introduced at opposite sides of the deformity

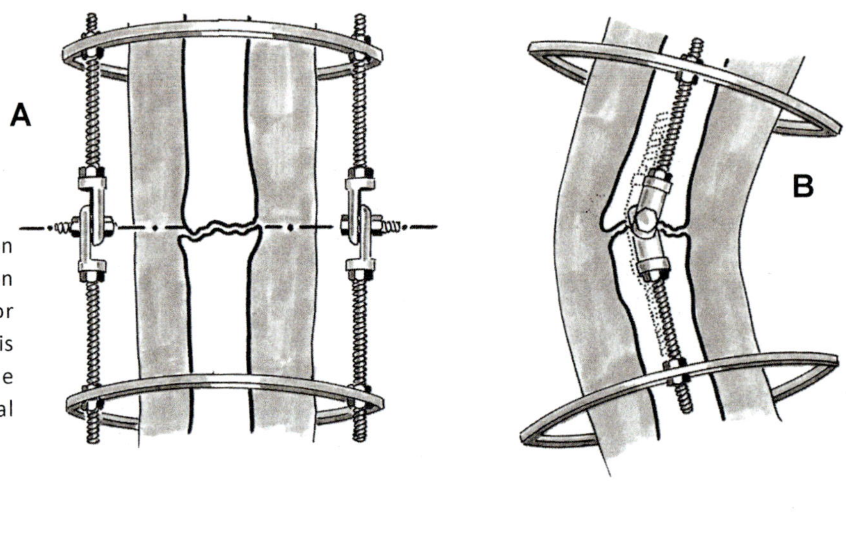

Figure 13.4: Positioning of the hinge rotation axis at the level of nonunion, with angulation deformity. A, frontal plane (anteroposterior view). The rotation axis of the two hinges is situated on the horizontal level of the deformity apex *(interrupted line)*. B, sagittal plane (lateral view)

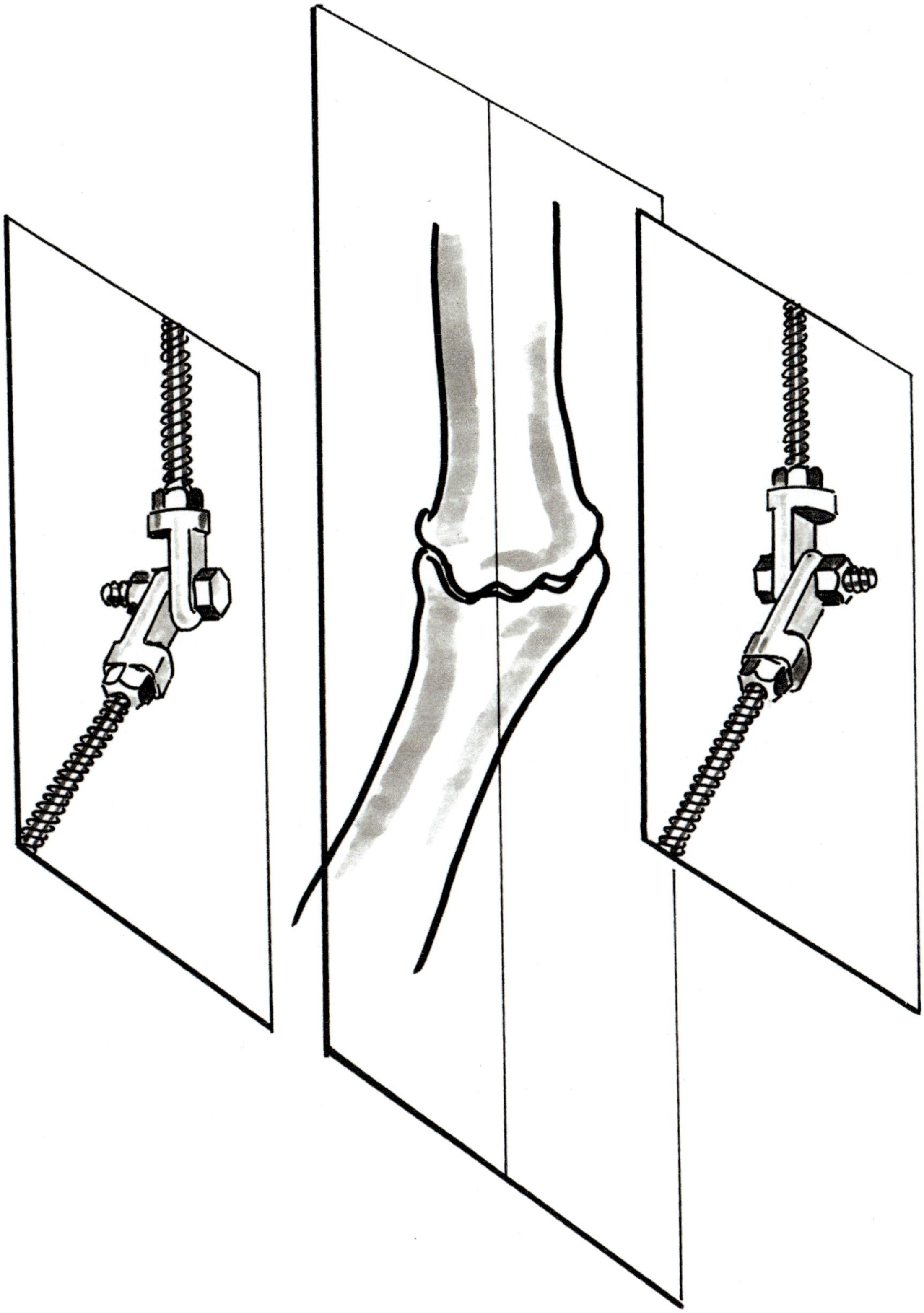

Figure 13.5: Hypertrophic nonunion with angulation deformity is shown in the sagittal plane. The two hinges situated on the level of the deformity apex also are oriented along the same sagittal plane

5. Movement of the axis of rotation of hinges to the concave or convex sides of a deformity produces corresponding compression or distraction of the fragments (Fig. 13.6).
6. The positioning of the hinges can be used to achieve different types of deformity correction, such as opening wedge, distraction, compression, translation, and derotation (Fig. 13.7).

If there is a gap between the angulated bone fragments it is always necessary to first correct the angulation, and then to apply compression or compression-distraction forces to the straightened fragments. This prevents slipping of the fragments, and prepares skin and soft tissue scars for transformation by influencing their neovascularization.

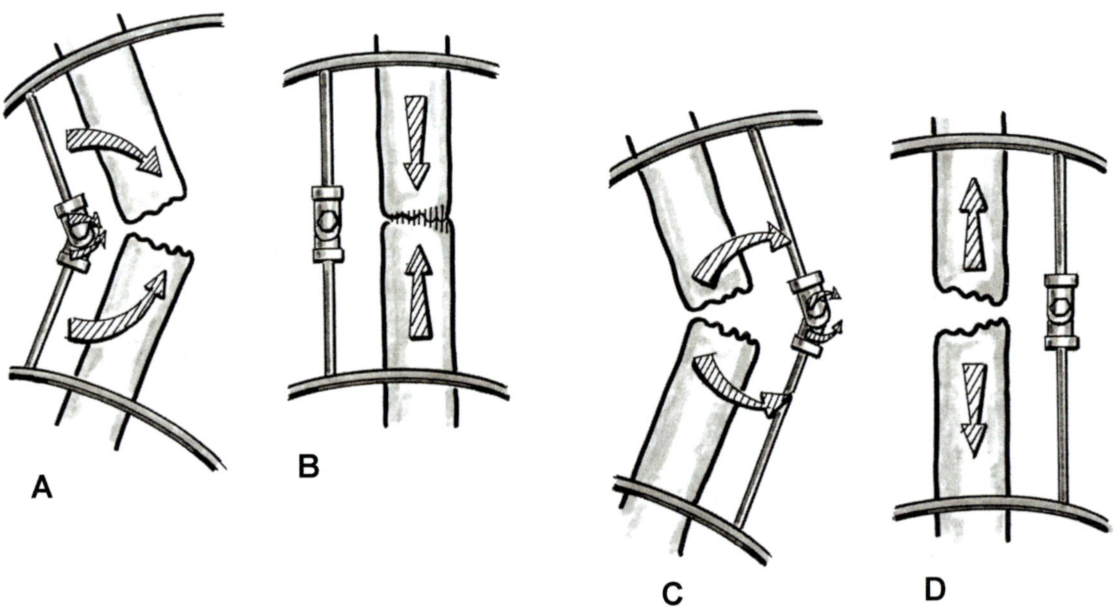

Figure 13.6: Effect of the hinge position on bone fragment movement. Section of the frame with hinge and bone nonunion is shown before and after correction. *Small curved arrows* indicate direction of hinge straightening; *large curved arrows* indicate direction of subsequent bone fragment movement during straightening; *straight arrows* indicate direction of the effective compression or distraction produced with straightening. **A,** hinge is situated at the concave side of the deformity. **B,** after straightening there is a compression effect *(shaded area)*. **C,** hinge is situated at the convex side of the deformity. **D,** after straightening there is a distraction effect

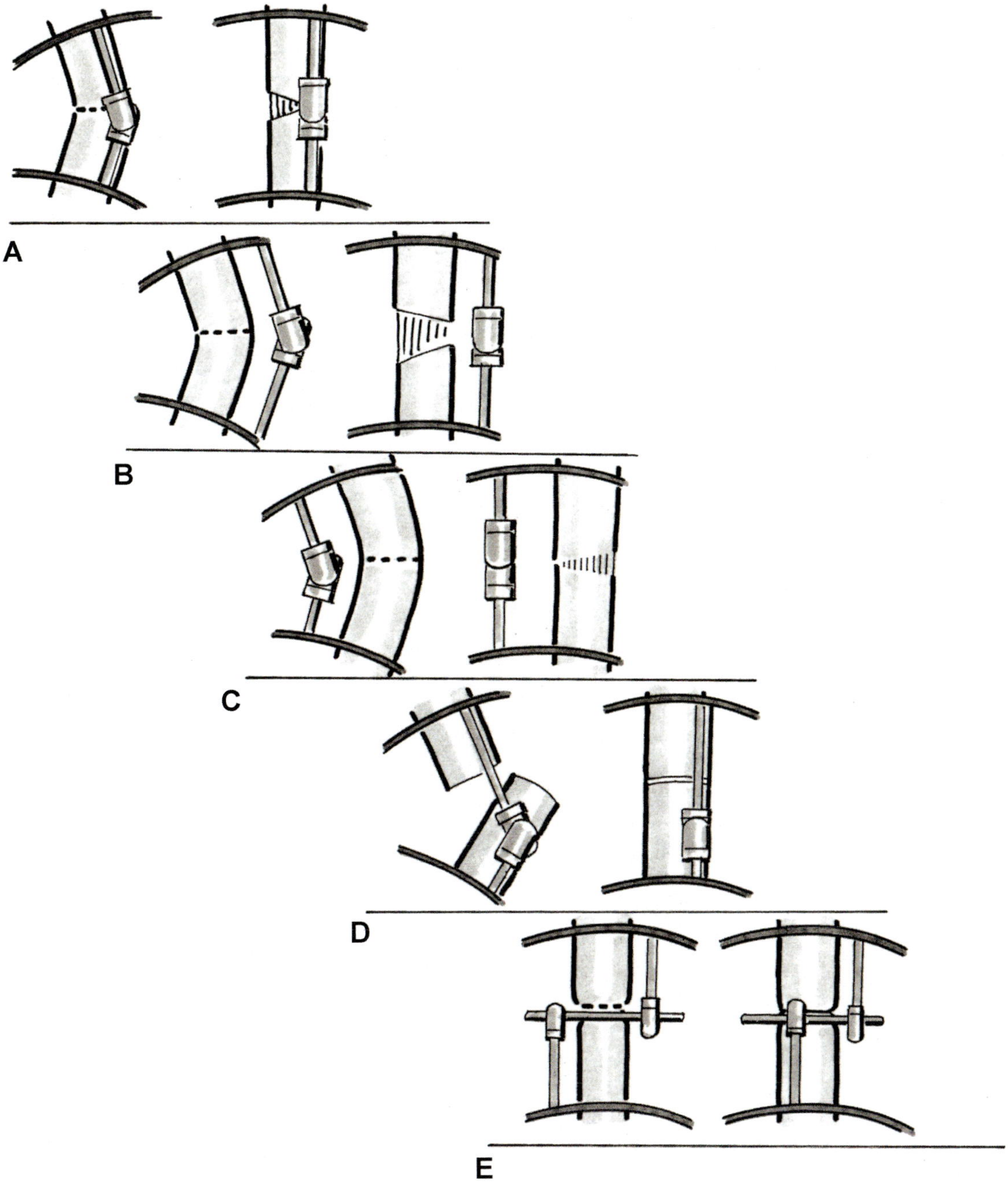

Figure 13.7: Different types of deformity correction achieved with various hinge positions. Schematic representation of the frame segment with two rings and the hinge shown before and after deformity correction. *Interrupted lines* indicate the site of osteotomy. A, with the hinge positioned at the edge of the convex side of the deformity the opening wedge type of correction is produced. B, with the hinge positioned at some distance out from the convex side of the deformity the distraction type correction is produced. C, with the hinge positioned at the edge or outside of the concave side of the deformity the compression type correction is produced *(shaded area)*. D, with the hinge positioned outside the level of the deformity apex the translation type of correction is produced. E, the derotation type of correction is produced without the use of hinges but with the help of connected half-hinges

OPENING WEDGE HINGE

The characteristic of this hinge is that the location of its rotation axis is situated on the concave side of the deformed bone. Because the majority of deformities require only straightening, this is the most common type of hinge. Practically speaking, it is difficult to determine how much the axis of rotation can be shifted within a relatively narrow bone contour. There are three possible positions for this hinge (Fig. 13.8):

1. The axis of rotation is on the projection of the bone wall at the concave side of deformity. Straightening with the opening wedge hinge produces a small opening at the concave side accompanied by compression of the bone at the convex side. This hinge is indicated chiefly in cases with osteoporotic bone fragments (in a hypotrophic type of nonunion) (Fig. 13.8B)
2. The axis of rotation is on the projection of the center of the bone contour. Straightening with this hinge creates the same opening at the concave side accompanied by a small amount of fragment compression at the convex side. This hinge configuration is indicated mainly in cases with normal bone structure (in a normotrophic type of nonunion) (Fig. 13.8C).

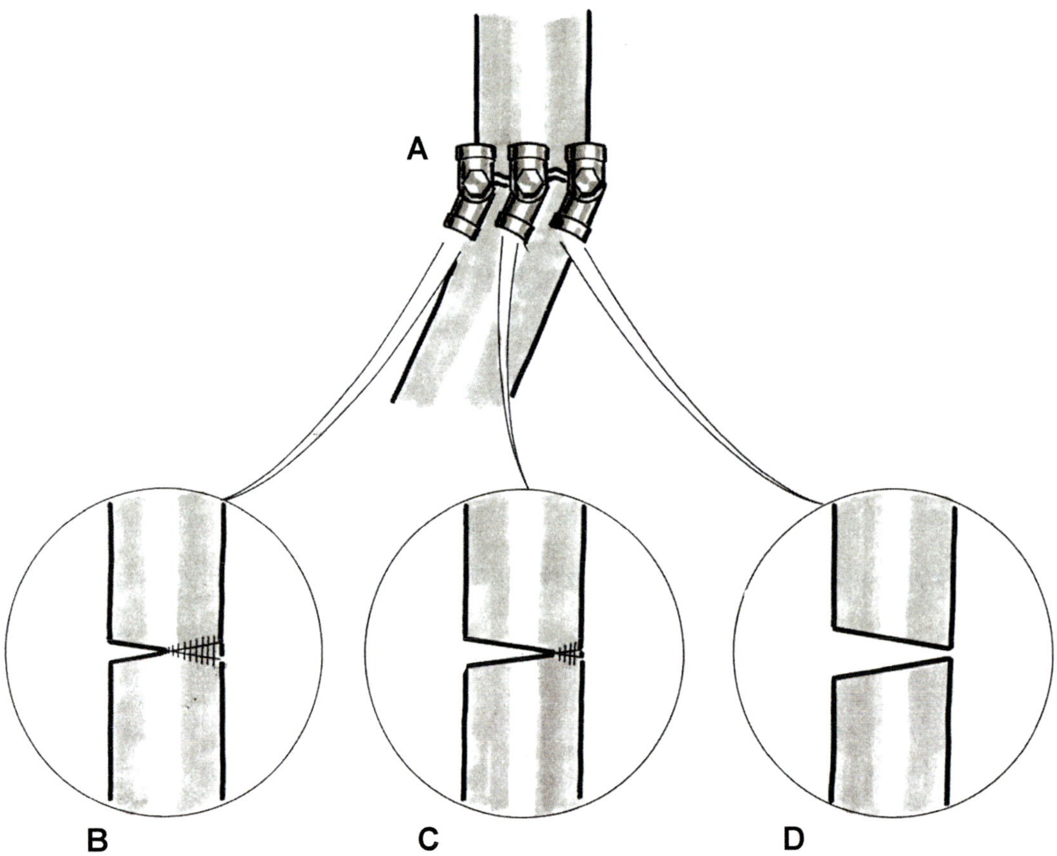

Figure 13.8: Three positions of the opening wedge hinge in relation to the bone cortex walls, and the effect of such positioning on deformity correction. A, segment of the bone with angular deformity and three positions of the hinges. B, small opening at the concave side and area of compression at the convex side *(shaded)*. C, small opening at the concave side and small area of compression at the convex side *(shaded)*. D, wider opening at the concave side and narrow opening at the convex side

3. The axis of rotation is on the projection of the bone wall at the convex side of deformity. Straightening with this hinge configuration produces a large opening at concave side accompanied by some opening at the convex side. Indications for this hinge configuration are chiefly in bone sclerosis, for example, in hypertrophic type of nonunion. Because sclerotic bone would be crushed by compression without stimulation of osteogenesis, it is recommended that compressive forces be avoided in such cases (Fig. 13.8D).

DISTRACTION HINGE

The chief characteristic of the distraction hinge is that the location of its axis of rotation is situated on the convex side of the deformity. Straightening with this hinge produces a wide opening on both sides of the deformity, sometimes equal to the creation of a distraction gap (Fig. 13.9). The size of this opened gap depends on the distance of the hinge from the bone. The greater the distance the larger the gap. There is a limit to the gap size, which is controlled by the distance of the hinge from the bone.

The distraction hinge is indicated chiefly in cases of deformity combined with Significant bone shortness. In such cases, the gap created by straightening must be filled by the bone fragment transport. This can be achieved subsequently with nonunion treatment.

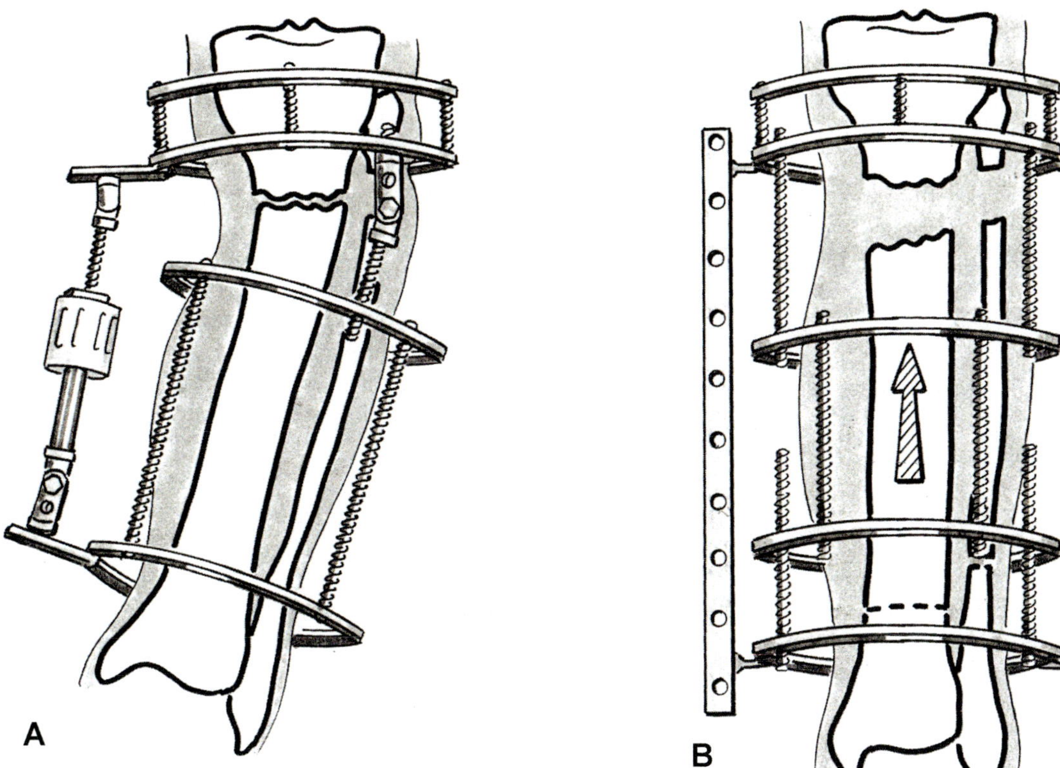

Figure 13.9: Correction of proximal tibial varus deformity combined with shortness, and subsequent bone transport technique for the closure of the distraction gap. A, frame is applied with the hinge axis of rotation situated outside the convex side of the deformity. The motor device (graduated telescopic rod) is situated at the side opposite the hinge and is connected to the frame proximal and distal components. B, after tibial straightening, the distraction gap was developed at the site of the corrected deformity. To fill this gap the external bone transport technique is planned. For this an additional ring is incorporated onto the distal frame component, two long plates are connected to the frame, and a distal tibial corticotomy is performed *(interrupted line)*. *Arrow* shows direction of shifting of the bone fragment

COMPRESSION HINGE

With the compression hinge the location of the axis of rotation is situated outside of the concave side of the deformity. Straightening with this hinge produces contiguous but not direct contact of the bone fragments. The compressive force of their contact depends on the distance of the hinge from the bone contour. The greater the distance the straighter the force of the fragment compression that can be achieved (Fig. 13.10). There is a limit to this force, due to the length of the hinge legs.

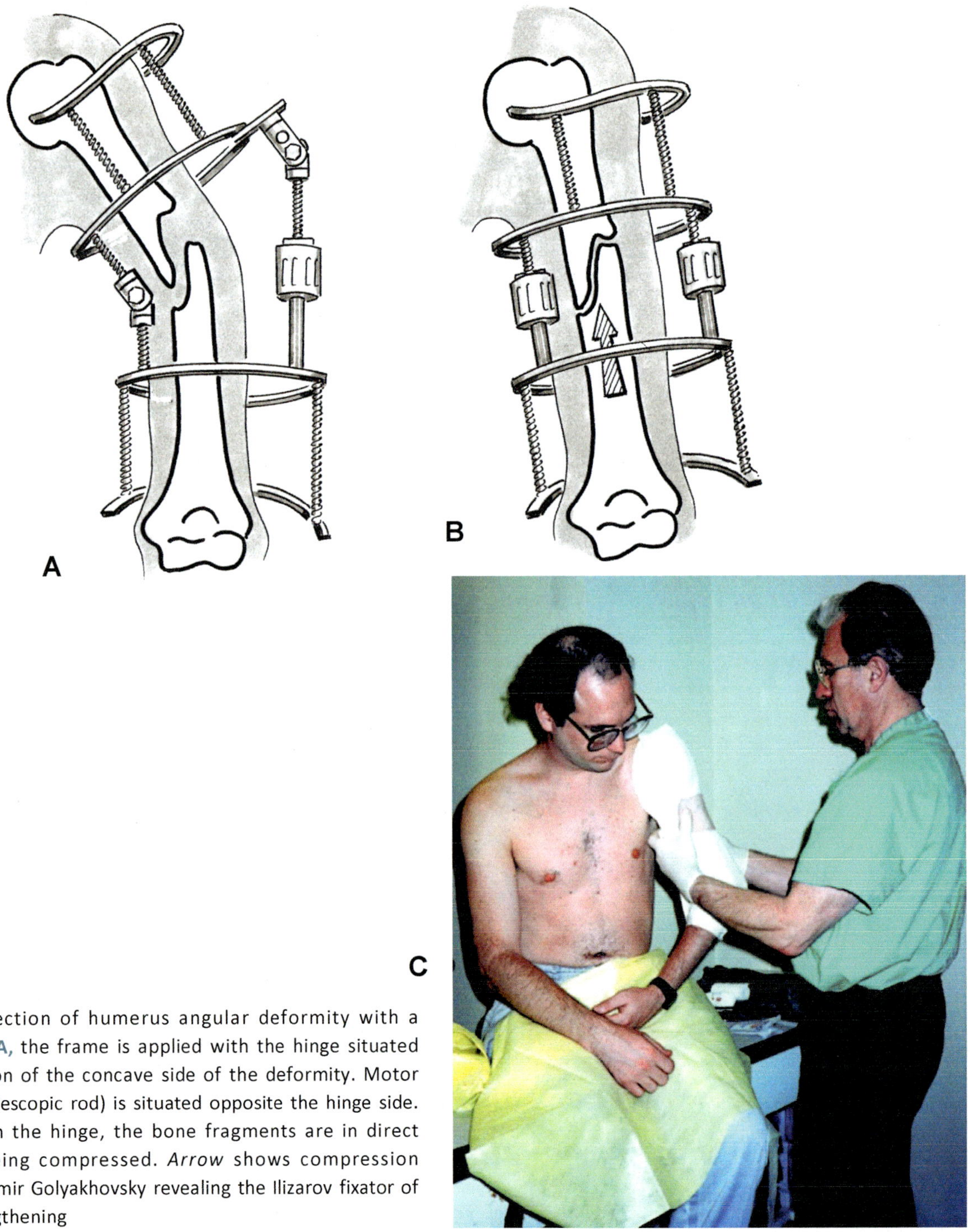

Figure 13.10: Correction of humerus angular deformity with a compression hinge. A, the frame is applied with the hinge situated outside the projection of the concave side of the deformity. Motor device (graduated telescopic rod) is situated opposite the hinge side. B, straightened with the hinge, the bone fragments are in direct contact and are being compressed. *Arrow* shows compression direction. C, Dr Vladimir Golyakhovsky revealing the Ilizarov fixator of the left brachial lengthening

The compression hinge is indicated in cases of deformity combined with bone loss. In such cases the fragment ends approach each other, and their compression creates closing of the bone defect. The most suitable situation for this hinge is in treating osteoporotic bone ends, particularly with icicle-type protrusions.

TRANSLATION HINGE

The translation hinge is used to simultaneously correct the combined deformity of angular bending and transverse displacement. The characteristic of the translation hinge is that the location of its axis of rotation is situated outside the level of the deformity apex.

There are two possibilities for treatment of this type of combined deformity. If the distal fragment is displaced toward the concave side, the rotation axis of the hinge must be placed above the deformity apex at the convex side of proximal fragment (Fig. 13.11).

If the distal fragment is displaced toward the convex side, the rotation axis of the hinge must be placed below

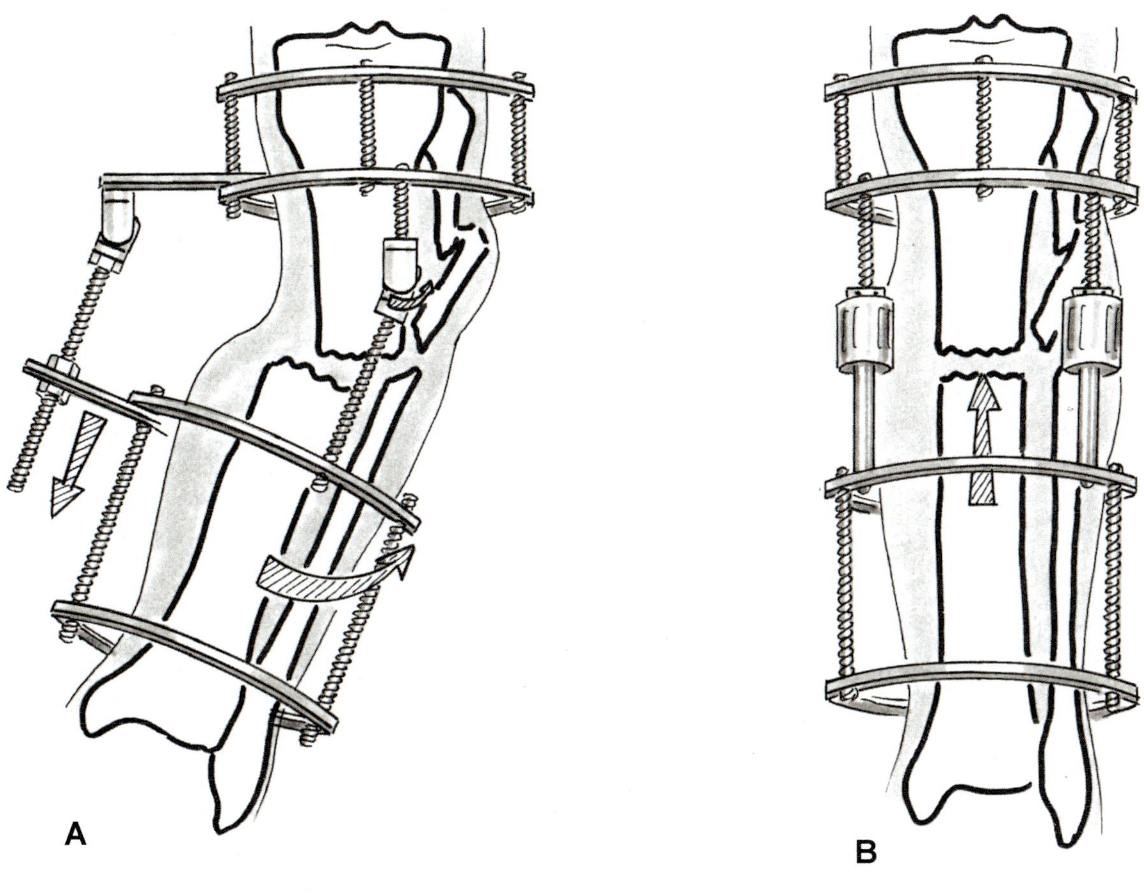

Figure 13.11: Correction of tibial angular bending combined with transverse displacement via the translation hinge. The distal fragment is displaced toward the concave side. **A,** frame is applied with the hinge situated above the deformity apex, at the convex side of the proximal bone fragment. Motor device (threaded rod with nuts) is situated opposite the hinge side. *Straight arrow* shows direction of the correcting forces; *small curved arrow* shows direction of the distal half-hinge motion; large curved arrow shows direction of the distal fragment motion. **B,** straightened bone fragments are in contiguous association, and are being compressed. *Arrow* shows direction of compression

the deformity apex at the convex side of the distal fragment (Fig. 13.12).

Straightening with these hinges produces a contiguous association of the fragment ends but does not bring them closer together because they are a type of opening wedge hinge. The greater the translation displacement the farther the hinge axis must be positioned from the apex of the deformity.

TRANSLATION CORRECTION DEVICE

In a translation deformity without fragment angulation there is no need to use hinges. In such cases hinges are replaced by devices assembled from supports or posts and threaded rods. The horizontal bars of these devices are placed at the level of the deformity apex. They must be strictly parallel to the rings above and below the deformity and to each other (Fig. 13.13).

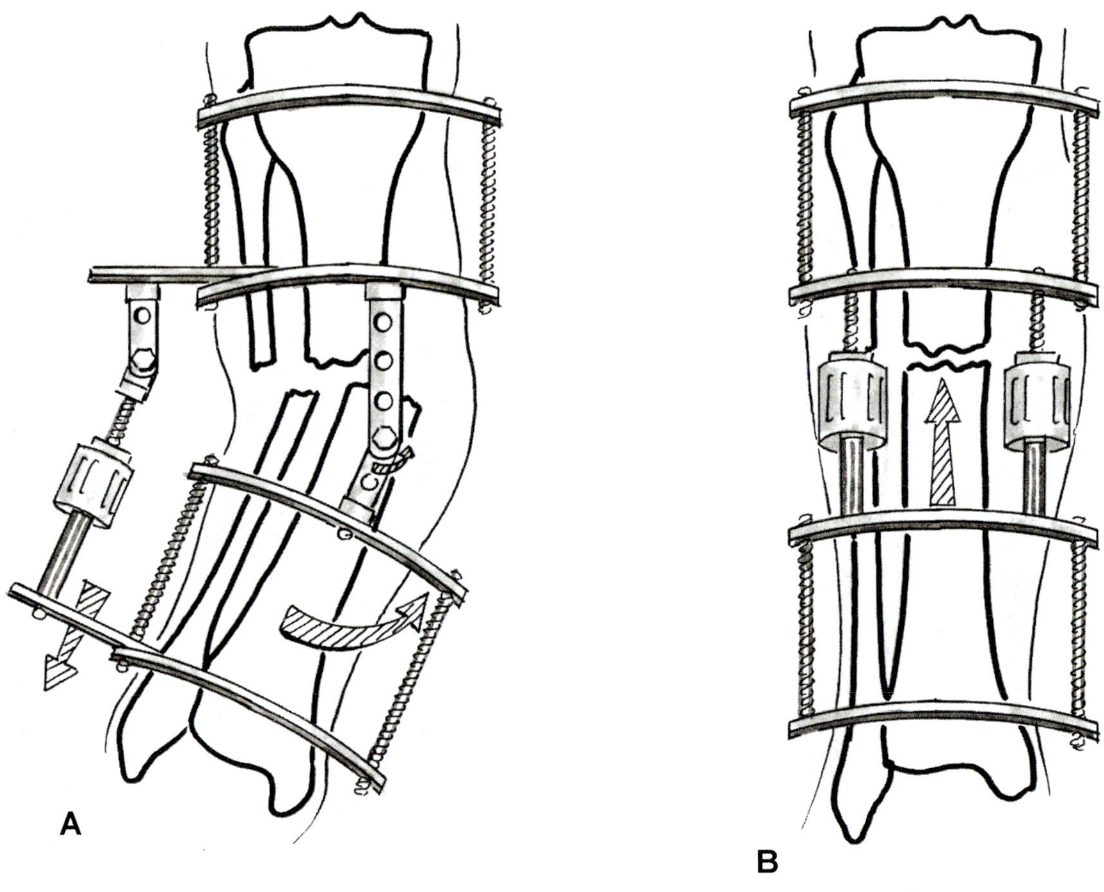

Figure 13.12: Correction with the translation hinge of tibial angular deformity combined with transverse displacement. Distal fragment is displaced toward the convex side. **A,** frame is applied with the hinge situated below the deformity apex, at the convex side of the distal bone fragment. Motor device (threaded rod with nuts) is situated opposite the hinge side. *Small curved arrow* shows direction of the distal half-hinge motion; *large curved arrow* shows direction of the distal fragment motion. **B,** straightened bone fragment ends are in contiguous association, and are being compressed. *Arrow* shows compression direction

To preserve and restore local blood circulation, the translation deformity correction should be carried out as early as possible, before distraction is begun. Side displacement of the bone fragments squeezes the bone marrow and periosteal vessels, and even with distraction, in a position of translation deformity, those vessels still may be constricted. This will delay or stop development of regenerate and produce nonunion, hypoplastic regenerate, or pseudocyst at the site of distraction.

To ensure stability, at least three or four devices must be incorporated between the rings, all of them located along the same horizontal plane.

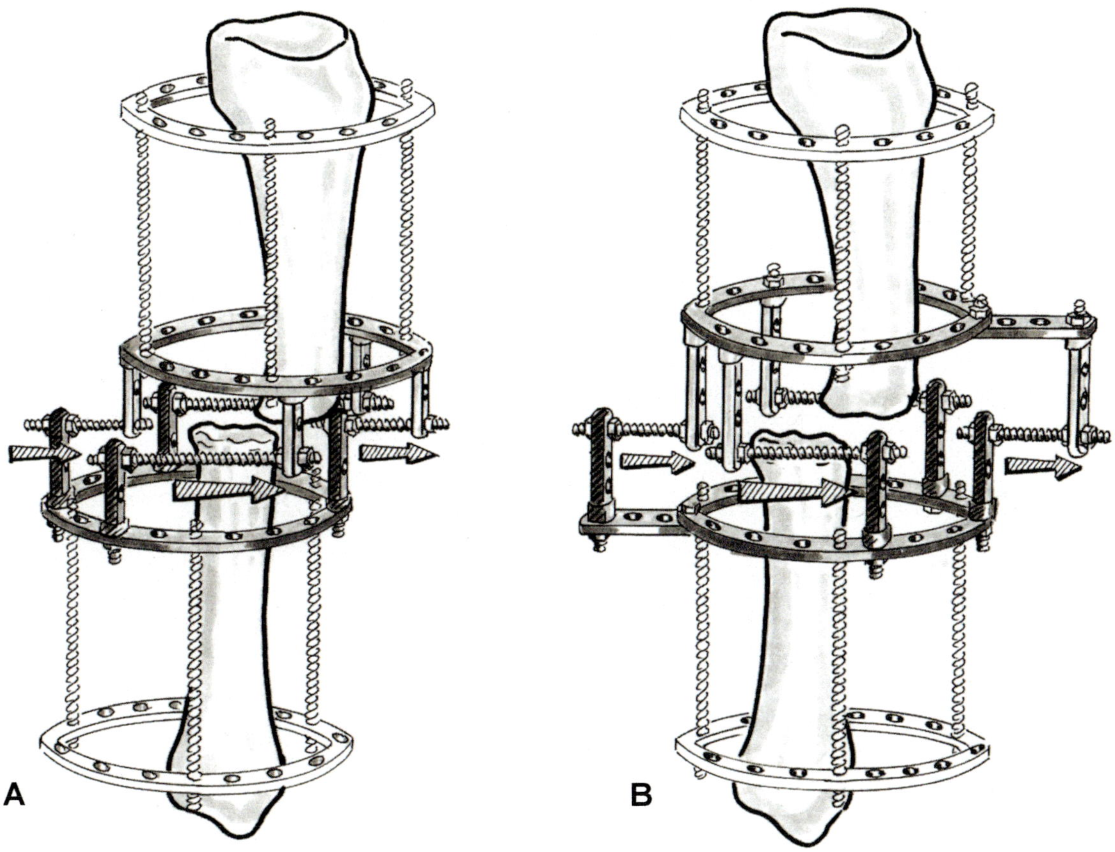

Figure 13.13: Translation device for correction of deformity. Four-ring frame is applied to the tibial fragments malaligned in translation deformity, with the distal fragment displaced posteriorly. Translation correction devices are connected to the proximal and distal frame components. Horizontal threaded rods of these devices are situated at the level of displacement and are set in the same direction. Motor forces (turning nuts) are applied to the supports, which are attached to the distal rings *(shown shaded). Arrows* indicate direction of the translation deformity correction forces. There are two possible frame construction corrective techniques for treating these displaced fragments. A, two-axis frame. When both frame components are centered around the corresponding displaced bone fragment axes, and therefore are placed in the displacement positions, the four translation devices are assembled with supports attached to the rings and are connected by short threaded rods. These short rods and nuts provide the motor forces to correct or translate the deformity. When the distal frame component is aligned exactly with the proximal component the deformity is corrected. B, one-axis frame. When both frame components are centered around the proximal bone fragment axes, and therefore are situated along the same axis, two of the four translation devices are assembled by incorporating short plates and supports with threaded rod. These are the anterior and posterior devices. Correction of translation deformity is completed when the distal frame component is brought forward anteriorly

ROTATION CORRECTION DEVICE

In rotation deformity without fragment angulation, derotation devices assembled from the supports or posts and threaded rods are incorporated between the rings. The horizontal bars of these devices are placed at the level of the deformity apex, and must be strictly parallel to the rings above and below. In contrast to the translation devices, they cannot be parallel to each other, but must be placed so that their horizontal bars are at similar angles to each other (Fig. 13.14).

DEROTATION MANEUVER

As an alternative to gradual correction with the help of devices, rotation deformity can be corrected instantly with the aid of a special maneuver. Indications for this are that the rotation deformity is not more than 10 to 15 degrees, that correction of all other deformities is performed in advance, and that the surrounding soft tissues are in good condition.

The rotation correction maneuver is produced by the four threaded rods connecting two rings proximally and

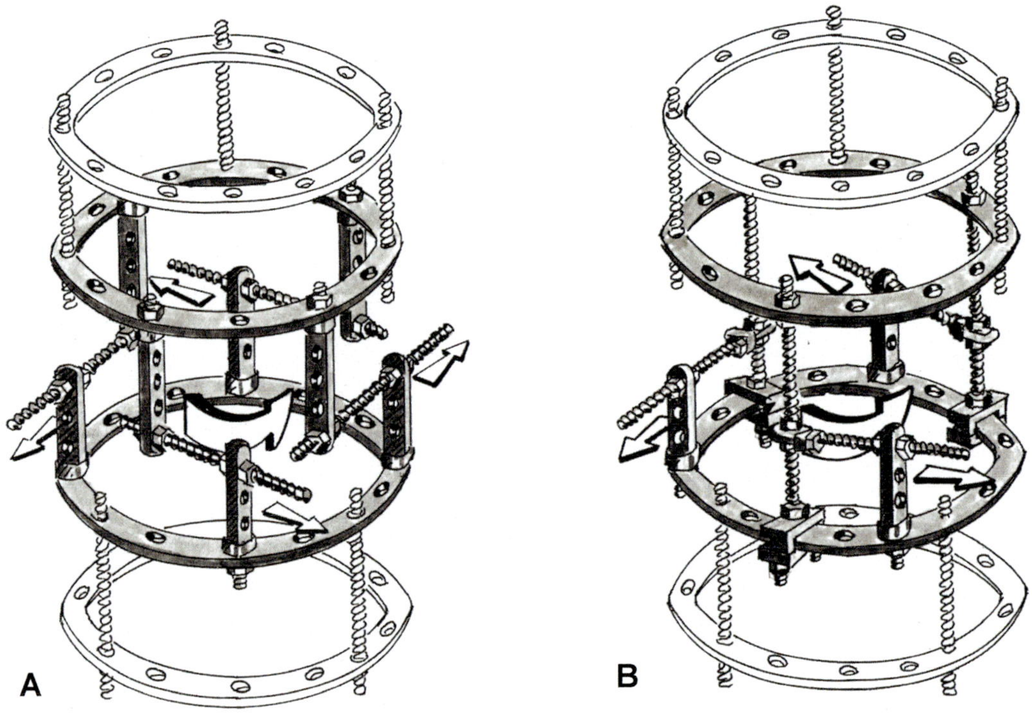

Figure 13.14: Two types of rotation correction devices, incorporated between proximal and distal components of the four-ring frame. Horizontal threaded rods of these devices must be situated at the level at which the bone fragments are derotated, and they are set in the direction with angulation to each other. Motor forces (turning nuts) are applied to the supports, which are attached to the distal ring *(shown shaded). Straight arrows* indicate direction of those forces; *curved arrows* indicate direction of rotation resulting from the simultaneous movement of all motor nuts. A, four derotation devices are assembled with supports attached to the rings and are connected by short threaded rods. These short rods and nuts provide the motor forces to correct rotation deformity. Ninety-degree angulation between the forces provides smooth derotation. B, three derotation devices are assembled with vertical threaded rods connecting two rings. At the distal end these rods are fixed to the detachable wire-fixation buckles, which are attached to the ring without tightening. Horizontal rods are connected to the vertical rods by the tightened female half-hinge and are connected to the supports attached to the distal ring. One hundred twenty-degree angulation between the force direction provides smooth derotation

distally to the deformity (Fig. 13.15). All rods are introduced obliquely, being *inclined to the side opposite the planned derotation side* and placed parallel to each other. Derotation is performed by tightening the distal nuts, which vertically straightened the rods. This shifts the distal ring by approximately 10 degrees per ring hole.

In contrast to the translation deformity correction, it is recommended that the derotation be carried out only after distraction is performed. This prevents the newly developed bone regenerate blood vessels from being squeezed and disrupted.

DEROTATION COMBINED WITH LENGTHENING

If there are indications for both lengthening and derotation of the same limb, it is recommended that these

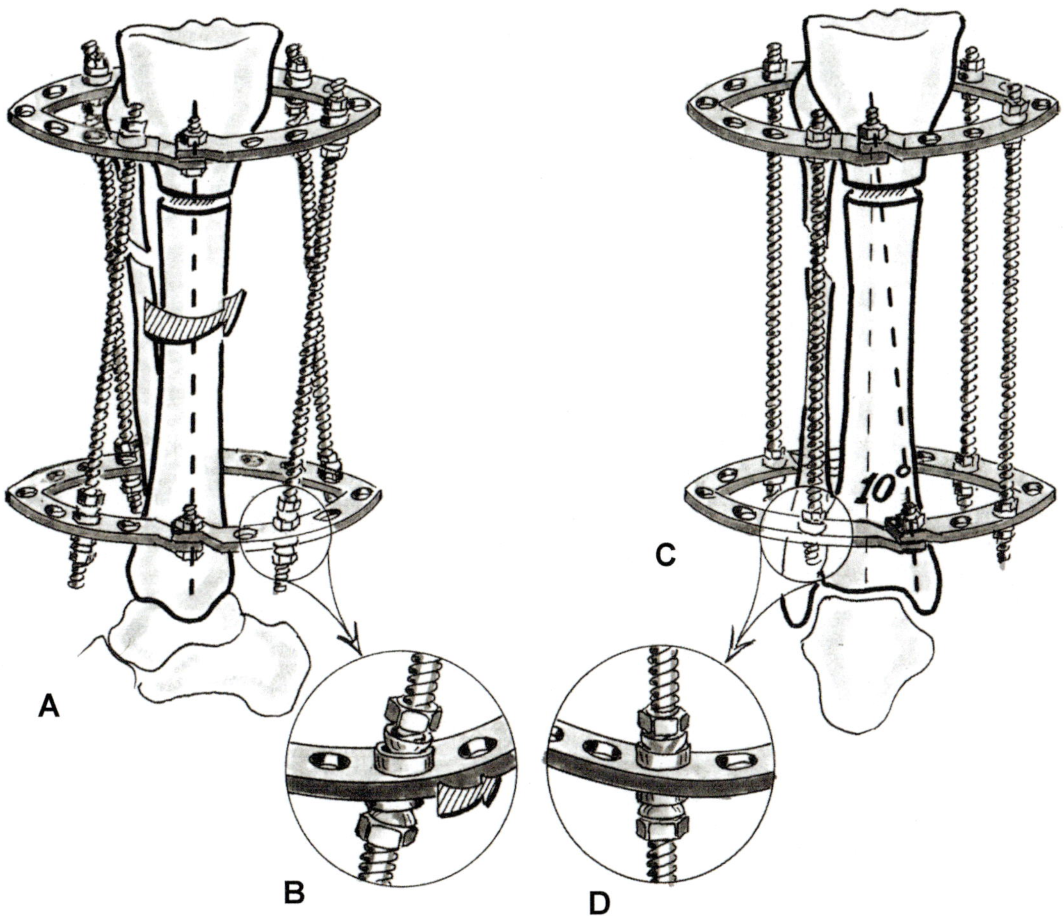

Figure 13.15: Derotation maneuver technique. Two-ring frame is applied to the tibia, and a proximal tibial corticotomy with fibular osteotomy is accomplished. *Straight broken line* indicates alignment of the half-ring connection sites relative to each other. A, tibia and fibula in external rotation position. Four threaded rods are introduced obliquely and are shifted at the distal ring. *Curved arrow* shows direction of the planned derotation, and all rings are shifted one hole toward the opposite direction of the derotation and parallel to each other. The half-ring connection sites, however, are situated in a straight vertical line. B, magnified segment of the distal ring with an obliquely introduced rod fixed by the loosely applied pairs of conical washers at both walls. Simultaneous tightening of all of these washers by the nuts produces straightening of the rods. C, tibia and fibula are in neutral position. Four rods have been straightened by tightening the nuts and washers, which produces shifting of the distal ring approximately 10 degrees. This is shown by the oblique shifting of the *interrupted line* passing between the half-ring connections. D, threaded rod final position at the site of the fixation of the distal ring

procedures be performed separately. First, lengthening is accomplished, and derotation is started 2 to 3 weeks later, after appearance of the initial bone regeneration signs on a regular radiograph or sonogram. The reason for performing these procedures separately is to preserve optimally the newly formed blood vessels from excessive mechanical coercion during the course of combined tissue stretching and torsioning.

SPEED OF CORRECTION WITH HINGES (RULE OF TRIANGLES)

Because the distraction-compression device (in most cases the graduated telescopic rod) is placed at some distance from the hinge axis, the speed of distraction produced is translated to the hinge at a slower rate. To determine the rate of angulation correction at the site of the axis, one is guided by the rule of triangles (Fig. 13.16). According to this rule, the speed of distraction-compression of the motor device is transferred to the hinge axis by a factor of 3: 1. In this example, for 1 mm of movement at the axis there must be 3 mm at the motor site. The distraction rate is not uniform for the soft tissues; it is much greater on the side opposite the hinge. This must be taken into consideration when calculating the speed of angulatory correction.

The speed of derotation correction is subject to a similar rule, because the derotation device itself forms a triangular figure with the bone center. The speed of correction with translation devices is not, however, subject to the rule of triangle; 1 mm of movement at the site of the device is translated to 1 mm of movement at the site of deformity.

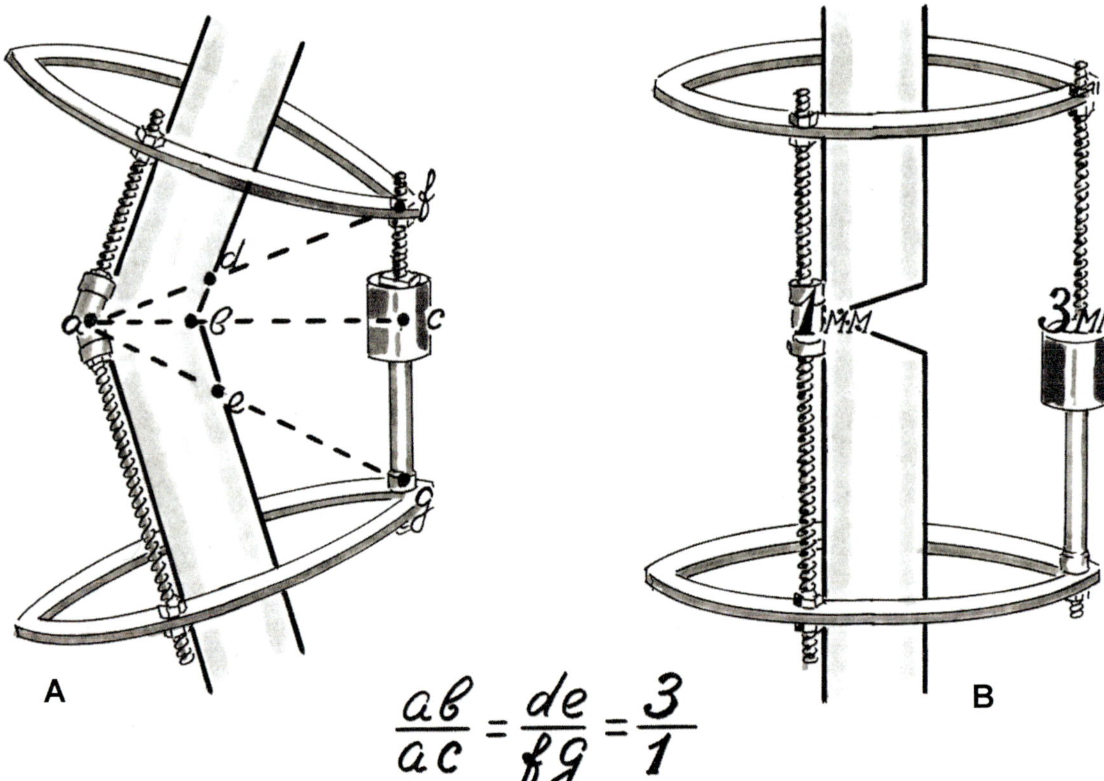

A B

$$\frac{ab}{ac} = \frac{de}{fg} = \frac{3}{1}$$

Figure 13.16: Segment of the frame with the hinge and motor device. **A,** letters *a, f,* and *g* represent three points of fixation between the hinge and device, producing a triangle. **B,** speed of distraction (compression at line *b-c*) is passed to the hinge axis *a* at a ratio of 3: 1 (3 mm to 1 mm)

TWO-AXIS HINGES

The two-axis hinge consists of a single unit that permits rotation around two orthogonal axes. These hinges are used for the simultaneous correction of two concurrent types of deformity. For example, they can be used in the case of recurvation or antecurvation combined with side angulation. Although they make it possible to shift a bone fragment in two directions, they are limited by the restricted ability of the distraction-compression devices to act in both directions simultaneously. Thus complex configurations of these devices are required to achieve the desired movement. In addition, both axes of the two-axis hinge are not located at exactly the same position (Fig. 13.17).

Depending on the clinical situation, the distraction-compression forces have to be directed initially to correct the preponderant deformity. Again, care must be taken to ensure motion only about the desired axis of the hinge. After this is achieved, the direction of forces is changed by reattachment of the motor devices to correct the other aspect of the deformity.

In large frames such as those used for the femur, leg, and arm, the weight and size of the corrected segment may cause destabilization in the second plane of the hinge. Thus the two-axis hinges are used mostly in the smaller frames, for foot and hand deformity correction. In clubfoot they can be used to correct varus and equinus deformities, and in the wrist they can be used to treat Madelung deformity by correcting angulation and subluxation. This type of frame also must have an increased number of ring connectors, which prevent undesirable instability in the hinge second axis (see Fig. 13.17).

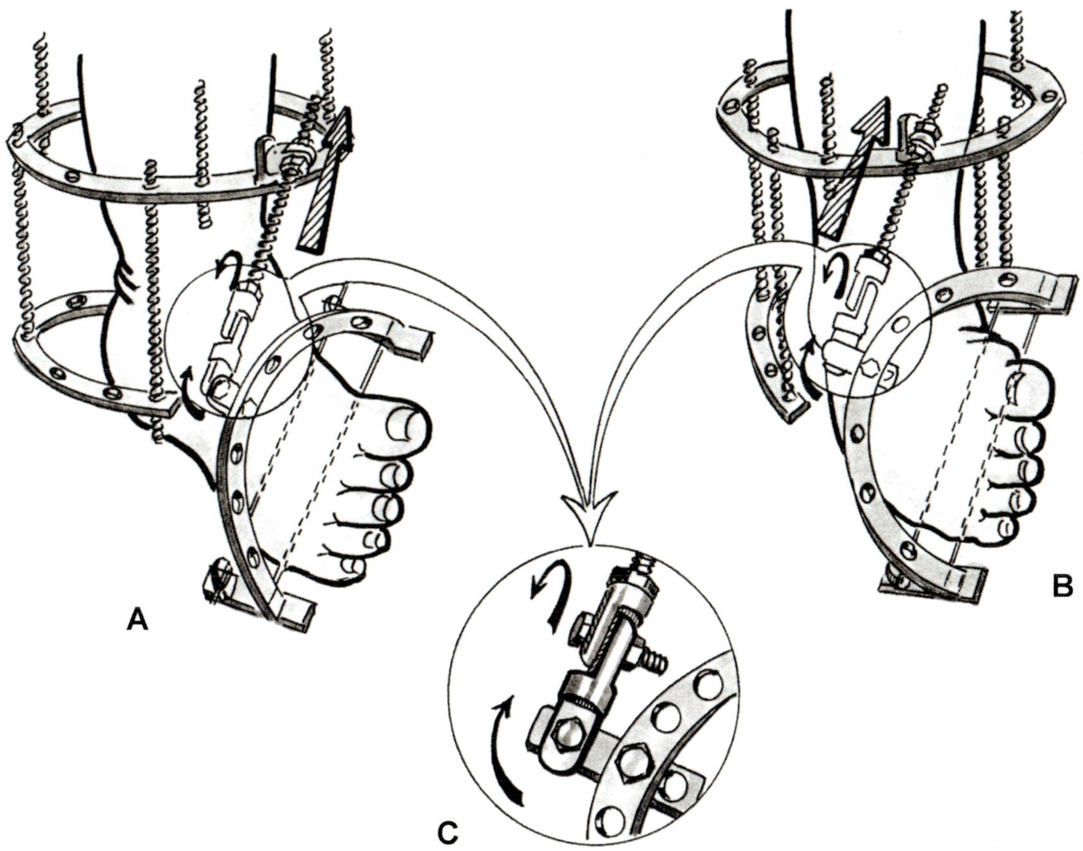

Figure 13.17: Simultaneous correction of foot equinus and varus deformities using the two-axis hinge. Section of the foot frame is shown. *Straight shaded arrows* indicate direction of the pulling device force; *black curved arrows* indicate directions of the forces within the hinges by the incorporated two-axis device. A, foot in lateral position. B, foot in straight position. C, magnified view of the two-axis hinge, connected by a short plate to the forefoot half-ring and to the pulling device

14 Chapter

General Principles of Ilizarov Technique

TECHNIQUE OF BONE DISTRACTION

Distraction is used for bone lengthening (primarily), for correction of bone deformities, for bone segment transport, as a stimulus for nonunion and pseudoarthrosis healing, as a stimulus for neovascularization, and for joint contracture correction.

Motor forces of distraction are achieved by movement of the nuts fixed to the ring or by turning of the graduated telescopic rod, and are translated to the tensioned wires introduced into the bone. Three parameters of these forces produce the full effect of distraction: *speed, rhythm,* and *distribution* on the bone circumference.

The optimum speed is 1 mm/day, and the optimal rhythm is four times per day. Thus there must be four distraction adjustments daily, at intervals of 6 hours, with each adjustment being 0.25 mm, or one-fourth of the thread pitch.

The speed and rhythm of distraction are adjustable; in some cases they must be increased, in others reduced.

The chief indications for increase in distraction speed and rhythm include: (1) young age of the patient, usually children up to 12 to 14 years; (2) when the X-ray control image indicates a tendency to premature bone consolidation at the site of distraction; and (3) when the X-ray control image indicates an uncompleted bone cut at the site of corticotomy.

The chief indications for reduction of the distraction speed and rhythm include: (1) severe pain at the site of distraction, especially after creating a 3- to 4-cm gap; (2) clinical signs of peripheral vascular and/or neurologic deficiency; (3) X-ray control image indicates slow development of bone regeneration.

In any event, the increase in distraction speed and rhythm cannot exceed 1.5 mm/day, in increments of six turns of 0.25 mm. The reduction of distraction cannot be less than 0.25 to 0.50 mm/day. In some cases a situation may arise in which distraction may be halted for 2 to 3 days, and even may be reversed with a slower speed (see compression technique description, later in this chapter).

The motor forces must be distributed evenly on the moving bone fragment circumference. Even distribution requires that these forces be applied with consideration to the number and positioning of wires attached to the ring. The resistance of the surrounding soft tissue to distraction also is easier to overcome with the even distribution of forces. Undesirable bone angulation also may develop because of asymmetric distraction.

Provided that on average two wires are introduced into the bone at a 60- to 90-degree angle to one another, the optimal distribution of distraction forces is four points of application with 90-degree angles between them (Fig. 14.1).

It is not recommended that distractional forces be applied to the ring fixed to the bone with half-pins. For distraction of more than 2 to 3 cm there are two reasons to avoid exertion of forces on the half-pin ring. First, the half-pins cut the skin, leaving gross scars. Second, the half-pins do not allow micromotion at the site of distraction, which is an important component of the regenerate bone stimulation.

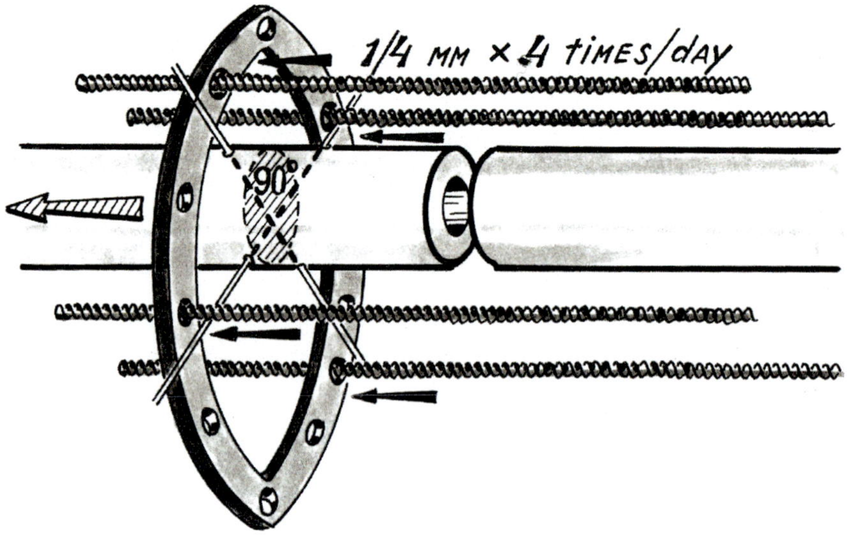

Figure 14.1: Three optimum parameters for distraction forces. Segments of the frame and the bone are shown with the corticotomy site to the right and the ring to the left. *Large arrow* indicates direction of distraction; *small solid arrows* indicate sites of application and direction of distraction forces. Four evenly distributed forces are applied to the ring four times a day, each producing 0.25 mm of ring motion each time. Together they produce 1 mm of bone distraction per day

Distraction Technique

There are three ways to perform distraction with the Ilizarov apparatus:

1. With the wrenches, by turning the nuts attached to the ring. This is done by loosening the nut at the ring wall situated farthest from the distraction site. Then the opposite nut is tightened to the ring wall, turned exactly one-fourth of the full turn. This produces 0.25 mm movement of the ring to the side opposite the corticotomy site and moves the bone. After this, the first nut must be tightened firmly to the ring wall to secure the new ring position (Fig. 14.2).

To be precise in turning the hexagonal nut for one-fourth of a turn, it is useful to compare the

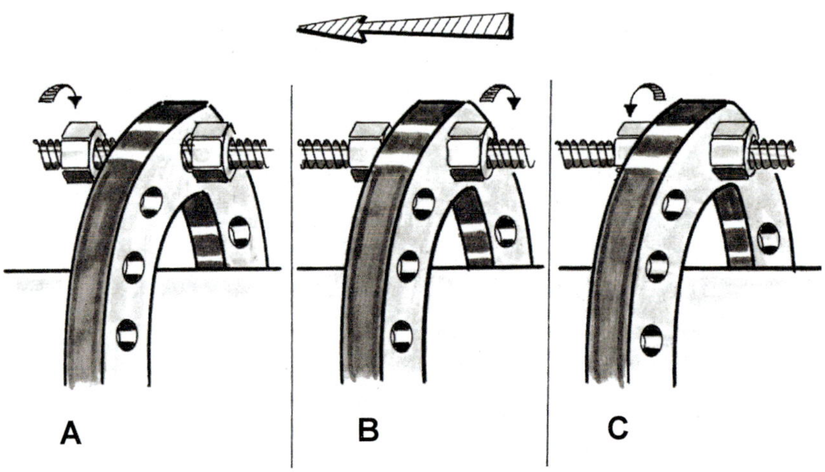

Figure 14.2: Distraction technique using the nuts. Segment of the pushing-pulling ring of a frame is shown with a threaded rod and nuts attached to the ring. *Curved arrows* indicate direction in which nuts are turned; *straight arrow* indicates direction of ring movement. A, nut at the wall opposite the distraction site is loosened. B, nut at the distraction site is tightened one-fourth turn, producing exactly 0.25-mm movement of the ring. C, first nut then is retightened to secure the new (moved) ring position

wrench position with the position of a clock hand. This simplifies the procedure, especially for non-trained patients or for parents who must perform this for their children. Imagine the wrench as if it was a clock hand against a dial; the nut must be advanced 3 hours each time (Fig. 14.3). Another way to simplify the precise turning of the nut for one-fourth of a turn is to color one of its six sides (e.g. with nail polish or correction fluid) and to advance the marked side to the 12-, 3-, 6-, and 9-o'clock positions, respectively, with each turn. There also is a special combined nut for the same purpose.

Because the threaded rods are flexible, this technique is recommended only for short rods used between the supporting and pushing-pulling movable rings. It is useful for 7- to 10-cm rods, and for the distraction device.

2. With the increased length of threaded rods up to 12 to 20 cm it is expedient to use the hollow aluminum telescopic rod technique. These rods increase frame stability by increasing the outer rod diameter, and also allow frame expansion from within.

To carry out distraction, it is necessary first to loosen the bolt tightening the head of the telescopic rod, then to turn the nut fixing this head on the threaded rod. The one-quarter turn will produce 0.25 mm of distraction. The bolt must be tightened after each nut turn (Fig. 14.4).

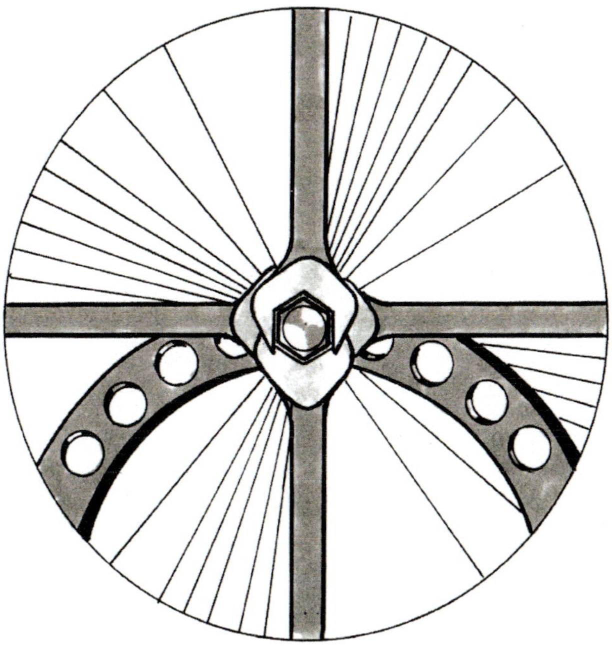

Figure 14.3: Wrench position in technique of distraction by turning of the nuts. The wrench is positioned according to the hands of a clock, and is turned "3 hours" with each turn. This produces 0.25 mm of distraction

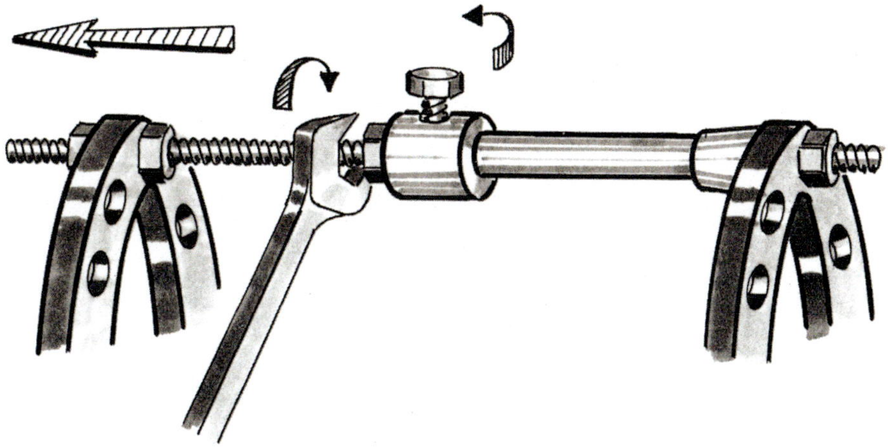

Figure 14.4: Distraction technique with the aluminum telescopic rod. *Straight arrow* indicates direction of distraction; *curved arrows* indicate directions in which the tightened bolt and fixing nut are turned

3. The most reliable, and the recommended method of performing distraction is by using the graduated telescopic rod. This device has a rotating head with a ratchet mechanism. This mechanism is released by depressing the lever, and it stops by itself after one-fourth revolution. With movement of the levers into locking position, a clicking sound is produced. Because of this sound the rod often is called the "clicker."

   The advantage of this technique is that the clicker may be turned with the fingers or with the special 19-mm wrench for telescopic rod, applied to the square part whose sides are calibrated in increments from 1 to 4 (Fig. 14.5).

4. In the 1980s Ilizarov developed the autodistractor, a mechanism programmed to produce a 1-mm revolution of the threaded rod, in 64 micromotions per day. In essence, this is a nonstop motor. Four autodistractors are attached to the threaded rods, and are powered by batteries carried on the patient's belt.

   This motor produces smooth distraction and is free of the constant need to be turned. Several companies in the United States now are trying to develop an analog of this system.

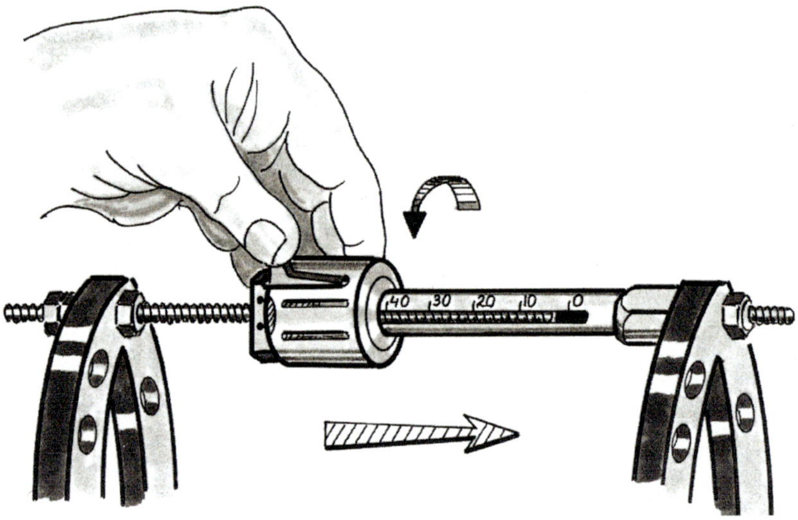

Figure 14.5: Distraction technique with the graduated telescopic rod. *Curved arrow* indicates direction in which the movable head is turned; *straight arrow* indicates the direction of distraction

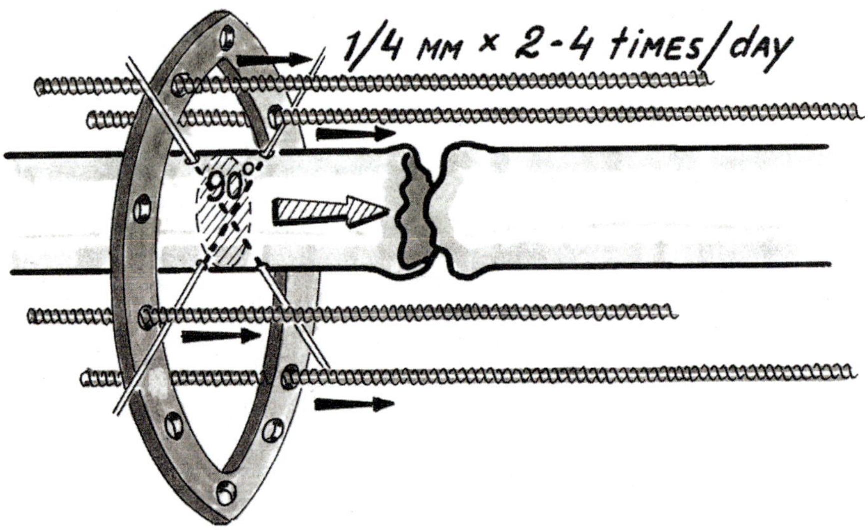

Figure 14.6: Three optimum parameters for compression forces. Segment of the frame and the bone are shown with the nonunion site on the right and the ring on the left. *Large arrow* indicates compression direction; *small arrows* indicate sites of application and direction of compression forces. Four evenly distributed forces are applied to the ring four times a day, each of them producing 0.25 mm of ring movement each time. Together they produce 1 mm of bone compression per day

TECHNIQUE OF BONE COMPRESSION

General Considerations

Compression is used in treatment of bone nonunion (primarily), correction of bone deformities, bone segment transport, arthrodesis technique, and reversing distraction.

The motor forces of compression are produced by the threaded rods fixed to the ring and are translated to the tensioned wires introduced into the bone or to the half-pins. Use of the thick half-pins for compression can be indicated in some cases of arthrodesis and for short compression (< 2 cm), but is not recommended for a large gap (> 3 cm) nonunion treatment for the same reasons that it is not recommended in distraction.

In most situations compression is produced in the same manner as distraction, but in the opposite direction. The same three parameters of operation effect compression: speed, rhythm, and distribution of forces on the bone circumference (Fig. 14.6).

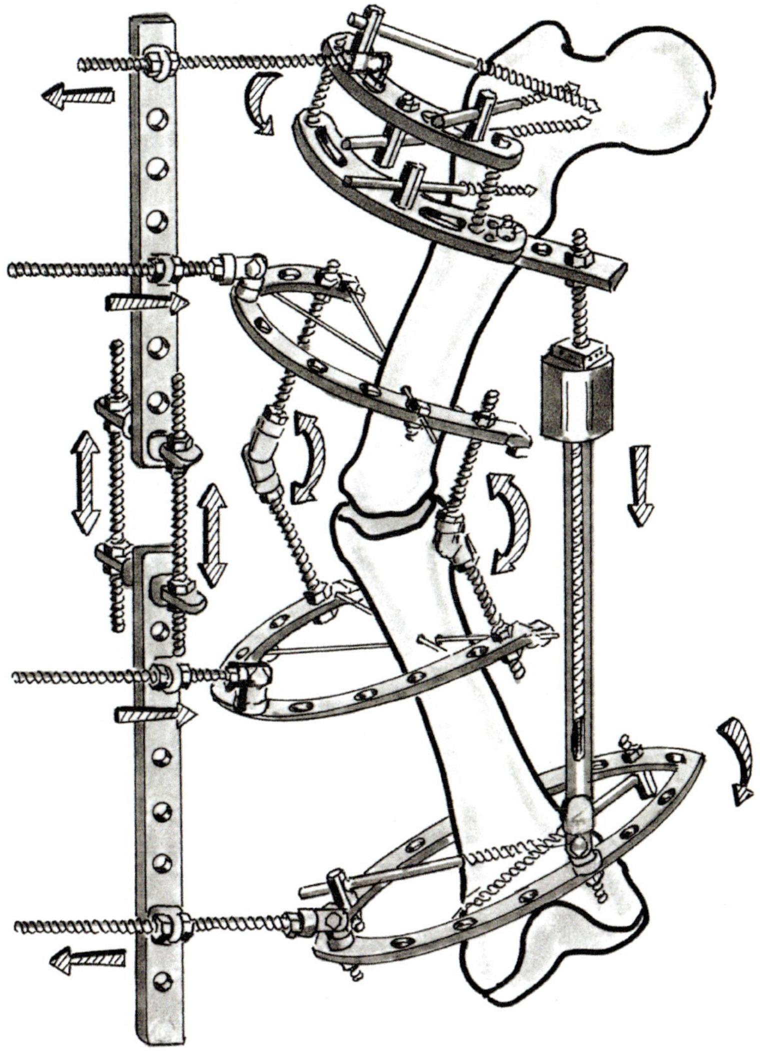

Figure 14.7: Compression-distraction technique (stage 1). Femoral bone pseudoarthrosis with angulation and shortness. The frame with the pushing component and multiple hinges is applied. The main supporting element of the frame consists of two connected long plates; additional support is provided by the telescopic rod. Pushing component consists of two half-rings connected with hinged rods and connected to supporting plates by hinged pushing devices. *Straight arrow* indicates direction of correcting forces; *curved arrows* indicate movement of the hinges. Note that the distal ring is fixed by two half-pins. This decreases risk of knee flexion contracture and is acceptable for a short distraction

The same three techniques used to produce distraction also are applicable to compression: (1) turning the nuts attached to the ring walls, (2) aluminum telescopic rod, and (3) graduated telescopic rod.

In contrast to the distraction technique, there are few indications for the increase of speed and rhythm in compression, but more indications for the reduction of compression speed and rhythm.

The chief indication for increased speed and rhythm in compression is the creation of a large bone loss after resection. In a situation in which 3 to 5 cm of bone tissue is to be resected, the speed of compression can be increased by up to 1.5 or 2 mm/day. But it is contraindicated to produce compression with full closure of such a large gap on the operating table. This can produce neurovascular deficiency. The chief indication for reduction of the compression speed and rhythm is severe pain at the site of compression.

Clinical signs of neurovascular deficiency must be monitored, with the X-ray control image indicating completed approximation of the bone fragments. In any event, the speed of compression cannot be reduced to less

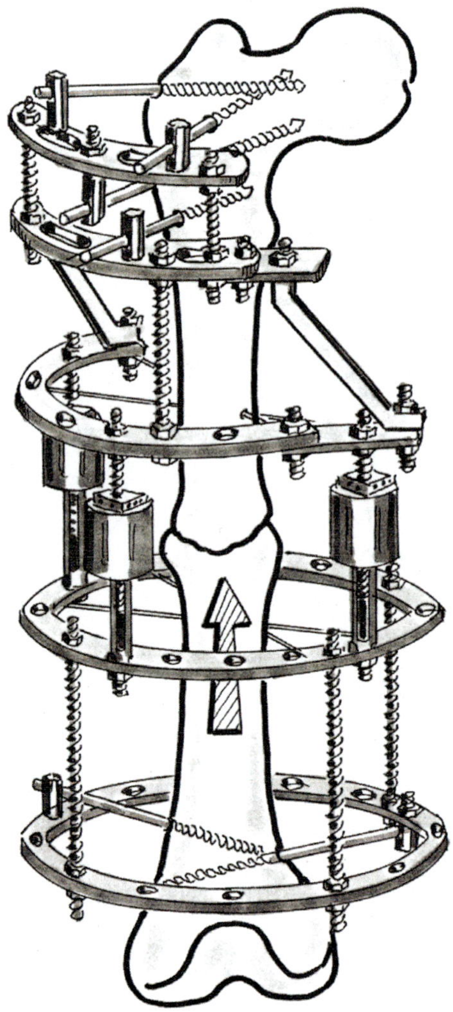

Figure 14.8: Compression-distraction technique (stage 2); same as in Figure 14.7 after accomplishment of angulation deformity correction. Frame now is adjusted for application of the straight compression-distraction forces. The following modifications have been effected: (1) distal half-ring of the pushing component is replaced by the full ring; (2) supporting long plates and telescopic rod are removed; (3) proximal frame component is reinforced by introduction of two oblique support connectors; (4) distal frame component is reinforced by the introduction of threaded rods; (5) both proximal and distal components are connected by three short graduated telescopic rods, which produce strong compression in the direction indicated by the *arrow*

than 0.25 to 0.50 mm/day. In some cases compression may be stopped for 2 to 3 days, then resumed at very slow speed.

Combined Distraction-Compression Technique

In certain cases of severe deformities with limb shortness and bone loss it is necessary to use distraction at one level combined with compression at another level. Depending on the predominant deformity, this may be primarily a case of distraction with compression as an additional treatment element, or vice versa. With significant bone loss this combined technique is called the segmental bone transport technique (see chapter 15).

In primarily compression cases, such as bone nonunion, distraction can be used as an additional treatment element to stimulate bone neogenesis and development not only of the nonunion healing but also of lengthening at the site of nonunion. This can be done without surgical intervention, with apparatus application, and with subsequent compression-distraction maneuvers. Professor Ilizarov calls this treatment "bloodless." Descriptively precise or not, this term reflects the idea of the technique. In many cases of hypertrophic and normotrophic nonunion, the alternating compression with subsequent distraction maneuver is used two or three times to stimulate bone neogenesis. Usually compression for

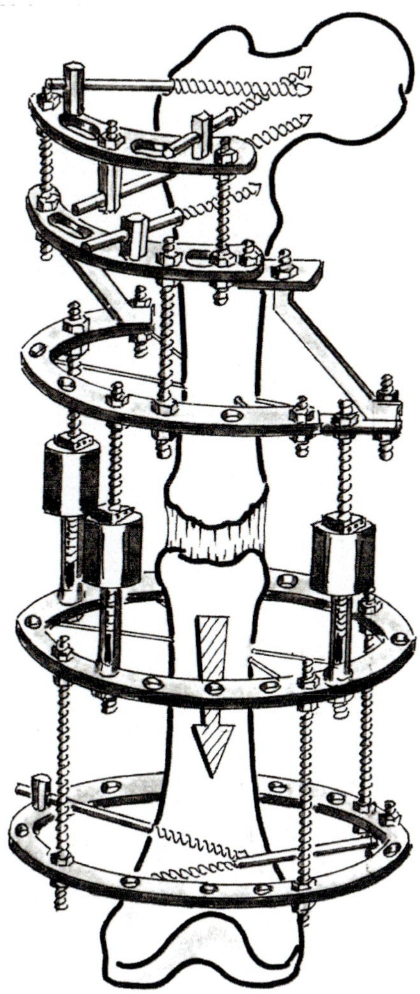

Figure 14.9: Compression-distraction technique (Stage 3); same as in Figure 14.8 after compression is accomplished. Compression forces applied to three graduated telescopic rods, were reversed and now are working as distraction forces in the direction indicated by the *arrow*. Slow distraction (0.25 mm twice a day) produces changes at the site of nonunion, which contribute to the bone tissue neogenesis with subsequent bone regeneration

10 days is followed by distraction up to 10 to 20 mm. In such cases distraction-compression is performed slowly, 0.25 mm twice a day (Figs 14.7 to 14.9).

After achieving this distraction, stop the procedure for 7 to 10 days, then proceed with slow compression, up to 7 to 10 mm. After a 5- to 7-day respite the distraction is performed a second time. Regeneration of tissue is monitored by frequent radiographic or ultrasound examination.

This maneuver is called the accordion technique, and is based on observations that the local scar tissues surrounding the nonunion site must be crushed to be transformed into tissues capable of neogenesis (Fig. 14.10).

Distraction as Stimulating Force for Development of Regenerate

Despite the generally accepted view of compressive forces as the only stimulus for bone neogenesis, Ilizarov demonstrated that stimulation of certain tissue growth and regeneration can be achieved by gradual distraction. The distraction forces create tissue stress capable of stimulating local metabolic activity with cell transformation.

With rigid bone fragment fixation, proper speed, and frequency of distraction, it is possible to stimulate the latent resources of scar tissue necessary for their potential neogenesis, bypassing the compression stage. This eventually leads to the development of bony regenerate.

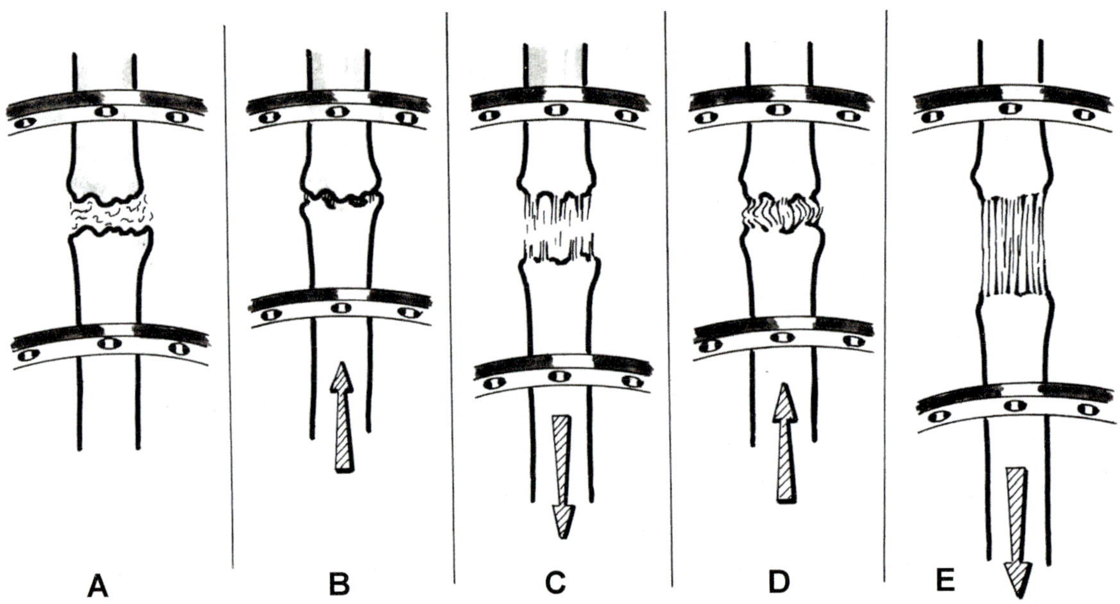

Figure 14.10: Monofocal compression-distraction (accordion technique) for nonunion treatment. Partial view on the segment of the apparatus with two rings above and below the nonunion site. *Arrows* indicate direction of the distal ring movement. **A,** view before start of treatment, with the scar tissue filling the gap between fragments. **B,** stage 1, compression, brings the bone fragments into contact and crushes the scar tissue. **C,** stage 2, distraction, produces the columns of fibrovascular tissue arising from the crushed scars and the bone surface. There is always a different degree of balance between the newly formed tissue and old tissue surviving the crush of compression. **D,** if the intensity of the regenerate development does not follow distraction, then stage 3, repeated very slow compression, helps stimulate tissue tropism and brings the balance between new and old tissues to the positive side. **E,** stage 4, repeated distraction, helps the collagen bundles consolidate within a bony matrix and stimulate the production of osteoblastic cells. This is seen on radiographs as the initial regenerate cloud with longitudinally oriented calcified columns

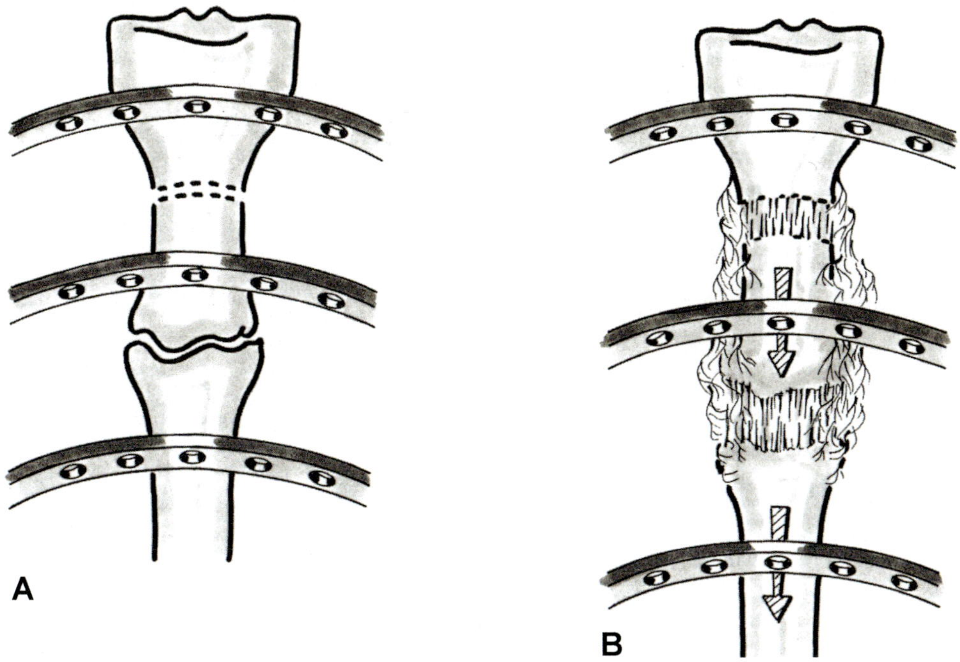

Figure 14.11: Corticotomy as a stimulus of osteogenesis in monofocal distraction treatment of hypertrophic nonunion. Partial view of the proximal tibia and the apparatus frame. *Arrows* indicate direction of distraction at the sites of corticotomy *(above)* and nonunion (below). A, corticotomy *(interrupted lines)* is performed not far from the nonunion site. B, distraction-stimulated neovascularization, which brings additional resources to the healing of the distracted nonunion site

The corticotomy of the same fragment near the nonunion site and simultaneous distraction of the nonunion and corticotomy sites increase the potential to stimulate tissue resources to healing at the nonunion.

In such cases distraction at the corticotomy site leads to increased local neovascularization, which in turn brings additional stimulus to the mechanical effect of tissue tension stress. In many cases of nonunion distraction this becomes a powerful tool for treatment (Fig. 14.11).

CORRECTION OF JOINT CONTRACTURES

General Considerations

Distraction and compression techniques are used for the treatment of joint contractures of a different origin, that is, acquired deformities and stiffness resulting from congenital malformations. The technique varies depending on what is superimposed: the periarticular soft tissue contracture or the intra-articular deformity and perhaps joint fusion. In most cases distraction must produce arthrodiastasis at first, transferring the correcting forces from the articular surface to the tubular bone and surrounding soft tissues. The distraction rods always are placed at the concave side of the deformity, and the compression rod at the convex side. Correct hinge placement is important; the hinge must be located strictly in the axis of joint rotation to avoid subluxation.

To maximize the lever arm, two rings (or two half-rings) should be applied at each segment above and below the joint. This also prevents drift of the bone within the rings.

The choice of full ring vs. half-ring depends on the extremity. It is more convenient to apply half-rings to the lower extremity and full rings to the upper extremity. They must be placed at 90 degrees to the bone axis.

When the wires are introduced, particular attention must be paid to the possible subsequent cut through the skin and soft tissues. With gradually changed joint

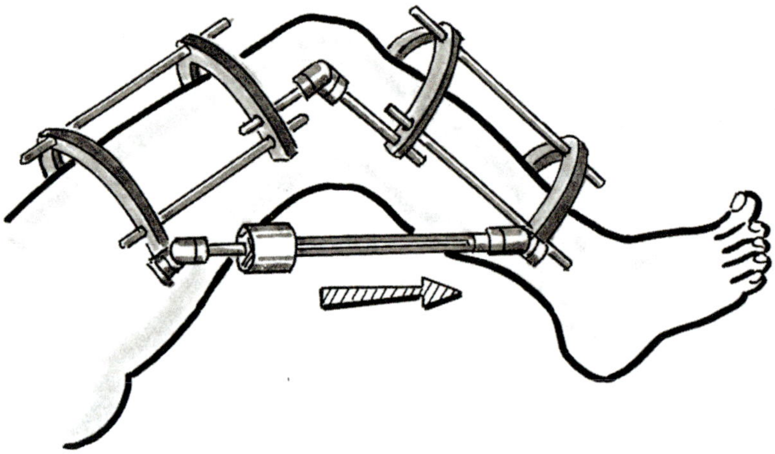

A

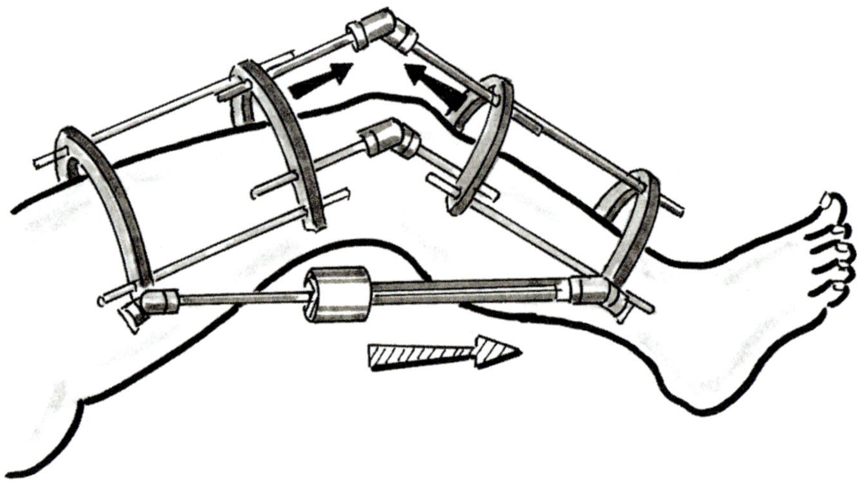

B

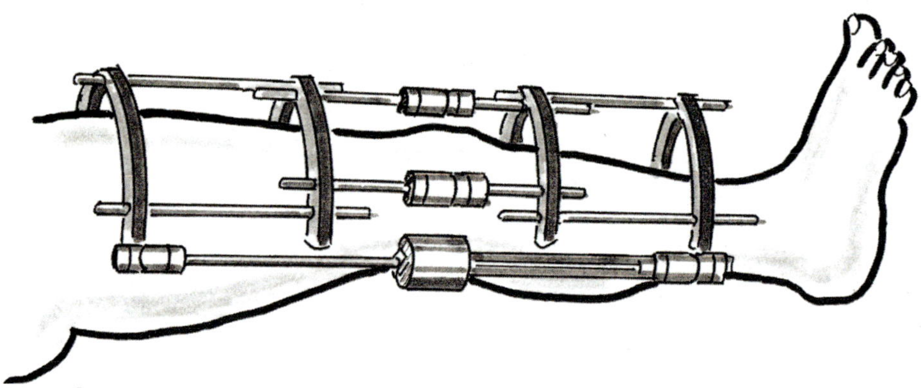

C

Figure 14.12: Knee flexion contracture correction. Right leg with 90 degrees of knee contracture and typical frame assembly. *Arrows* indicate directions of distraction and compression. A, appearance of the leg and fixator before distraction. B, with continuous distraction the frame is reinforced by the hinged compression device introduced at the convex side of the deformity. This stabilizes the knee and prevents tibial posterior subluxation. C, appearance of the leg and frame at the end of the treatment angulation, there always is a possibility that a cut through skin would extend the limit of its elasticity. Thus the skin must be pushed toward the joint site at the moment of wire introduction. The rate of distraction and/or compression is subject to the same rule of triangle as for angulation correction: for 1 mm of distraction at the joint site there must be 3 mm of distraction at the "motor" device site. For correction of most joint contractures the acceptable rate is 1 to 3 degrees per day, divided by three to four times.

In joint deformity with severe intra-articular changes or bony fusion there is an indication for the wedge-type resection with subsequent simultaneous or gradual correction. In planning a type of correction the condition of the local soft tissues must be considered. The wider the base of the resected wedge the slower the angulation correction.

Clinical signs of peripheral blood circulation and neurologic deficiency should be checked everyday during contracture correction. The joint surface alignment must be checked at least every other week. In the case of a subluxation, it must be corrected by application of the translation devices.

Soft Tissue Distraction in Joint Contracture Correction

This technique is performed chiefly to straighten the knee joint. Because of the large masses of the thigh and leg, the frame consists of two levels of fixation for each segment. It is more convenient to use half-rings on the leg frame because the patient easily can position the leg on the bed. In some cases distraction at the concave side must be reinforced by compression at the convex side (Fig. 14.12). Bilateral knee contracture correction must be performed simultaneously, and requires 2 to 3 months, on average. During this treatment there is a need for frequent monitoring, at least every other week. With gradual joint straightening the speed of motor devices has to be adjusted to the new angle. Because the distance from the axis of joint rotation to the threaded rods of distraction and compression motor devices decreases, the speed and rate of the movement of these rods has to be decreased accordingly.

The typical complication of severe knee flexion contracture correction is posterior tibial subluxation. In this situation, the anterior translation of the tibia, with the creation of more arthodiastasis can substitute temporarily for angulation correction. But to continue translation the frame must be reinforced with more hinged components.

Correction of Joint Contracture Combined With Deformity

In most clinical situations this combination consists of subluxation that has resulted from congenital or acquired malformation, with restricted range of motion as the consequence. This is typical in radial clubhand and wrist contracture, clubfoot with ankle contracture, and fibular hemimelia with foot contracture.

Elimination of the deformity must precede contracture correction. To accomplish this, the main supporting part of the frame is applied to the affected limb; in addition, the hinged correcting component is connected (Fig. 14.13).

Correction of Joint Fused in Malposition

For functional and cosmetic reasons, the joint fused in malposition can be corrected by a combination of osteotomy with gradual distraction, and then can be fused again in a more acceptable position. In this type of treatment three major factors must be considered:

1. Severity of malposition.
2. Projected correction, with moderate malposition. It is possible to achieve correction by simple transverse osteotomy and an opening wedge type of distraction. In this treatment, the local blood circulation and nerve tropism usually are not disturbed much.
3. Surrounding soft tissue preservation.

With severe malposition it is more rational to perform the wedge osteotomy followed by gradual compression, With this treatment there is risk of local blood circulation and nerve tropism disturbances. To avoid this, gradual correction is recommended.

In both types of treatment the main supporting part of the frame is applied to the affected limb and the hinged correcting component is connected to it. In many situations the fused joint correction must be combined with simultaneous lengthening and/or straightening of the limb (Fig. 14.14).

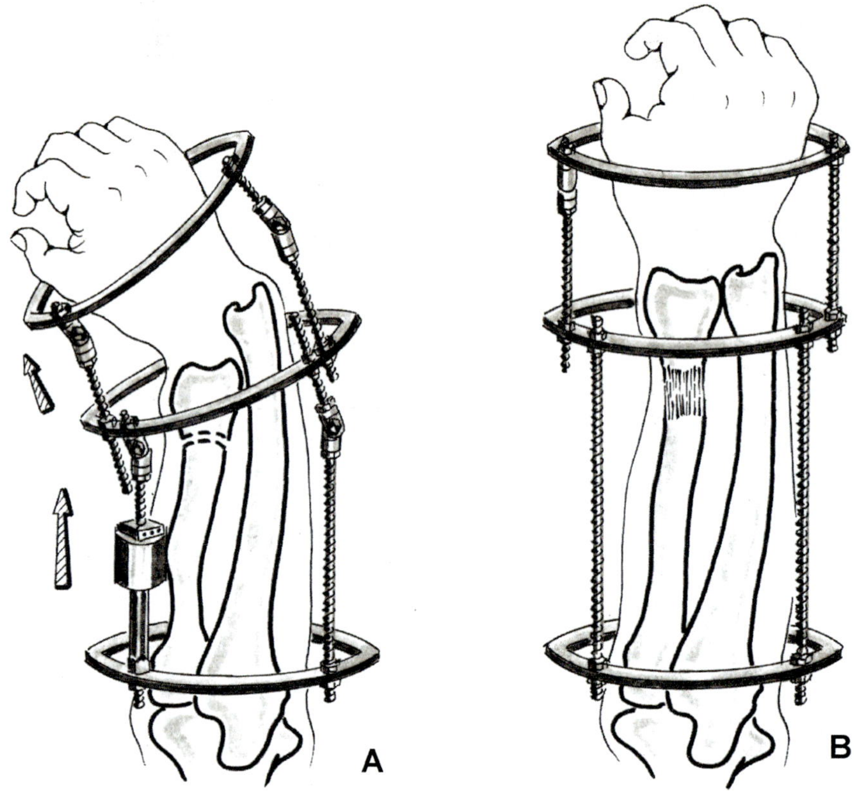

Figure 14.13: Correction of wrist joint deformity combined with clubhand. Two-ring main supporting frame is applied to the forearm and connected with the hinged correcting hand component. Radial bone corticotomy is indicated by *interrupted line. Arrows* indicate direction of distraction. **A,** view before distraction. **B,** corrected radial bone and wrist deformities

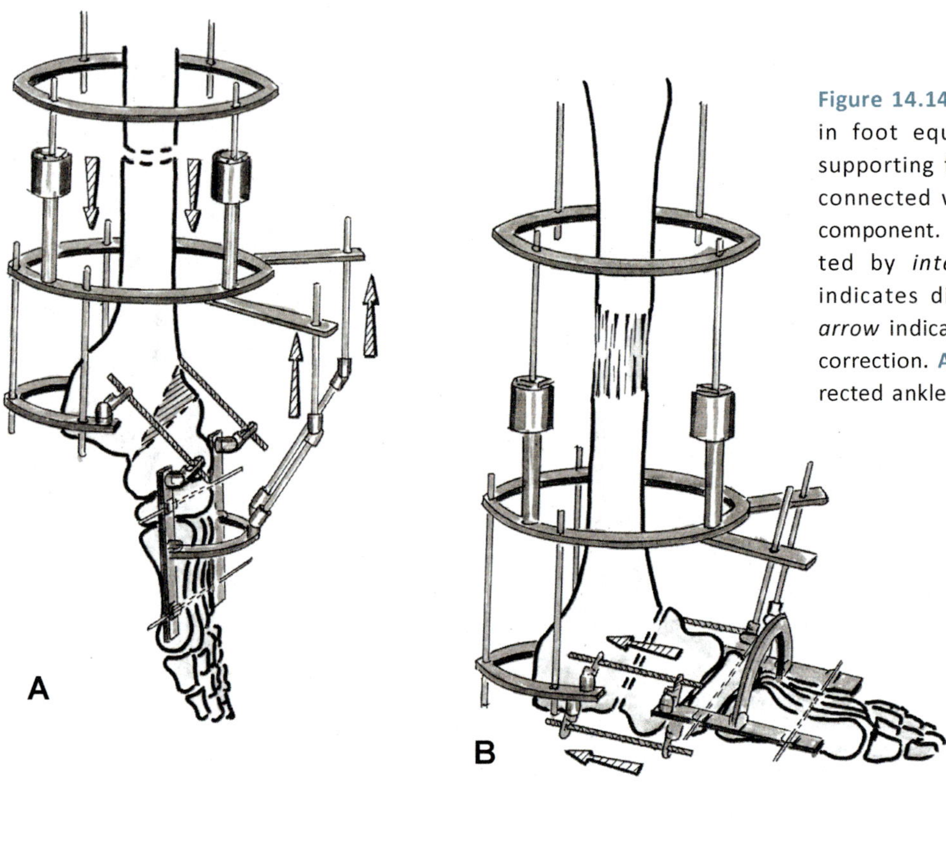

Figure 14.14: Correction of ankle joint fused in foot equinus position. Two-ring main supporting frame is applied to the leg and connected with the hinged correcting foot component. Wedge-type osteotomy is indicated by *interrupted line. Straight arrow* indicates direction of distraction; *curved arrow* indicates direction of ankle deformity correction. **A,** view before distraction. **B,** corrected ankle and foot position

CASE ILLUSTRATIONS

Figures 14.15 to 14.24 illustrate cases in which distraction-compression techniques were used.

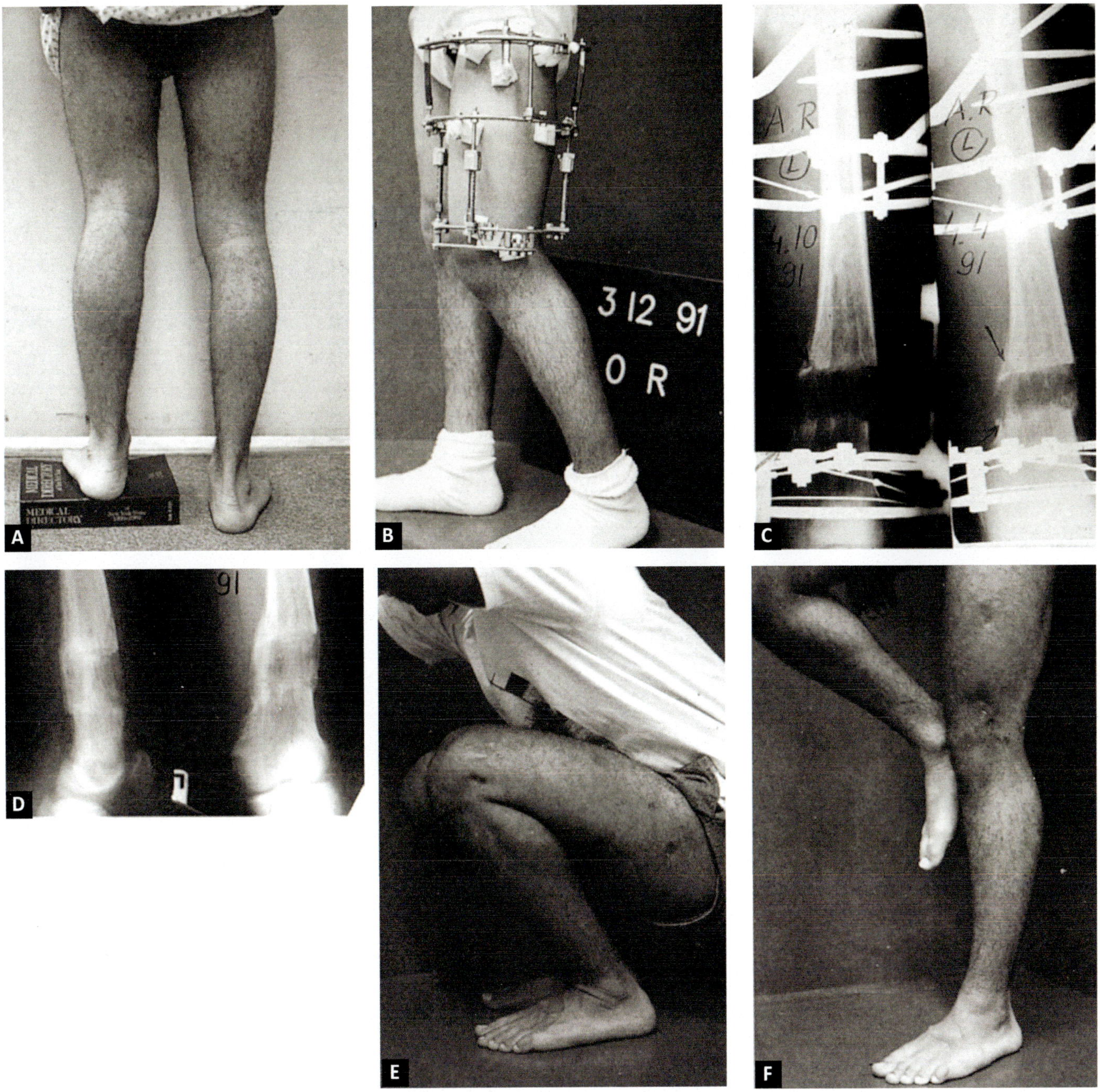

Figure 14.15: Femur Lengthening. Fourteen-year-old youth with 5 cm of congenital left femur shortness caused by Ollier disease. A, appearance of legs before treatment. B, left leg with Ilizarov apparatus 14 days after surgery. C, lateral and anteroposterior radiographs of the femur 40 days after distal corticotomy and distraction of 3 cm. D, lateral and anteroposterior radiographs of left femur after removal of the apparatus 3 months after surgery show 5 cm of distraction and calcified bone regenerate development. E and F, appearance of legs and functional result at 18 months after treatment

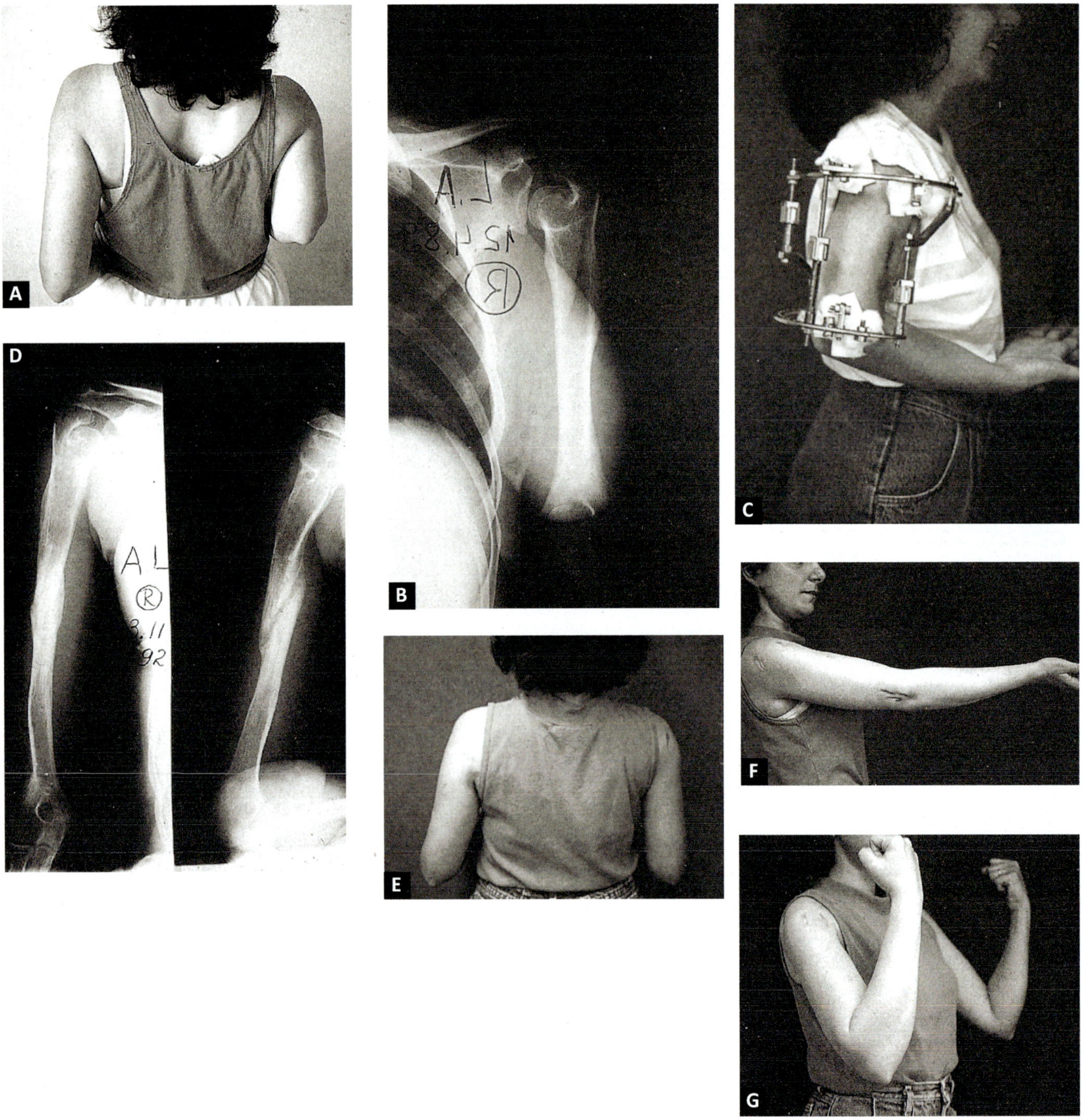

Figures 14.16: Humeral Lengthening. Thirty-one-year-old woman with 9-cm shortness of right humerus as a sequela of infection when the patient was 3 months of age. **A,** appearance of upper arms before treatment. **B,** radiograph of the right humerus before treatment. **C,** right upper arm with Ilizarov apparatus 15 months after surgery. **D,** lateral and anteroposterior radiographs of the right humerus 2 years after surgery, with 9 cm of distraction. Healed oblique stress fracture is seen at the regenerate site. **E,** appearance of both upper arms 2 years after treatment. **F** and **G,** functional results of treatment

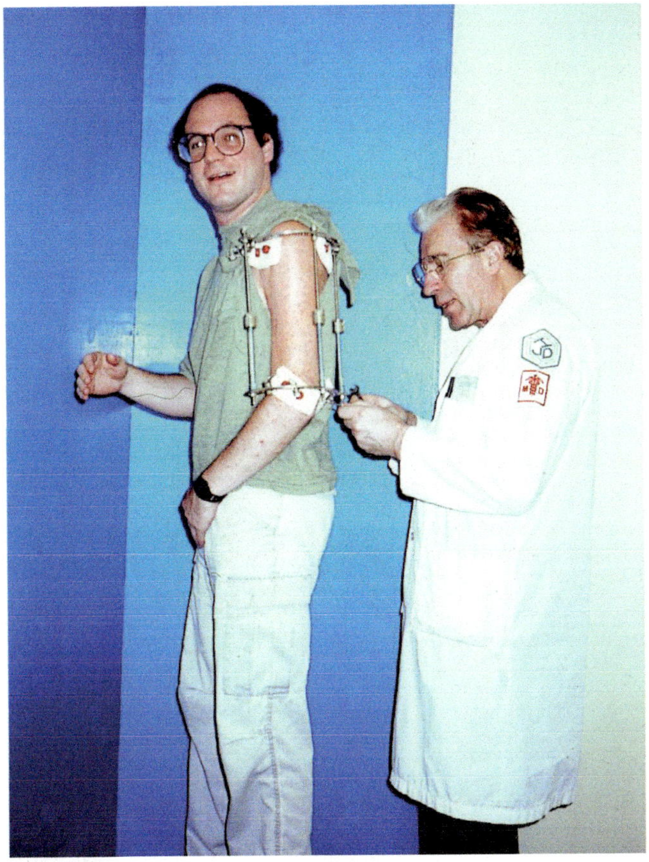

Figures 14.16H: Dr V Golyakhovsky with a patient after lengthening his left upper arm

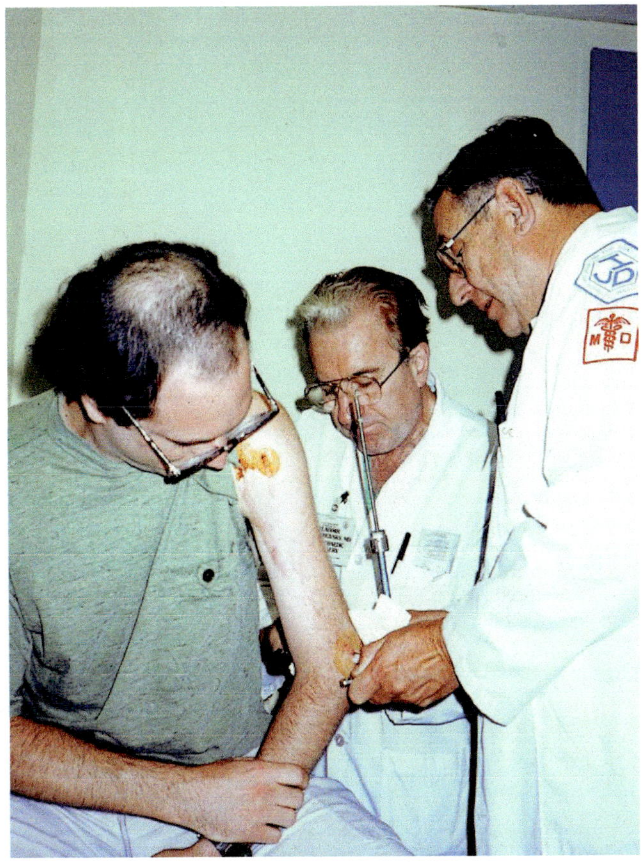

Figures 14.16I: Drs V Golyakhovsky (left) and V Frankel removing the Ilizarov apparatus from the patient's left upper arm after lengthening

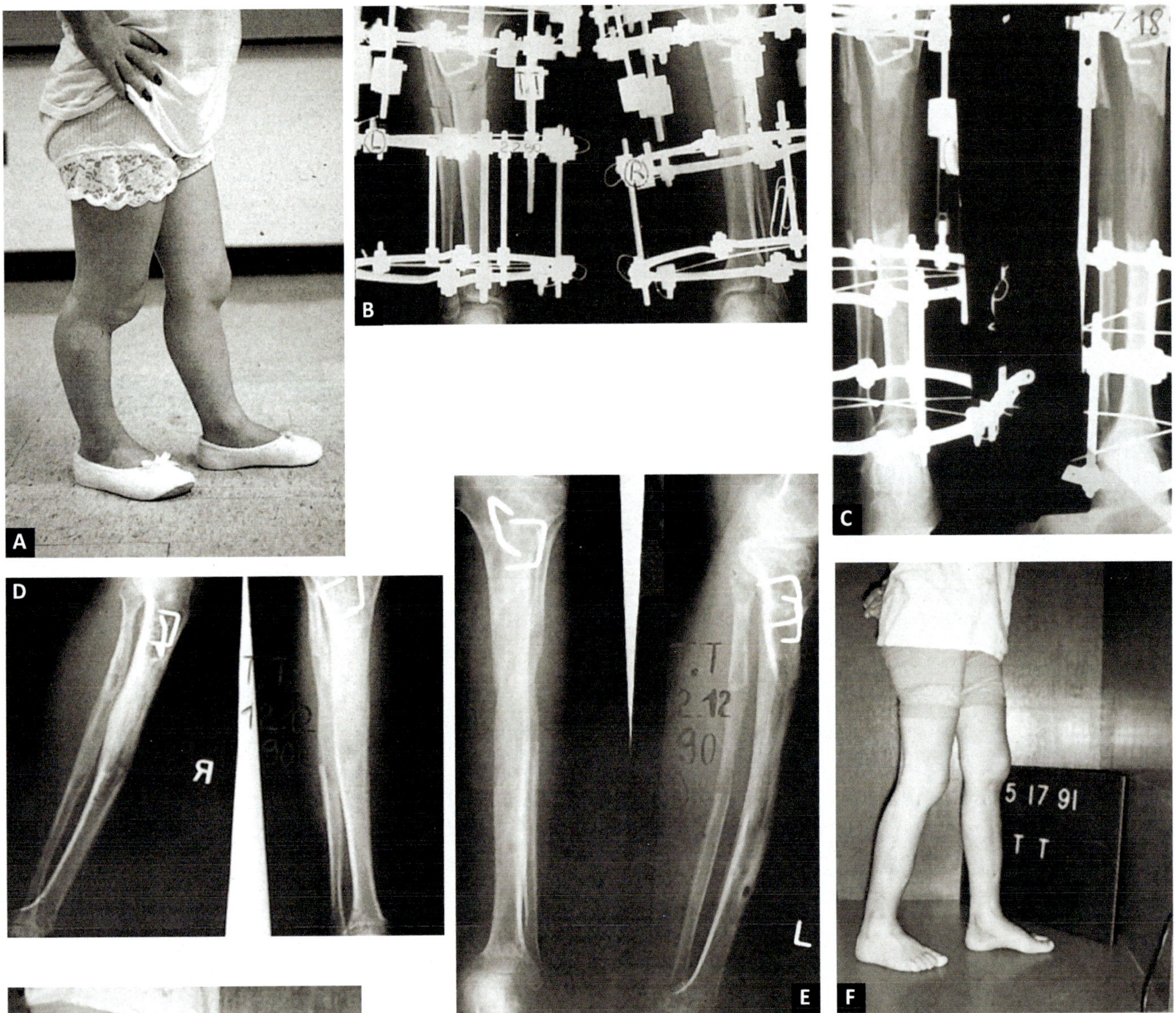

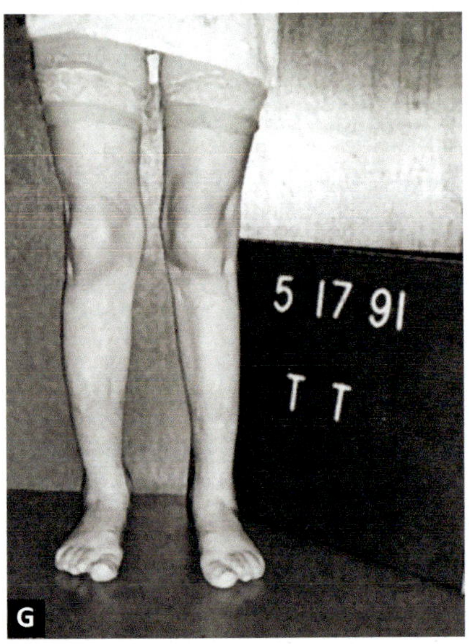

Figure 14.17: Bilateral Leg Lengthening. Twenty-year-old woman with multiple epiphyseal dysplasia, status post-tibial osteotomy for genu varum of the legs (performed elsewhere), and shortness of both legs. **A,** appearance of legs before surgery. **B,** anteroposterior radiographs of both legs immediately after proximal corticotomy and application of Ilizarov apparatus to both tibias. **C,** anteroposterior radiographs of both legs 6 months after surgery, with 12 cm of distraction. **D** and **E,** anteroposterior and lateral radiographs of both legs 10 months after surgery, with 12 cm of distraction, immediately after apparatus removal. **F** and **G,** appearance of legs 16 months after treatment

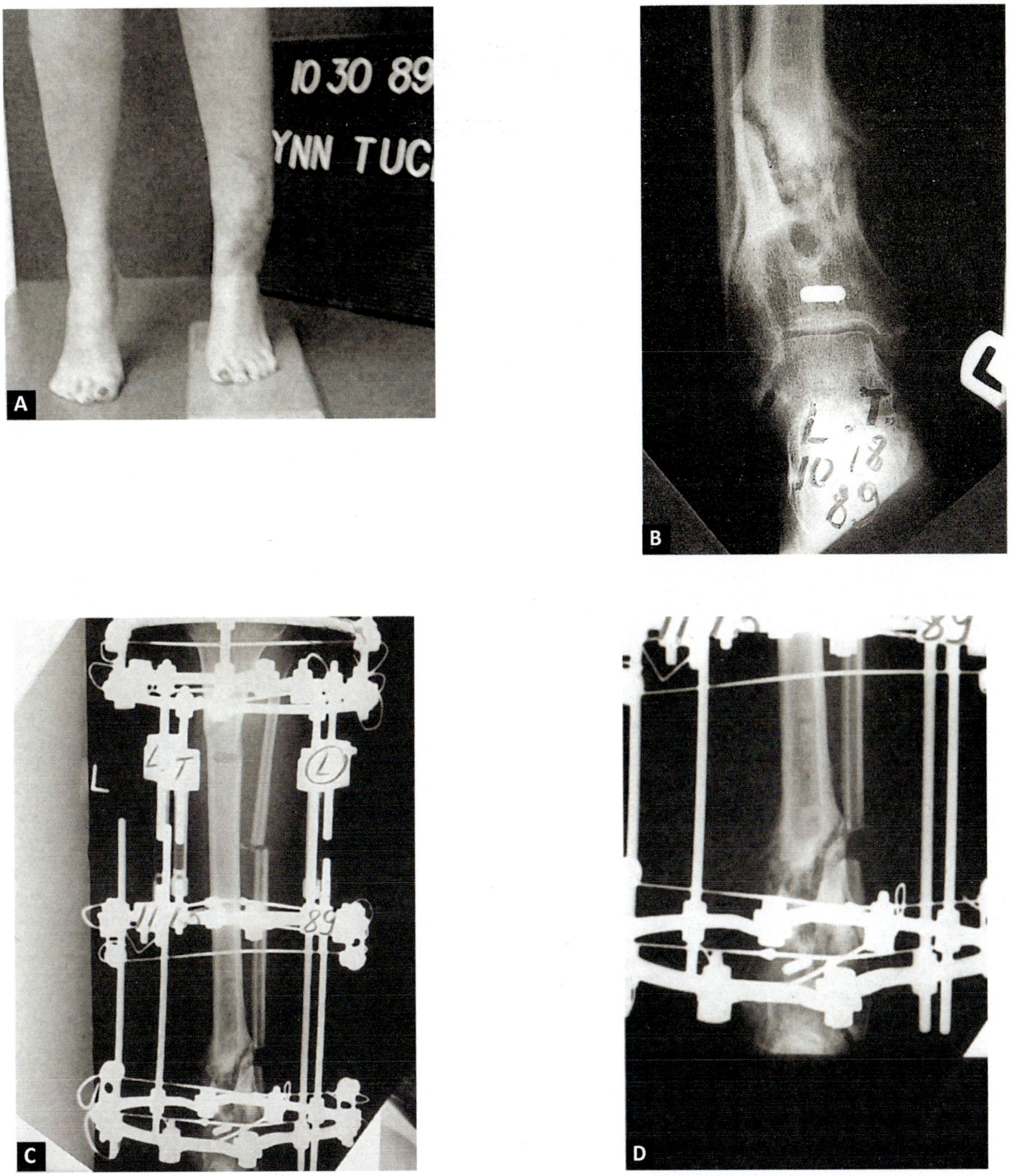

Figure 14.18: Tibial Nonunion with Compression Distraction. Thirty-seven-year-old woman with infected nonunion of the distal left tibia, shortness of 2 cm, varus deformity, and persistent pain syndrome. Patient had a history of unsuccessful multiple surgeries of left leg performed elsewhere. A, appearance of legs before surgery. B, anteroposterior radiograph of distal part of left leg shows hypertrophic type of tibial and fibular nonunion, with varus angulation and multiple cavities post screws, and bone infection. C, radiograph of left leg after proximal tibial corticotomy with distal fibular resection, medial fibular osteotomy, and application of Ilizarov fixator, Compression-distraction technique was used, with simultaneous distraction at the corticotomy site and compression of the nonunion site without opening and resection. D, anteroposterior radiograph of left leg 15 days after surgery. Compression is defined by concave appearance of the wires above and below the nonunion site

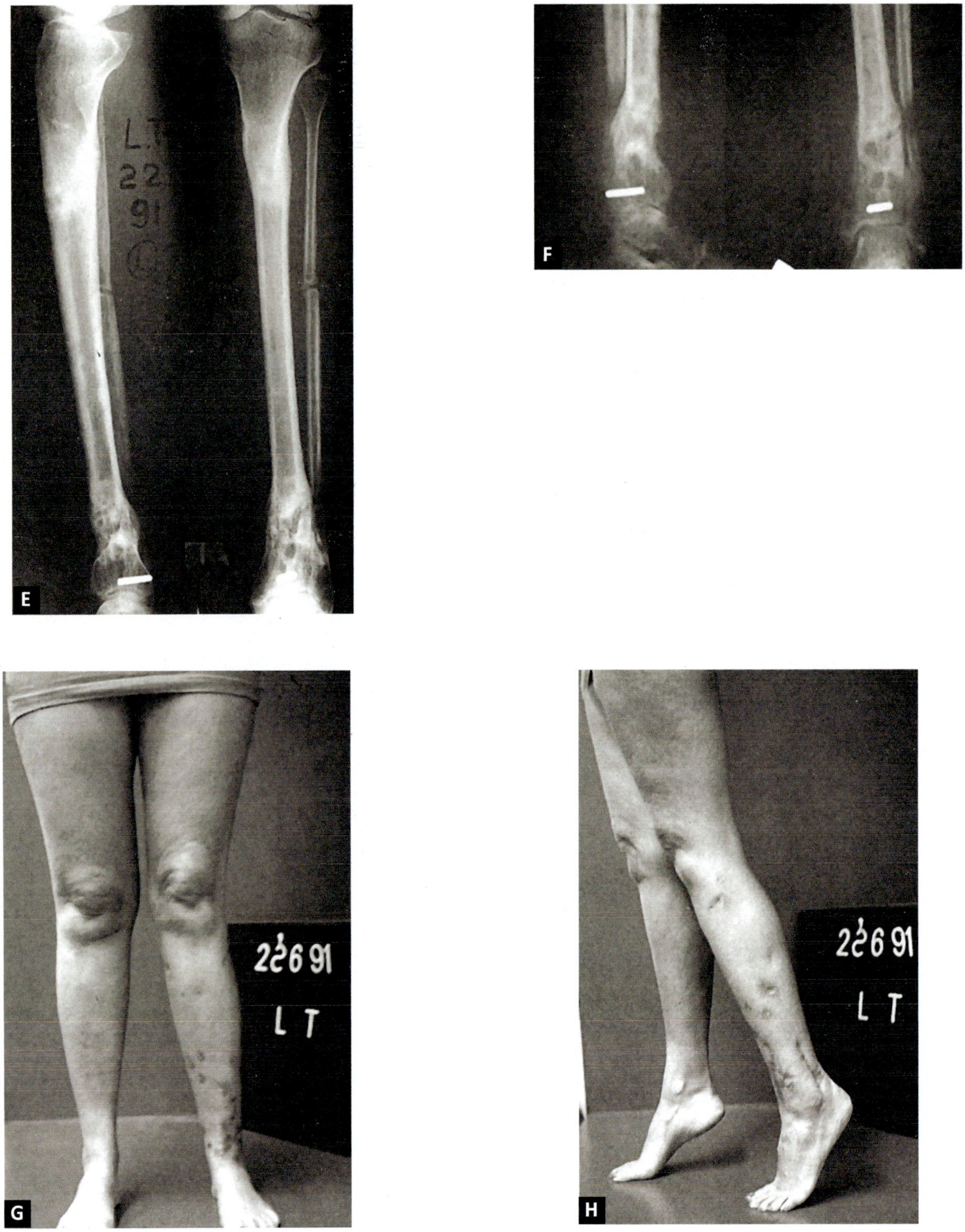

Figure 14.18 (Contd): E, lateral and anteroposterior radiographs of the left leg 16 months after surgery and 12 months after apparatus removal, with 2.5 cm of distraction and regenerate development at the proximal corticotomy site, and healed distal nonunion at the compression site. F, lateral and anteroposterior radiographs of distal part of left leg 16 months after treatment. G, appearance of legs 16 months after treatment. H, functional results of treatment

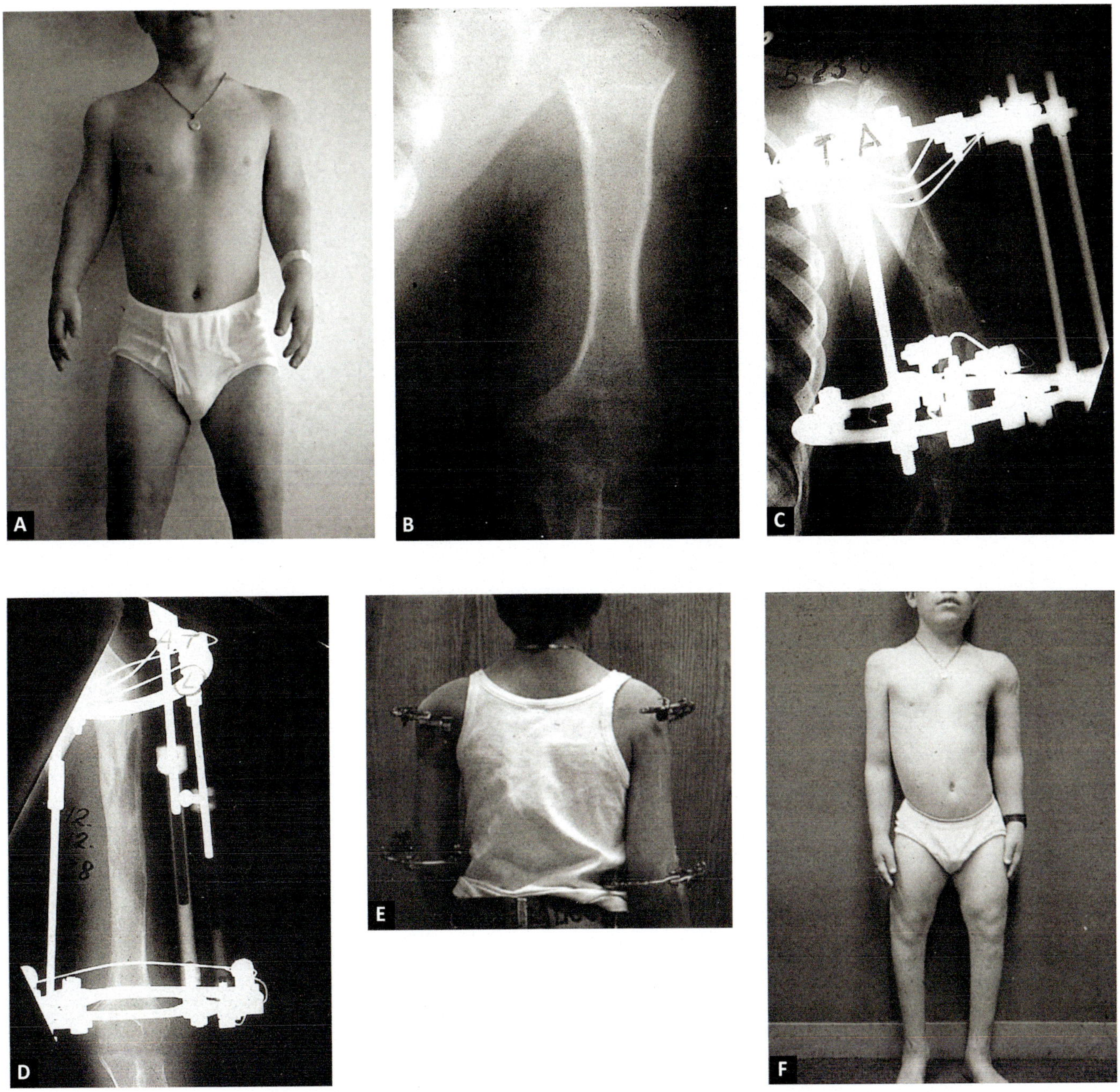

Figure 14.19: Humeri and Femora Lengthenings for Achondroplasia. Thirteen-year-old boy with achondroplasia, status post-bitibial lengthenings performed elsewhere, and short upper arms and femurs. Six limb lengthenings were performed in this patient using the distraction technique. A, appearance before treatment. B, AP radiograph of the left humerus. C, radiograph of the left humerus 6 weeks after proximal corticotomy, Ilizarov apparatus application, and 3.5 cm of distraction. Identical procedure was performed on the right humerus 1 month later. Distraction forces can be defined clearly by the convex appearance of the wires. Note premature healing at the site of corticotomy. Rate of distraction (0.25 mm four times per day) was too slow for this patient. D, radiograph of the left humerus 8 months after the first surgery and 6 months after the second corticotomy was performed to continue distraction. Rate of distraction was increased to 0.25 mm six times per day on both arms. Distraction of 16 cm of both humeri was achieved. E, patient with apparatus on both upper arms just before removal, 6 months after surgeries. F, appearance after lengthening of both legs (performed elsewhere) and both upper arms. Short thighs can be seen clearly

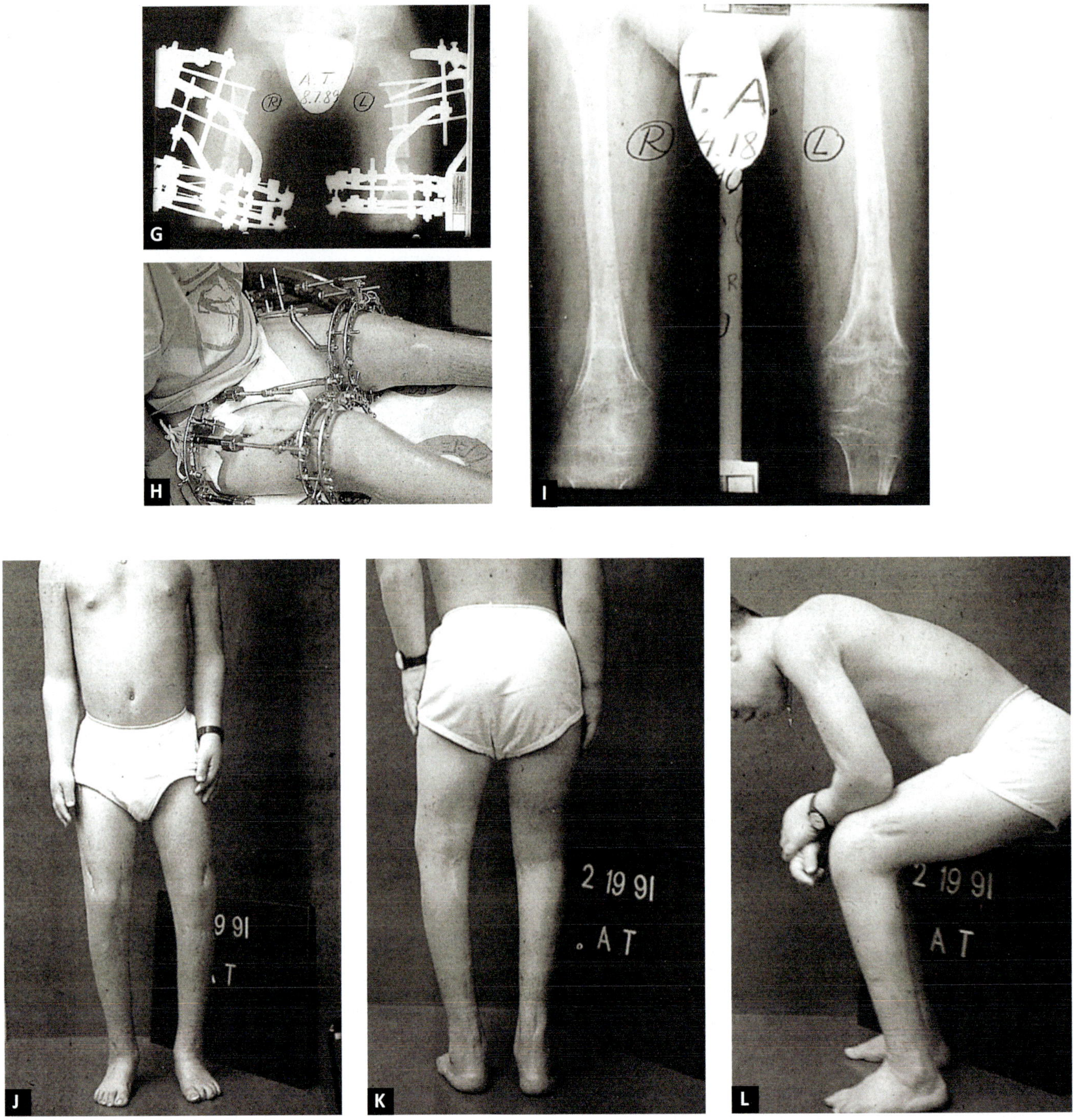

Figure 14.19 (Contd): G, AP radiograph of both femurs after distal corticotomies had been performed simultaneously, with application of two Ilizarov frames. H, appearance of both legs after 6 weeks of distraction at a rate of 0.25 mm, six times per day. I, AP radiographs of both femurs 8½ months after surgery and 1½ months after apparatus removal. Distraction of 12 cm was achieved, with development of completely calcified bone. J—L, results 3 years after treatment of both upper arms and 1½ years after treatment of both femurs

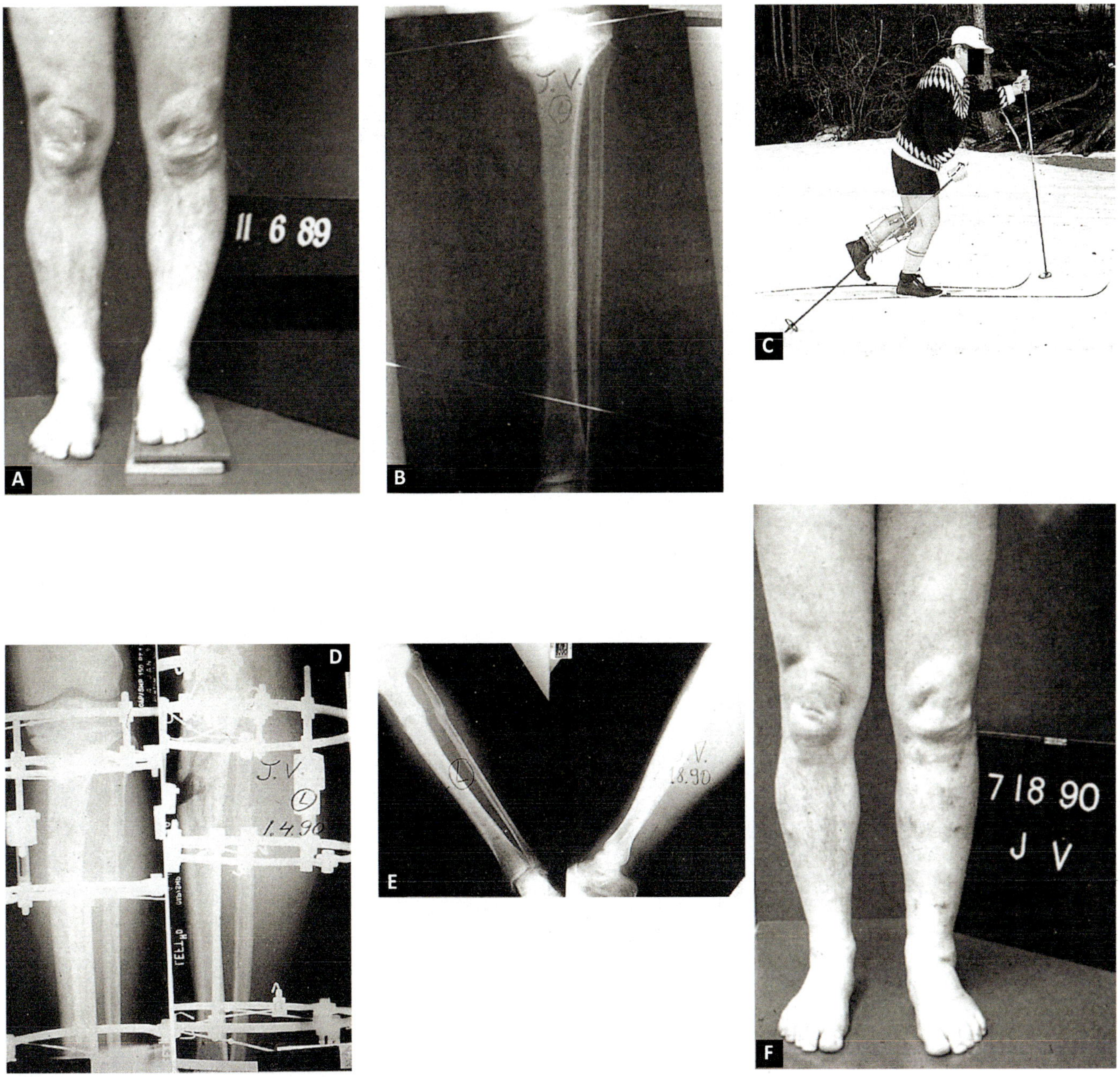

Figure 14.20: Correction of Nonunion with Deformity and Shortness of Tibial Plateau. Fifty-two-year-old man with nonunion of the proximal left tibia after tibial plateau fracture and 3 cm of shortness and varus deformity, status post-open reduction and internal fixation with high tibial opening wedge osteotomy performed elsewhere. **A,** Appearance of legs before surgery. **B,** AP radiograph of left leg on the operating table, with two K-wires introduced before procedure to determine proper position and inclination of the rings. **C,** patient activity 2 weeks after surgery. **D,** AP and lateral radiograph of left leg 2 months after proximal tibial corticotomy, fibular osteotomy, and Ilizarov fixator application. Simultaneous compression at the nonunion site was combined with distraction at the corticotomy site and correction of varus deformity **E,** AP and lateral radiographs of left leg 8½ months after surgery and 2 months after fixator removal show good healing at the sites of nonunion and corticotomy, and straight fragments alignment. **F,** appearance of legs 8½ months after surgery

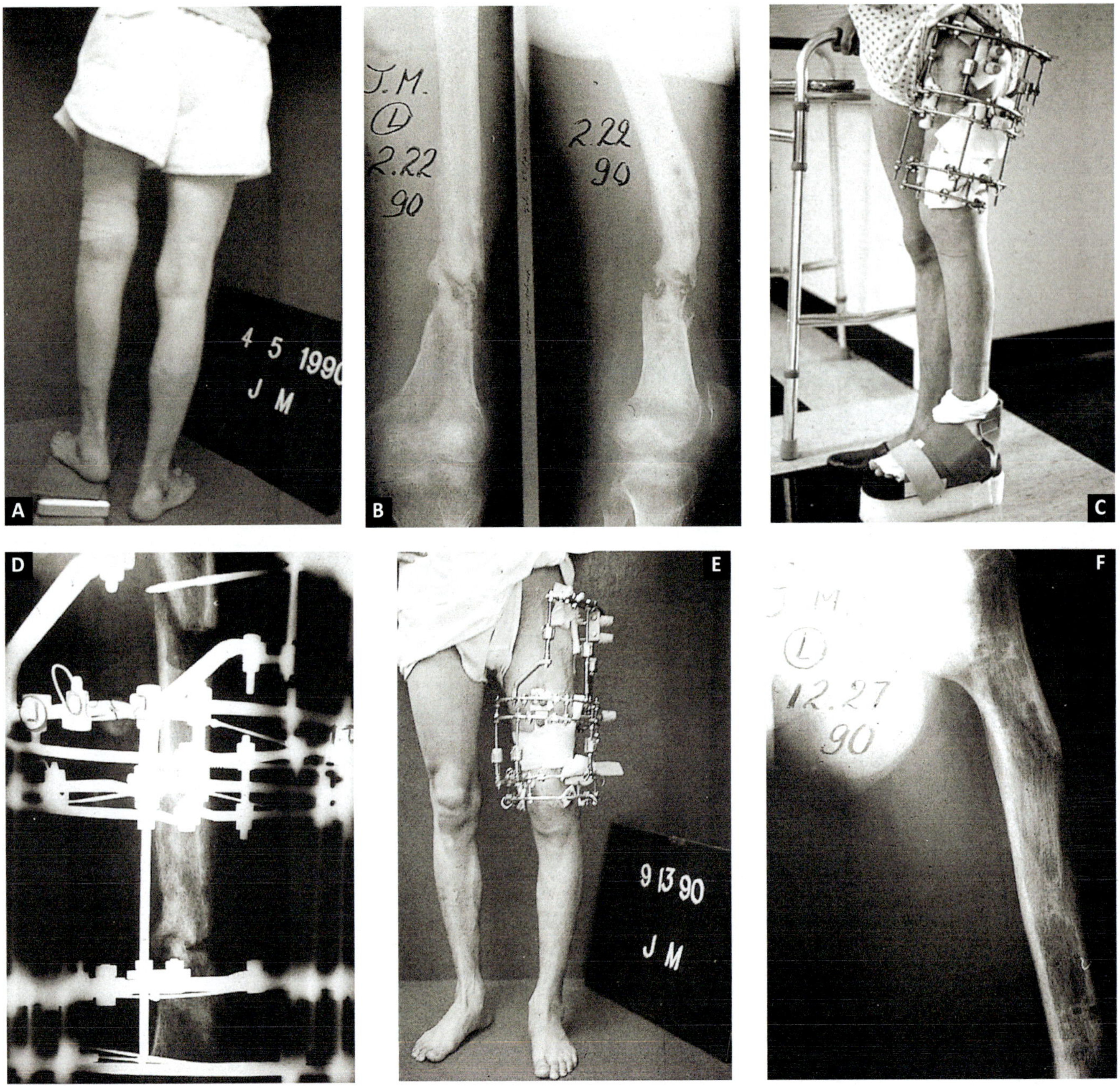

Figure 14.21: Bone Transport for Infected Femoral Nonunion. Eighteen-year-old man with infected nonunion of the left femur, active drainage at the nonunion site, and shortness of 5 cm. Patient had a history of unsuccessful multiple surgeries of the left femur performed elsewhere. A, appearance of legs before surgery. B, AP and lateral radiographs of left femur before surgery. C, appearance of the left leg 1 week after surgery, with an Ilizarov four-ring, one-arch fixator. D, AP radiograph of the left femur 1½ months after subtrochanteric corticotomy with subsequent distraction, combined with open reduction, partial resection, and debridement at the nonunion site, with subsequent compression (simultaneous with distraction). E, appearance of the legs 5 months after surgery. Combined simultaneous compression-distraction of the left femur is accomplished, and length of both legs equalized. F, AP radiograph of the proximal part of left femur 8½ months after surgery and 2 months after apparatus removal. Seven centimeters of lengthening was achieved by distraction at the site of subtrochanteric corticotorny, with development of well-calcified regenerate

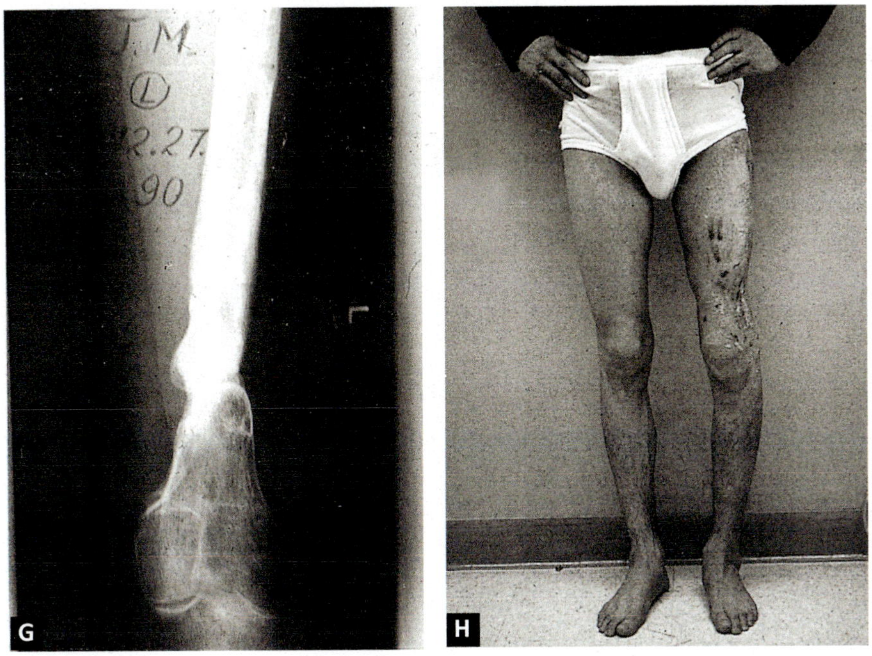

Figure 14.21 (Contd): **G,** AP radiograph of the distal part of left femur 8½ months after surgery and 2 months after apparatus removal. Complete nonunion healing is achieved with compression simultaneous to distraction of the proximal part. **H,** appearance of legs 1 year after surgery

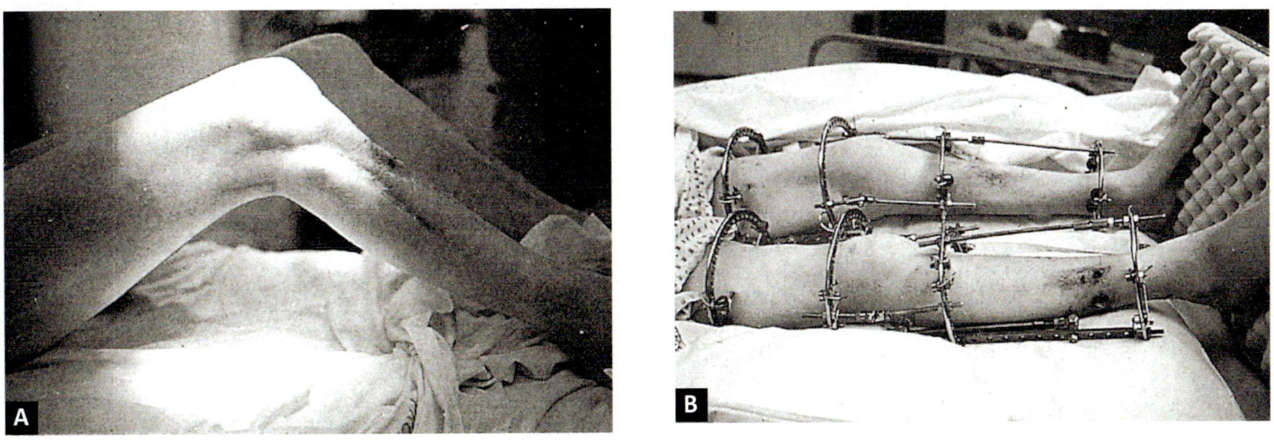

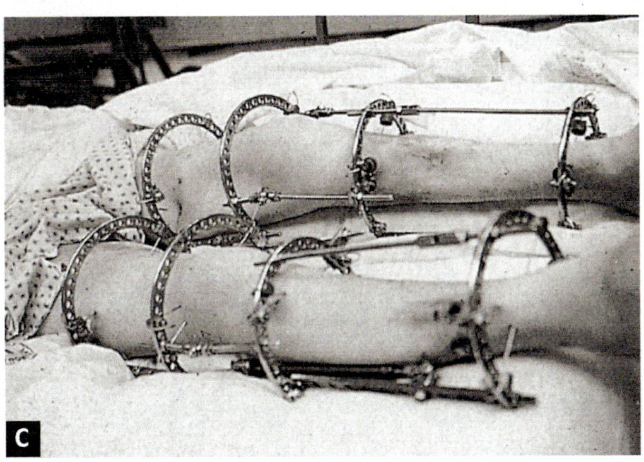

Figure 14.22: Correction of Bilateral Knee Flexion Contracture. Thirty-three-year-old woman with flexion contracture of both knees secondary to prolonged bedrest following severe head trauma. Range of motion in both knees was 70 to 110 degrees (extension to flexion). **A,** appearance of legs before procedure. **B,** 2 months after Ilizarov fixator application to both legs and gradual correction of flexion contracture without incisions or tendon lengthening. **C,** 4 months after apparatus application, just before removal. Extension up to 180 degrees was achieved at the right side and up to 175 degrees at the left side. After removal of the apparatus, custom plastic braces with knee hinges were made for both legs

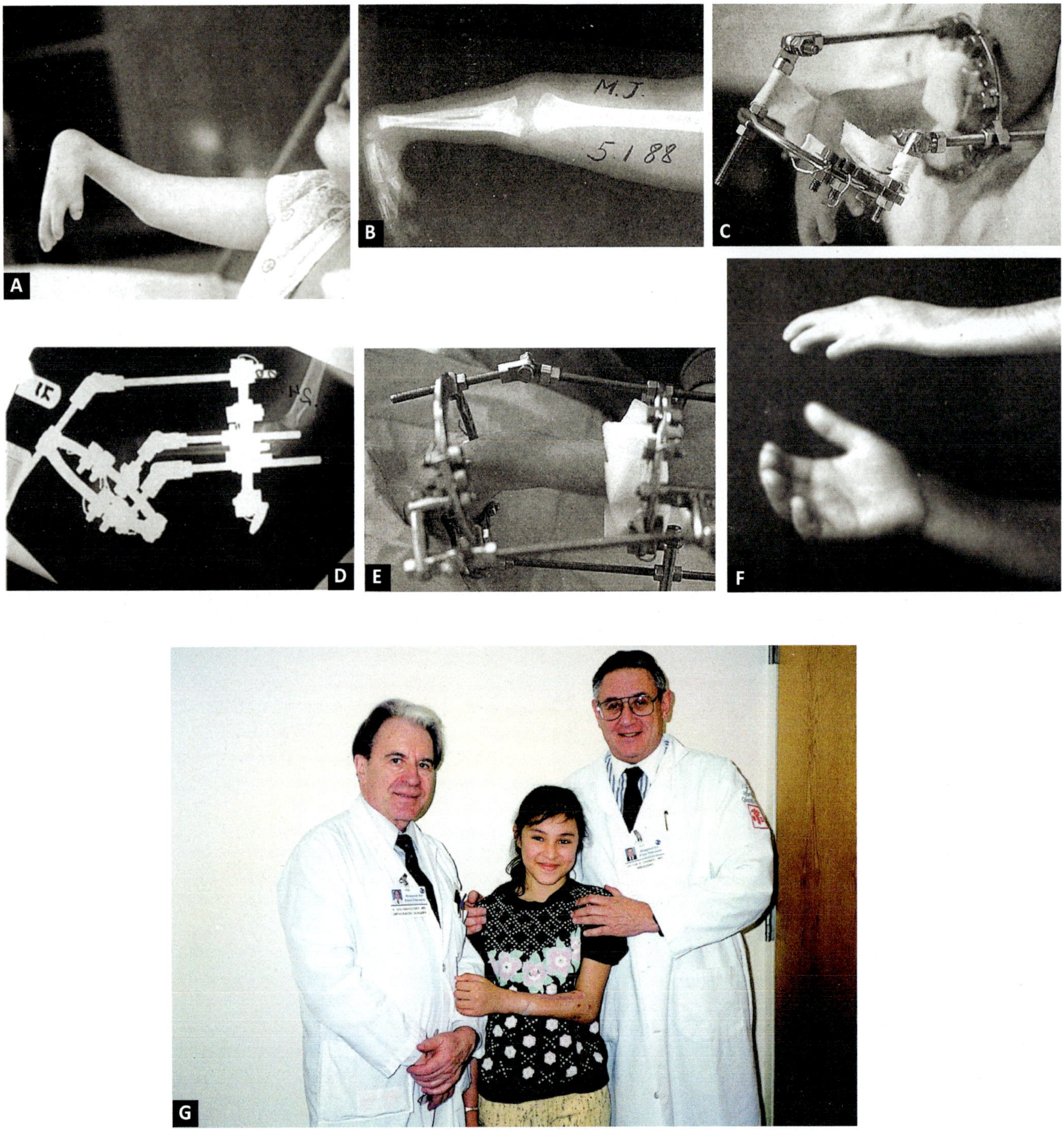

Figure 14.23: Correction of Wrist Contracture. Seven-year-old boy with Pollard syndrome and flexion contracture of right wrist. A, appearance of the right upper extremity before surgery. B, radiograph of right upper extremity before surgery. C, right upper extremity with Ilizarov fixator 1 week after application. No incisions or tendon lengthening was performed. Three hinges are situated at the wrist axis: one upper hinge and two side hinges. D, radiograph of the same forearm during gradual distraction and wrist straightening 1½ months after apparatus application. E, forearm during gradual soft tissue distraction 2 months after apparatus application. Two side hinges have been replaced by threaded rods. F, appearance of both hands and wrists 1½ years after treatment. Stable right wrist extension was achieved. G, Drs V.Golyakhovsky (left) and V Frankel with a patient after correction nonunion and lengthening her left forearm (the X-ray films of this patient are not presented in the book)

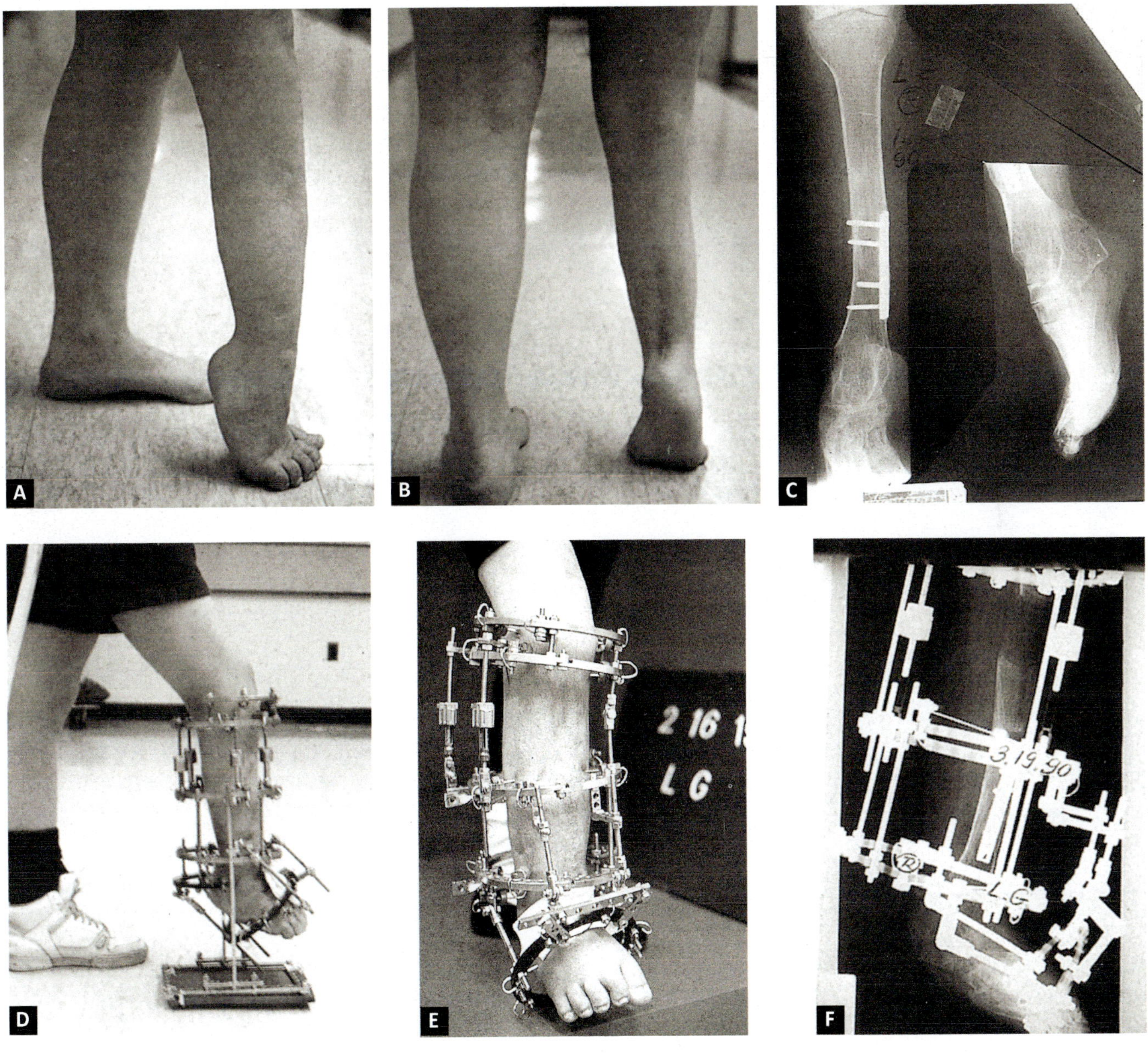

Figure 14.24: Lengthening of Tibia and Correction of Ankle Ankylosis. Twenty-year-old woman with congenital clubfoot and fibular hemimelia of the right leg, accompanied by the shortness of 8 cm, and ankle ankylosis in position of 170 degrees plantar-flexion. Patient had a history of unsuccessful multiple surgeries of the right foot performed since early childhood, and an unsuccessful attempt at lengthening of the right leg. A, B, appearance of legs before surgery. C, lateral radiograph of the right leg. D, appearance of right leg 2 weeks after corticotomy of proximal tibia with application of the four-ring Ilizarov fixator, and the wedge-shaped osteotomy of right ankle with application of the hinged foot component of the apparatus, with subsequent simultaneous tibial lengthening and foot position correction by gradual combined distraction and compression. Foot platform was connected to the apparatus for axial leg loading. E, appearance of the right leg 2½ months after surgery, with leg lengthening achieved and the foot brought into neutral position. Correction of the valgus deviation can be noted by the hinges at the upper medial site. F, lateral radiograph of the distal part of the right leg 3½ months after surgery. Delayed regenerate formation can be noted at the upper part of the film, and neutral position of the foot with development of initial healing at the ankle site at the lower part of the film

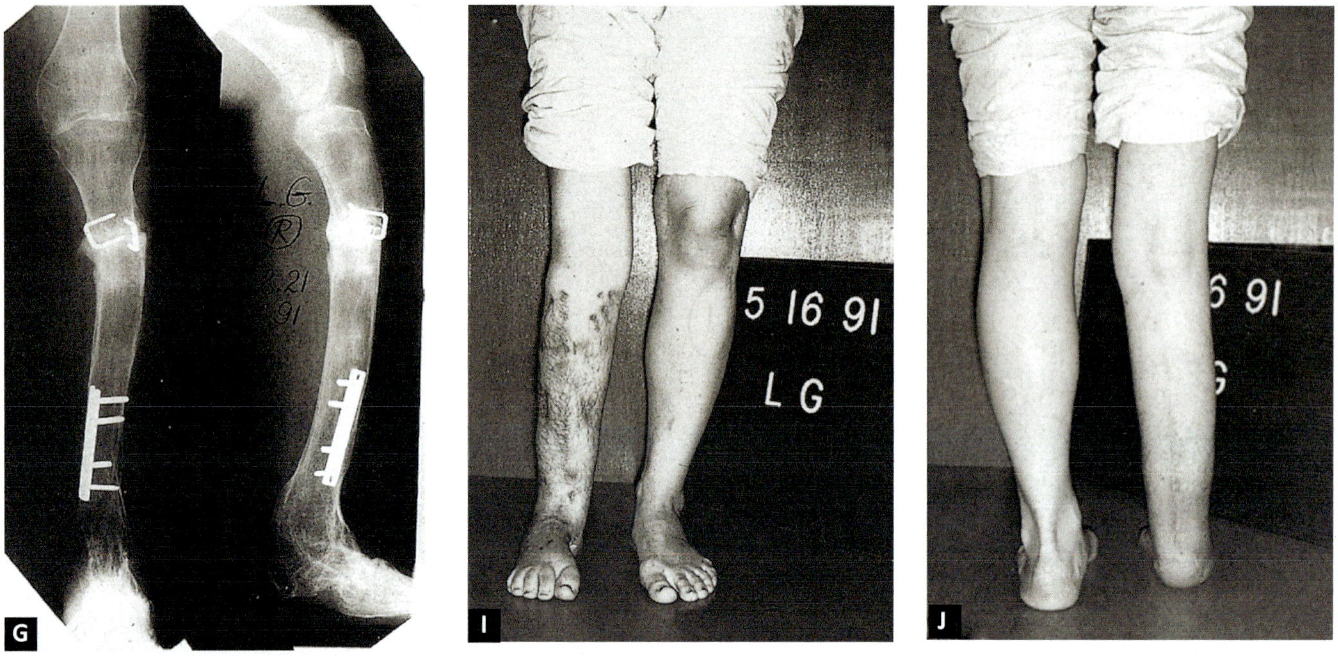

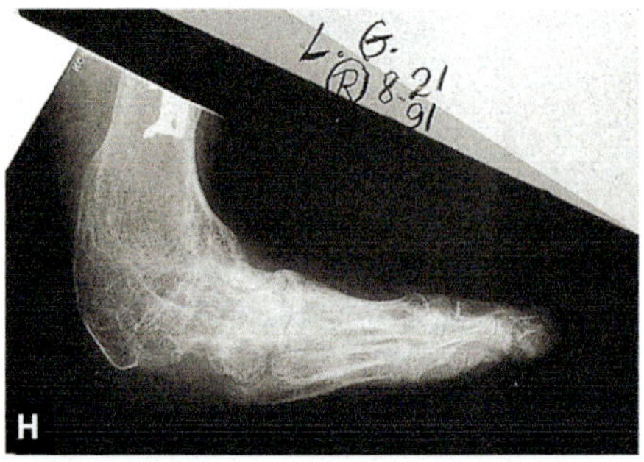

Figure 14.24 (Contd): G, AP and lateral radiograph of the right leg 8½ months after surgery and 2 months after apparatus removal shows stress fracture of the partially collapsed tibial regenerate with two-staple fixation. **H,** lateral radiograph of the right foot 8½ months after surgery. **I** and **J,** appearance of legs 15½ months after surgery

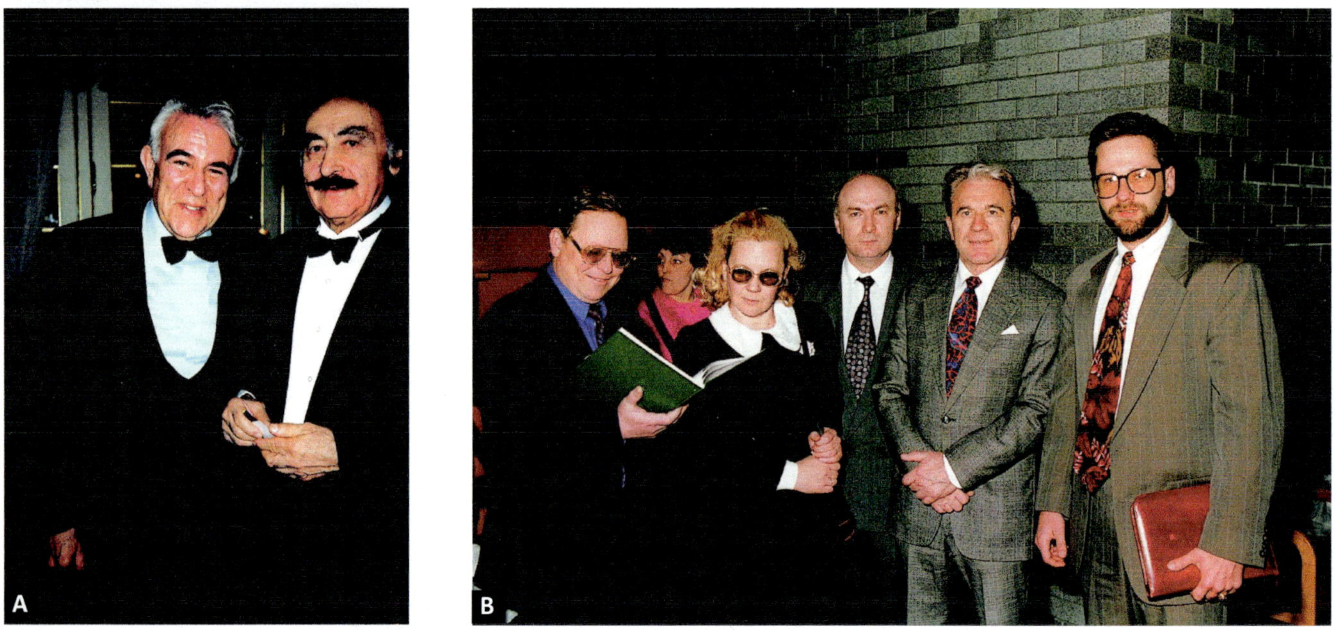

Figure 14.25: A, Dr Gavriil Ilizarov (right) with an American representative at the reception on his honor in New York. **B,** Dr V Golyakhovsky (second from right) with a group of Russian doctors of the Ilizarov Hospital from city of Kurgan at the reception in New York

15 Chapter

Segmental Bone Transport in Large Bone Loss and in Severe Infection

GENERAL CONSIDERATIONS

Treatment of large bone loss (3 cm and more) is one of the most complex problems in orthopedics. In many cases any or all of seven factors can be involved: bony defect, limb shortness, limb deformity, soft tissue scarring, local blood supply insufficiency, some degree of nerve insufficiency, or infection.

Ilizarov introduced a new technique of bone transport following corticotomy that consists of sliding a bone fragment internally to fill a defect and thus develop regenerate bone. This bone transport technique eliminates the need for bone grafting and makes possible simultaneous restoration of a bony defect, elimination of limb shortness, correction of deformity, improvement in the condition of the local soft tissues, increase in local blood circulation, improvement in nerve function, and possible elimination of infection.

The technique of bone transport provides a powerful tool for the treatment of large bone loss and severe osteomyelitis that require resection of a considerable piece of bone. The technique has become increasingly popular in the United States since first introduced in this country by Frankel in 1986.

The three types of bone transport technique are external, internal, and combined external-internal. They differ in the way that the bone fragments are transfixed to the frame and in how they are "transported" to the intended site. The external technique is indicated for combined bone loss replacement with correction of deformities and with lengthening of a limb, and the internal transport technique is indicated for bone loss replacement without deformity correction or limb lengthening.

EXTERNAL BONE TRANSPORT TECHNIQUE

The external bone transport technique consists of introducing K-wires transversely through the bone fragments and moving the fragments by shifting the rings to which they are transfixed. The distraction-compression forces act externally on the extremity. Depending on the presence or absence of limb shortness, the corticotomy is performed at one level (monofocal corticotomy) or two levels (bifocal corticotomy). In cases of major bone loss involving limb shortness, a bifocal corticotomy is performed and two bone fragments are transported simultaneously in the same direction (Fig. 15.1A). In a case of bone loss without limb shortness a monofocal corticotomy is performed and a single bone fragment is slowly transported into the desired position (Fig. 15.1B). In a case of major bone loss (e.g. following resection of an osteomyelitic bone of 10 cm or more) without limb shortness, a bifocal corticotomy is performed and two fragments are transported toward each other from opposing positions (Fig. 15.1C).

The external bone transport technique is more useful when the distance that each bone fragment is transported

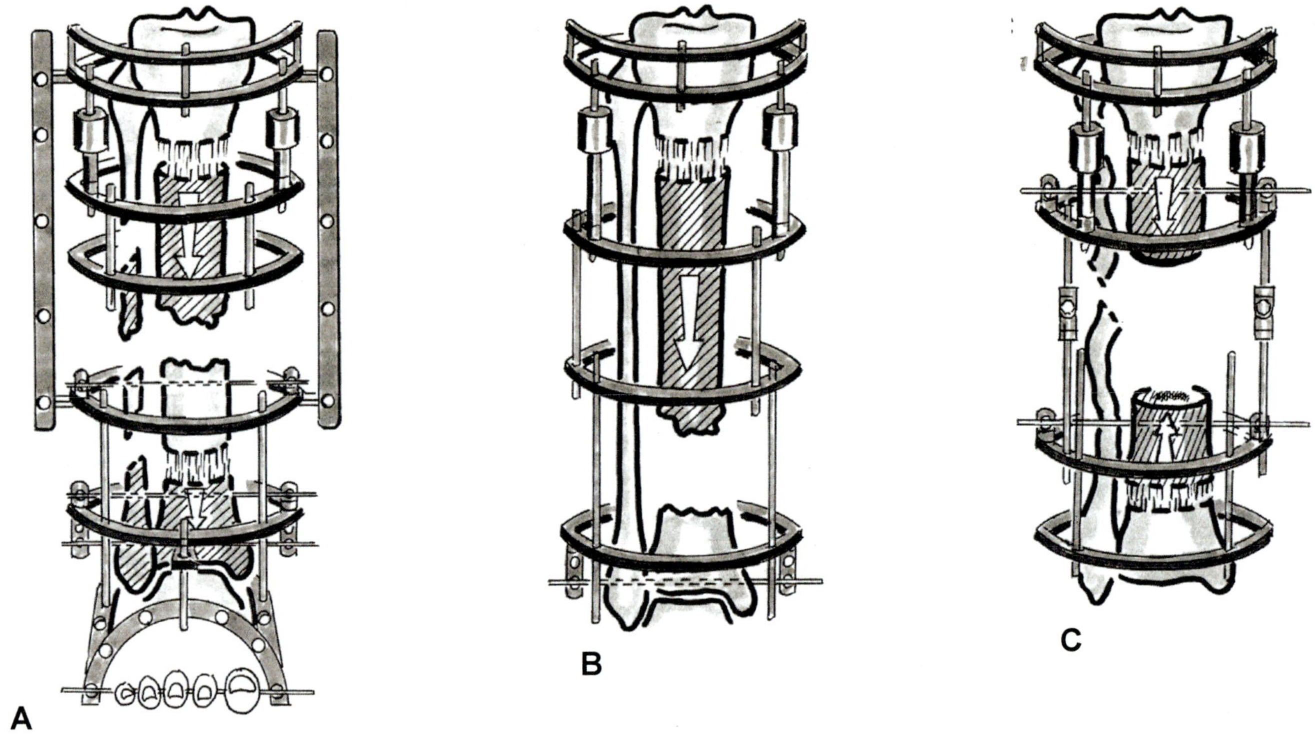

Figure 15.1: Three versions of the Ilizarov external bone transport technique. The transported bone fragments are *shaded*, the transport directions shown with *arrows*, the corticotomy sites with *interrupted thick lines*. A, for major tibial bone loss with substantial limb shortness, bifocal corticotomy and the transport of two fragments in the same direction distally are performed. Because the distal bone fragment is very short, the distal part of the frame is reinforced with the addition of a foot component. The proximal part of the frame is fortified by the addition of two long bars. B, in tibial bone loss without limb shortening, monofocal corticotomy and transport of the fragment distally are performed. No reinforcement of the frame is required. C, major tibial bone loss after bone shaft resection but without limb shortness requires bifocal corticotomy and the transport of two bone fragments toward each other. A correcting fibular osteotomy and insertion of correction hinges at the same level are performed

is no more than 5 to 7 cm. The frame of the apparatus consists of two or more connected but independently movable components. This is convenient for the correction of angulation and rotation because it allows insertion of corrective hinged devices.

INTERNAL BONE TRANSPORT TECHNIQUE

Internal bone transport consists of the introduction of K-wires obliquely to the bone fragments and the gradual sliding of those fragments to the desired position by distraction devices fixed to an immovable ring. The distraction-compression forces act internally, within the extremity. Depending on the size of the bony defect to be filled, a corticotomy is performed at one or two levels.

The frame of the apparatus differs from that of the external transport frame in that its components are not movable and are fastened to each other by long connecting bars, the rings remain fixed, fewer rings are required, and distraction devices are attached to the ring. Two types of K-wires are used for transport: olive wires and hooked wires.

This technique is more useful in cases of bone loss of 7 to 10 cm and larger. The frame of the apparatus consists of nonmovable rings. It is not convenient for the correc-

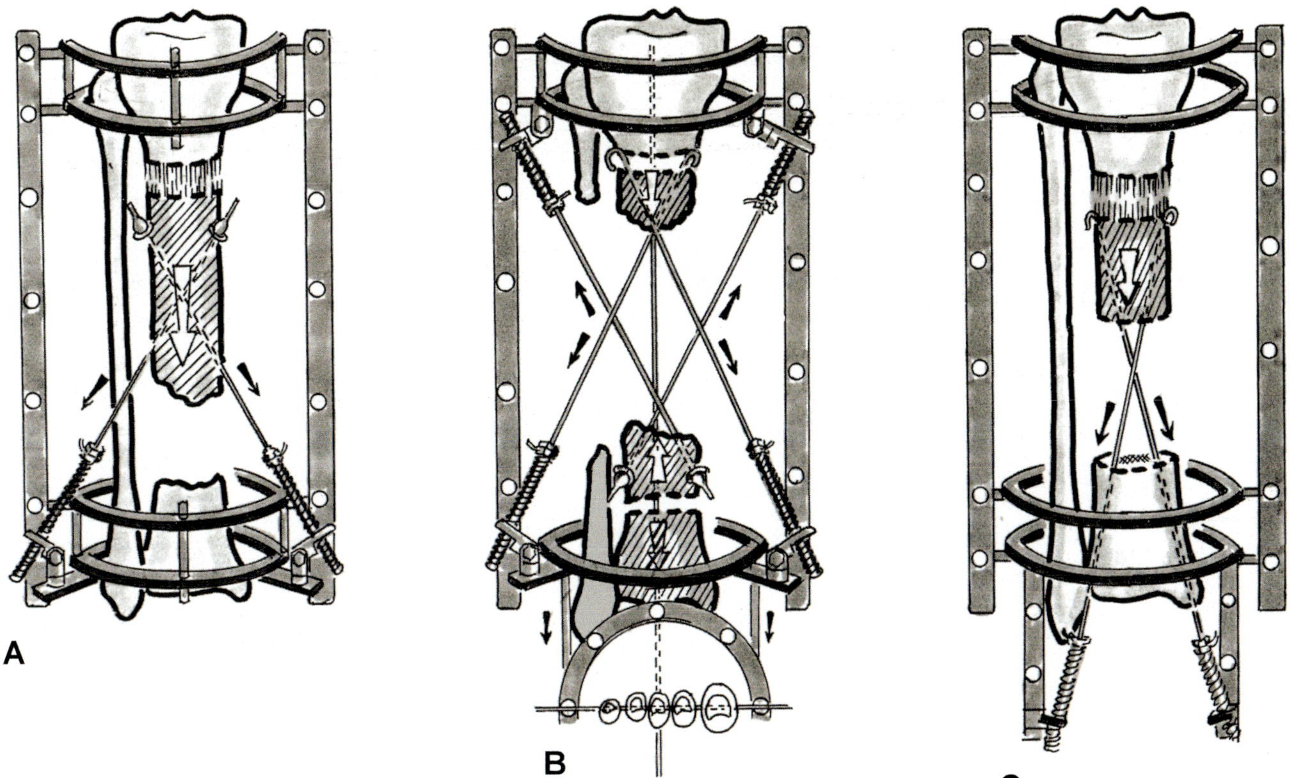

Figure 15.2: Three versions of the Ilizarov internal bone transport technique. Direction of the transporting forces is shown by *black arrows*. A, correction of a tibial bone loss without limb shortness requires monofocal corticotomy and transport via two obliquely introduced olive wires. Two inclined directions of the transporting forces turn into one resultant straight force *(large arrow)*. The distal end of each wire is fixed to a distraction device. B, major tibial bone loss is treated with bifocal corticotomy and transport of two bone fragments toward each other by four obliquely introduced wires. The hooked wires are shown proximally and the olive wires distally. An additional directing straight wire has been introduced through the calcaneus and through both tibial bone fragments. Because the distal bone fragment is very short, it is reinforced by the addition of a foot component. C, major tibial bone loss (e.g. following resection for osteomyelitis) without limb shortness requires monofocal corticotomy and transport of the fragment by two hooked wires. These wires are introduced obliquely through the two bone fragments and serve as transporting and directing forces, eliminating the need for an additional directing wire

tion of angulation and rotation because it does not allow insertion of correcting hinged devices. Without limb shortness, the transport is accomplished by using two crossed oblique wires (Fig. 15.2A).

In cases of major bone loss, transport is achieved in opposite directions, with the sliding fragments approaching each other. To avoid deviation of the fragments being transported, introduction of an additional straight guidewire into the bone marrow canal is recommended (Fig. 15.2B).

In cases in which bone loss is combined with significant limb shortness an additional corticotomy of a distal fragment is performed, and distraction at this level is produced simultaneously with bone transport. The distal part of the frame is reinforced by addition of a foot component, and the rate of distraction must be half the usual 1 mm/day, because it is being performed in opposite directions.

In cases of major bone loss (more than 15 cm) without limb shortness the transport is performed by two wires introduced obliquely through two fragments. This maneuver helps prevent deviation of the transported fragment (Fig. 15.2C).

COMBINED EXTERNAL-INTERNAL TRANSPORT TECHNIQUE

The combined external-internal bone transport technique consists of the introduction of K-wires transversely to one fragment of the bone, as in external transport, and obliquely to the opposite fragment, as in internal transport. The distraction-compression forces act externally and internally to the extremity.

This technique is indicated mainly in cases of major bone loss (more than 10 cm) combined with limb deformities, deep soft tissue scars, and local blood supply insufficiency. The choice of a site for external or internal transport depends on the size of the transported fragment and the presence or absence of deformity. External transport is more convenient for large bone fragments and deformities (Fig. 15.3A), and internal transport for a site with deep scars (Fig. 15.3B).

Depending on the presence or absence of limb shortness, external transport is applied to either the distal or the proximal side. In cases involving limb shortness there must be reinforcement by a foot component on the distal side similar to that shown in Figures 15.1 and 15.2.

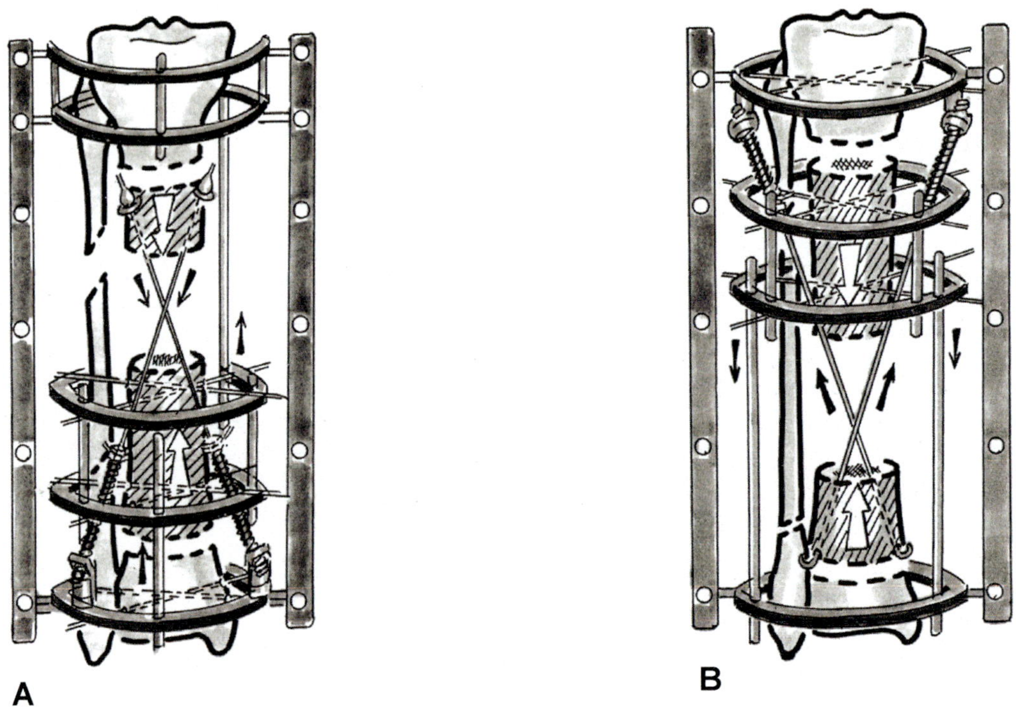

Figure 15.3: Two versions of the Ilizarov combined external-internal bone transport technique. Both frames have been stabilized with long bars. Only variants of major bone loss without limb shortness are presented. The same bifocal corticotomy and transport of two fragments toward each other are shown in both versions. The transported bone fragments are *shaded,* the transport directions shown by *arrows,* and corticotomy sites by *interrupted thick lines.* **A,** external transport is best for large bone fragments and deformities. **B,** internal transport is used in sites with deep scars

ADVANTAGES AND DISADVANTAGES OF THE TECHNIQUES

The main advantage of the external transport technique is that it is easier to perform and can be used for simultaneous correction of shortness and deformity. Its main disadvantage is that it is not always adequate in cases involving major bone loss (10 cm or more). The distraction process is, moreover, complex because multiple wires are used.

The main advantage of the internal transport technique is that it produces better results in cases of major bone loss and leaves less skin scarring. The distraction is easier for the patient because fewer wires are involved. The main disadvantage is that it is more difficult to perform and cannot always be used if limb lengthening is required. The internal transport technique also does not produce a compression force strong enough for bone fusion to occur between two transported fragments. In internal bone transport the bone fusion requires use of additional transverse wires and of additional rings to achieve adequate external compressive forces after the fragments have been transported.

SPECIAL CONSIDERATIONS IN SEGMENTAL BONE TRANSPORT TECHNIQUES

During the long course of treatment that the Ilizarov technique of bone transport entails (10 to 12 months), a considerable number of complications can occur, including deviation of the transported bone fragment, transient nerve palsy, development of foot equinus, nonunion of transported bone fragment with the opposed bone, stress fracture of regenerated bone, and some shortness of limb. Most of these complications can be resolved during treatment. In the case of development of foot equinus the addition of a foot component to the apparatus frame produces an excellent final result. For stress fractures of the regenerate, the application of a long cast may produce good results. For nonunion, implantation of an intramedullary rod produces a good result.

BIOMECHANICS OF ILIZAROV EXTERNAL FIXATOR RELATING TO FRAME CONSTRUCTION IN LARGE BONE LOSS AND DISTRACTION AND TO ANATOMIC FACTORS

A variety of factors control the stability of the Ilizarov fixator during long distraction or large bone loss replacement. This multiplicity of factors allows for a wide range of bending, torsion, and axial stiffness of the construction. Many of these factors are influenced by the choice of components made by surgeons in frame construction; these factors are called extrinsic stabilizing factors. Other factors are influenced by the specifics of the surgical application.

The Ilizarov external fixator and other circular ring fixators offer certain advantages over unilateral and bilateral frames. In general, circular fixators have more isotropic mechanical properties in bending, nonlinear axial rigidity, and the ability to readily create configurations for complex corrections. For any fixator system there are two fundamental interrelated considerations: stability and rigidity. Stability is the ability of the fixator to maintain the necessary mechanical configuration during treatment; rigidity is a measure of the mechanical response of the fixator, which has importance in the healing response. For all fixators the desired aim is to achieve a stable frame (in general, rigid) and wire configuration coexistent with the specific requirements and limitations of the clinical situation.

Anatomical factors may or may not be controllable by the surgeon. These factors, called the intrinsic stabilizing factors, are also important for the stability of the bone fragments.

The first factor is the mechanical configuration of the bone ends. After contact of the bone ends, stability is greatly enhanced if two parallel surfaces meet (Fig. 15.4A). Contact of two oblique surfaces provides the least stability, and should be fixed with wire stoppers (Fig. 15.4B). Irregularities of the bone ends can allow interdigitation and firm contact such as invagination of a bone spike into the medullary canal (Fig. 15.4C). The area of tissue contact between the bone ends influences the amount of stability achieved.

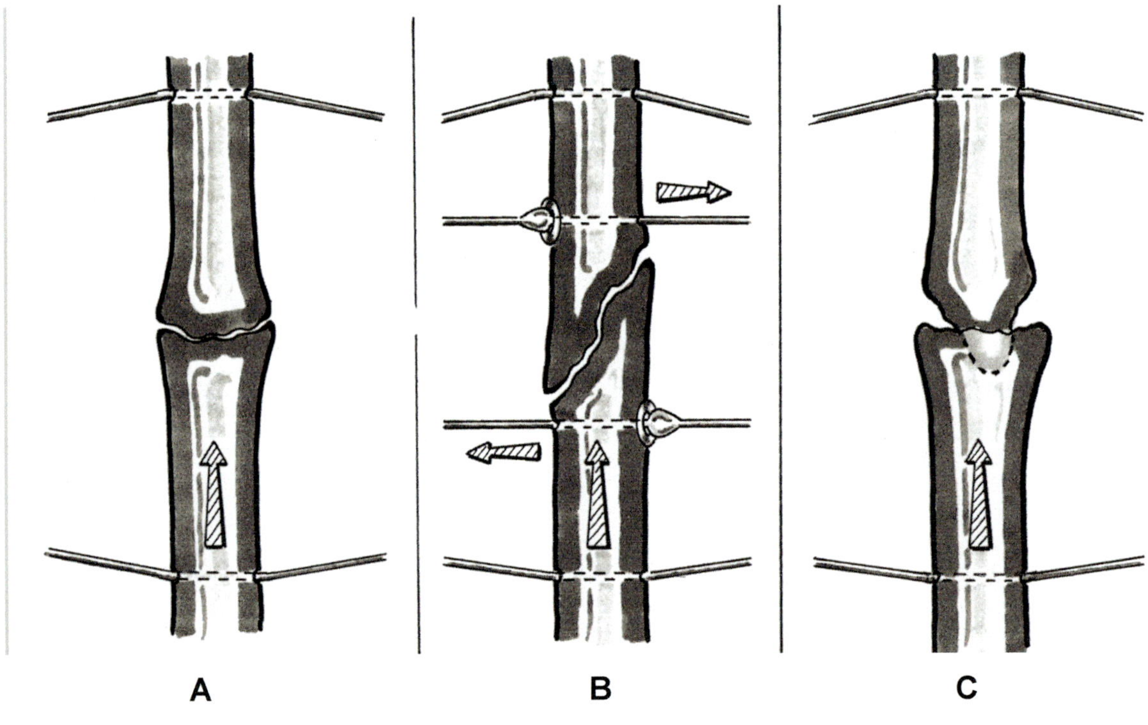

Figure 15.4: Three mechanical configurations of bone ends that influence stability of the fragments under compression. *Vertical arrows* indicate direction of compression. The bone fragments are shown with the frame segment consisting of two wires above and below the nonunion site. The wires are shown being bent with the concave side facing the nonunion. This confirms the tension from compression. A, stability is enhanced greatly if two parallel surfaces meet. B, contact of two oblique surfaces requires introduction of two wires with stoppers directed to the side of the nonunion or fracrure *(horizontal arrows)*. The wires are introduced above and below the contact surface but not through it, because they must not interfere with the vertical compression. It is recommended to use the stoppers with washers for better distribution of horizontal compression forces and prevention of penetration into soft bone (in case of an old nonunion with osteoporosis). C, invagination of a bone spike of one fragment into the medullary canal of the opposed fragment allows interdigitation and firm contact

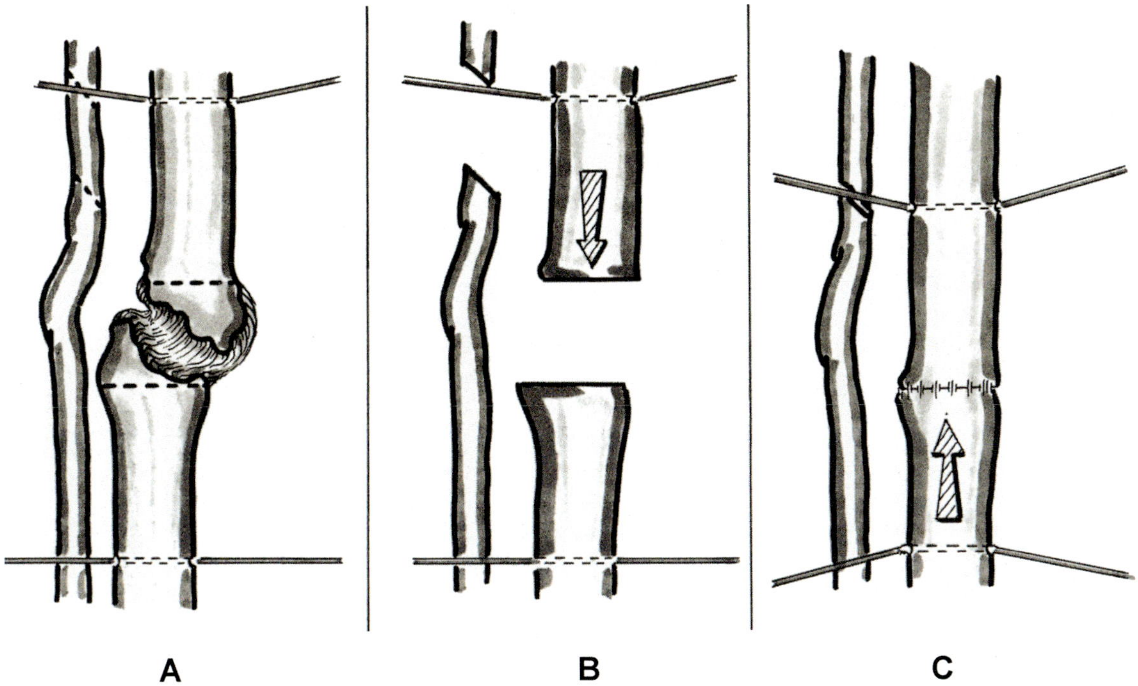

Figure 15.5: Influence of scar tissue on the compression of two opposed bone fragments, and recommended treatment tactic. The bone fragments are shown with the frame segment consisting of two wires above and below the nonunion site. The wires are bent in position; *arrows* indicate the direction of sliding distraction-compression. A, abundance of scar tissue produces fragment displacement and prevents healing. *Interrupted lines* indicate recommended sites of resection. The fibular resection must equal that of the tibia. The convex bending of the proximal wire indicates the fragment in a position of distraction. B, after bone resection, distraction for bone transport is continued. Fibular osteotomy always is performed at a different level than resection. C, resected bone fragments in contact and compression

Second, elasticity of tissue between bone ends can produce unequal displacement and prevent healing if a scar is present. In this case, nonunion site resection is recommended, but must be performed after bone transport and distraction are accomplished (Fig. 15.5).

Third, the presence of a gap between the bone ends requires reinforcement and additional stabilization of the bone ends. The Ilizarov technique obviates the need for a bone graft. The local segmental transport or defect filling transport technique is recommended instead (Fig. 15.6).

Fourth, tension of the soft tissues surrounding the bone must be considered to prevent neurovascular complications. Correction of the deformity immediately can produce pain, swelling, and numbness. Follow the golden rule of the Ilizarov technique: *Everything must be done gradually.*

The surgeon should assess all of these factors in any given situation and use the controllable elements to develop a suitable frame for each case.

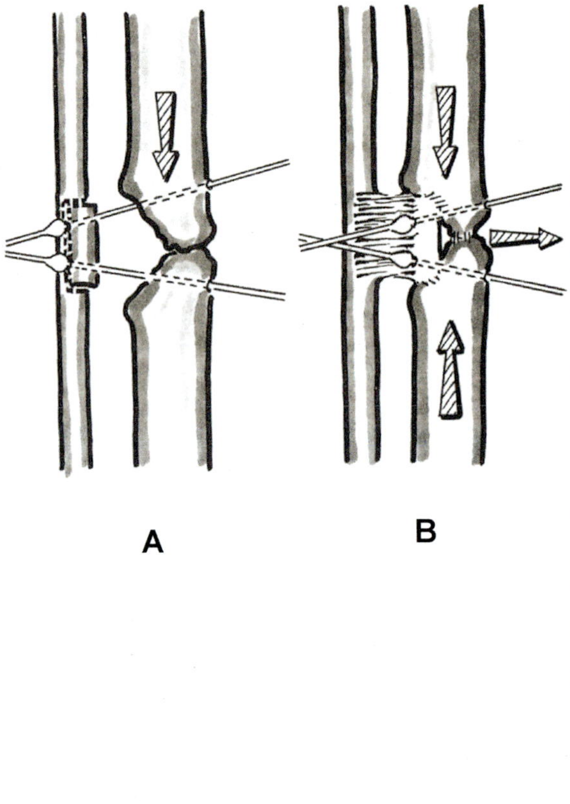

Figure 15.6: Two types of gap deficiency between the opposed bone fragments, and recommended treatment. The bone fragments with nonunion site are shown after they have been transported toward each other. *Arrows* indicate the direction of distraction and compression; *interrupted lines* indicate osteotomy sites. A, with the gap located at the fibular side, the segmental osteotomy of the fibula is performed with the introduction of two olive wires. B, gradual medial translation of the fibular segment is accomplished, with reinforcement of the nonunion site by synostosis and elimination of the tibial gap. C, with the gap located at the tibial medial side, longitudinal osteotomy of the tibia is performed with the introduction of an oblique olive wire, accompanied by fibular osteotomy (at a level different from that of the tibia). D, gradual defect filling of the osteotomized fragment is accomplished, with reinforcement of the nonunion site

TECHNIQUE OF SEGMENTAL BONE DEVIATION CORRECTION

The free bone segment, transfixed at both ends and transported a significant distance through soft tissues of different densities, will be influenced by many mechanical factors:

1. Incomplete corticotomy at the segment base (the posterior bone wall is most difficult to cut through).
2. Unbalanced distribution of distraction forces resulting from incorrect wire positioning.
3. Pulling forces of the muscle groups attached to the segment (flexors usually are stronger than extensors).
4. Retention forces of the surrounding scar tissues.
5. Inadequate performance of distraction technique (often due to patient noncompliance because of pain or incomprehensibility).

Depending on the prevalence of these forces and factors, deviation of the transported segment may occur. Resulting displacement of the leading bone end will produce deformity and prevent healing.

The best way to avoid bone segment deviation is to prevent it by introducing a guidewire or by using wires with stoppers (olive wires) on two levels of each segment. Technically this is not always possible. Often the segmental deviation is detected first on anteroposterior and/or lateral radiographs, and must be corrected as soon as possible. To accomplish this the pushing-pulling devices must be added to the reinforced Ilizarov fixator frame. One of many advantages of this fixator is that it can be used to correct displaced bone fragments by a relatively simple adjustment. Depending on the complexity of the adjustment, the speed and rhythm of distraction-compression must be adapted to the new frame.

Correction of One-Level Deviation

In the external bone transport technique bone-segment deviation is corrected by frame reinforcement and addition of the pushing-pulling device (Fig. 15.7). At least two long connection plates are fixed to proximal and distal rings, with angulation of 90 to 180 degrees between them. One of these plates has to be placed opposite the side of bone deviation. The pushing-pulling device is introduced at the level of the ring closer to the deviated segment end. Depending on the degree of deviation and the size of the segment, the correction maneuver requires one or two devices, one to act as a pulling mechanism and another as a pushing mechanism (Fig. 15.7). In the

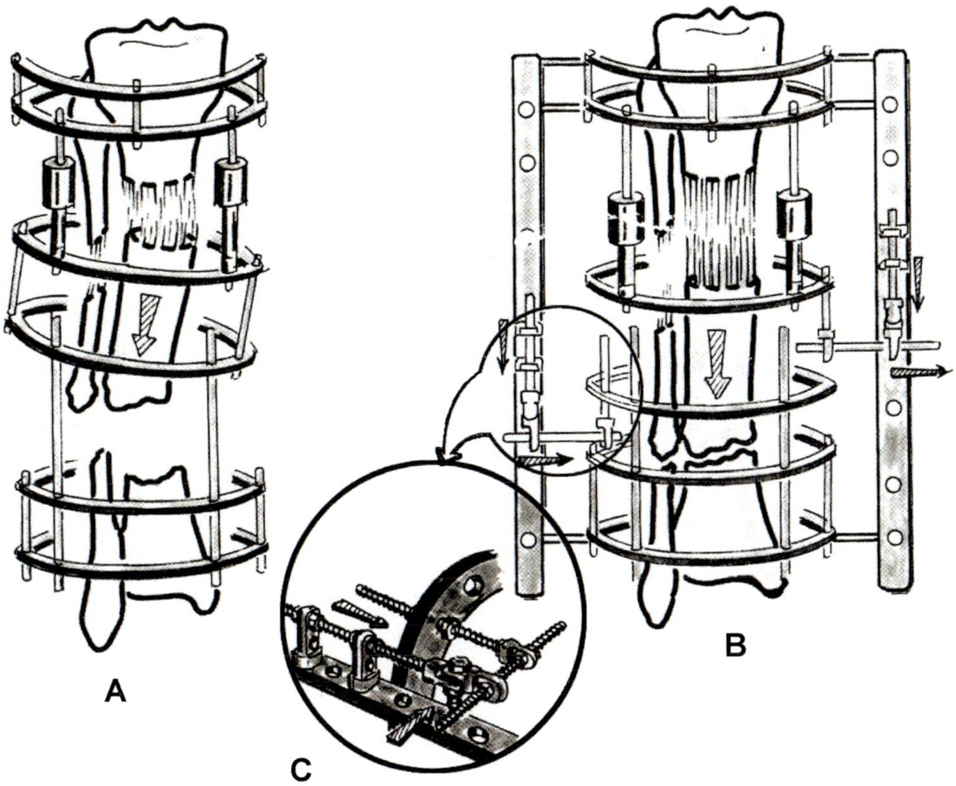

Figure 15.7: Technique of bone segment deviation correction during external bone transport. The six-ring frame is shown applied to the tibia with bone loss. Proximal corticotomy is performed, and transport of the proximal bone segment distally is in progress. *Arrows* indicate direction of the bone segment movement. A, sliding bone segment lateral deviation. B, frame is reinforced by two long connecting plates. The pushing device is introduced at the level of the transported segment leading end from the lateral side, and the pulling device from the medial side. C, enlarged view of the pushing device. To ensure continuation of distraction, both devices have long vertical threaded rods

internal bone transport technique one-segment deviation is corrected by adjusting the rate of distraction or by introducing an additional wire with stopper. If a bone segment is pulled by two hooked or olive wires, one at the backside is pulled faster, and the other slower. If a bone segment is pulled by only one wire, it is recommended that the transverse olive wire be used and the deviation corrected by gradual shifting with the pulling device (Fig. 15.8).

Correction of Two-Level Deviation

The technique of two-level deviation correction is performed the same way as described for one-level deviation. The difference is that with the pushing-pulling devices transverse olive wires are introduced at the levels of both deviated segments. The more complex the correction the slower the distraction rate should be. The reason for this is the influence that the change of distraction direction has on the maturity of the bone regenerate. Any change in direction of distraction brings about some changes in the orientation of the newly formed bone microcolumns. This can suppress the filling and the maturity of the cancellous regenerate. Bearing in mind that in any case of bone transport there are already significant changes in bone metabolism, all corrections must be performed in stages.

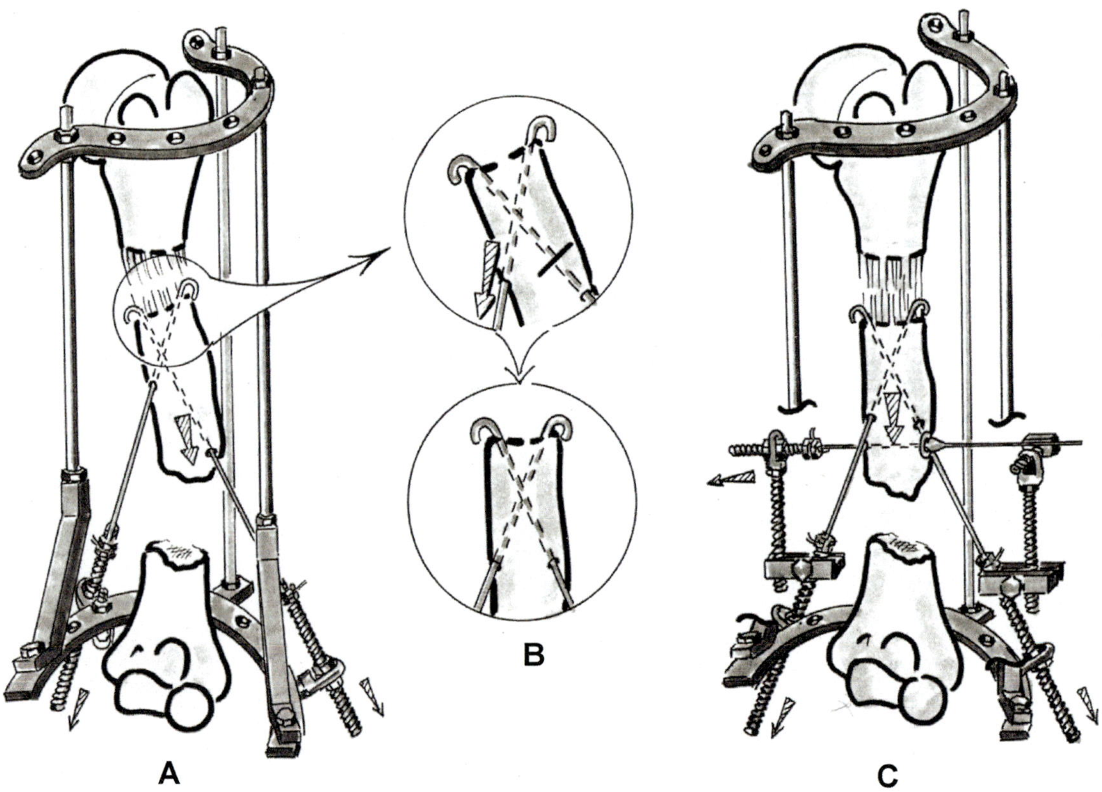

Figure 15.8: Technique of bone segment deviation correction during internal bone transport. The two-ring frame is shown applied to the humerus with bone loss. Proximal corticotomy is performed, and transport of the proximal bone segment distally is begun. The *arrows* indicate the direction of the bone segment movement. A, sliding bone segment lateral deviation. B, deviation is corrected by adjustment of the rate and rhythm of distraction. The hooked wire introduced from above, laterally to medially on the slower side is pulled twice as fast as the second wire. C, same deviation is corrected by introduction of the olive wire with a washer, connected to the pulling device

COMBINED DISTRACTION WITH CORRECTION OF INCONGRUENCY AND ROTATION DEFORMITY

In planning distraction combined with deviation or rotation deformity correction, the surgeon must take into account the same factors mentioned for rate adjustment and the complexity and order of correction. The newly formed longitudinally oriented bone microcolumns must mature before they are able to withstand derotation. Thus the recommended sequence is to first produce distraction with necessary corrections and then to stabilize the bone for at least 2 weeks. The next step is to produce gradual derotation at the level of the regenerate, which should be in the initial stage of maturity (Fig. 15.9).

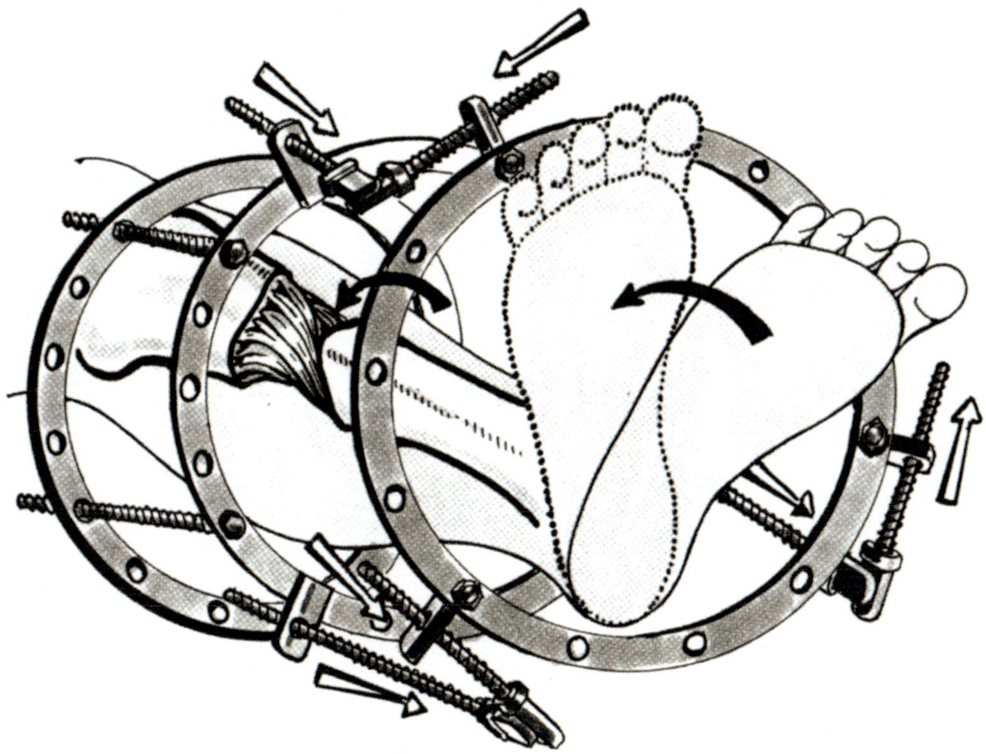

Figure 15.9: Technique of combined distraction with rotation correction. Distraction of the right leg with subsequent external derotation. The three-ring frame is applied, and a proximal corticotomy with distraction is accomplished. *Open arrows* indicate direction of distraction and derotation; *black arrows* indicate distal leg movement. Overrotation of the vertically oriented microcolumns at the site of distraction-derotation is shown

CASE ILLUSTRATIONS

Figures 15.10 through 15.14 illustrate cases in which segmental bone transport techniques were used.

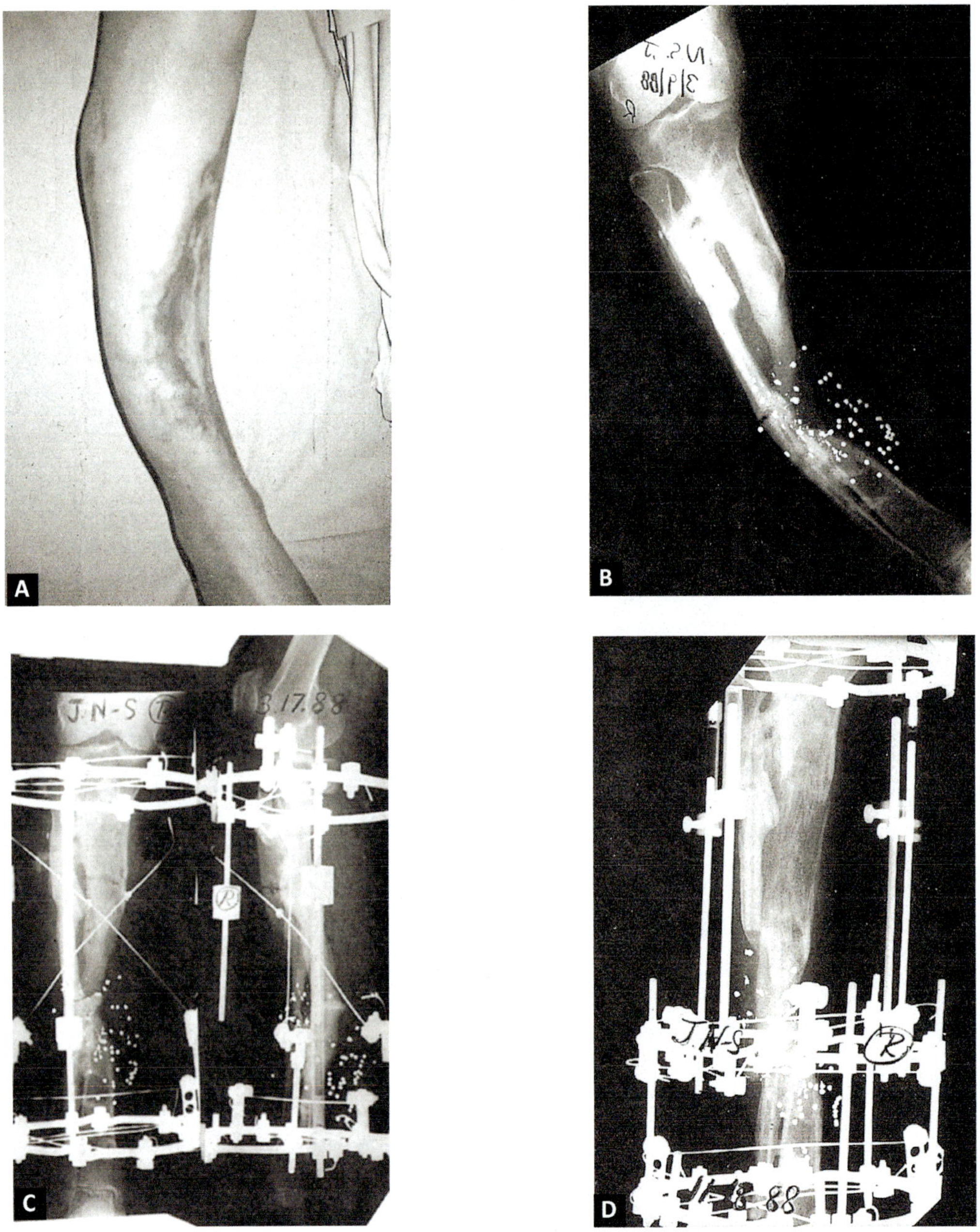

Figure 15.10: Internal Bone Transport for Infected Nonunion with Deformity and Lengthening. Twenty-seven-year-old man with a 5-year history of infected nonunion of the right leg (in an active drainage stage), 8 cm of tibial bone loss, varus deformity, only the posterior tibial artery functioning, and deep drawn skin scars. Status post-gunshot wound and unsuccessful multiple surgeries (12 procedures) performed elsewhere. **A,** appearance of leg before treatment. **B,** AP radiograph of leg before treatment shows buckshot and unsuccessful attempt at synostosis with a fibular graft from the other leg. **C,** AP and lateral radiographs of leg immediately after proximal tibia corticotomy, with application of the two-ring frame and introduction of two oblique olive wires for internal bone transport. **D,** AP radiograph of leg 8 months after surgery. Note 7-cm-long calcified bone regenerate. Frame is adjusted for compression of transported bone fragment with the opposed distal end

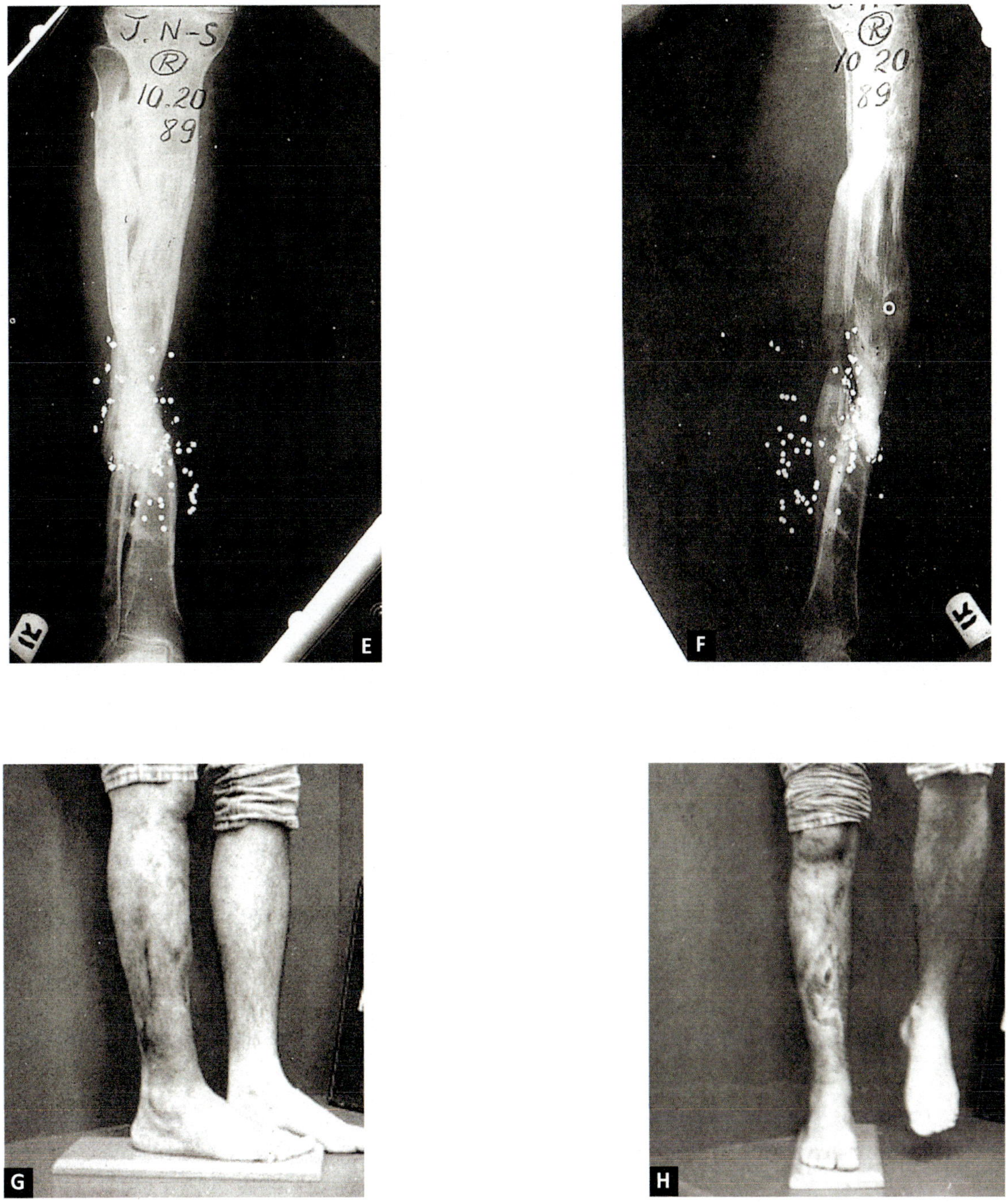

Figure 15.10 (Contd): E and F, AP and lateral radiographs of leg 19 months after surgery show complete healing and restoration of tibial length and shape. G and H, appearance of legs 2 years after surgery. There was a functionally and cosmetically insignificant leg shortness of 1 cm

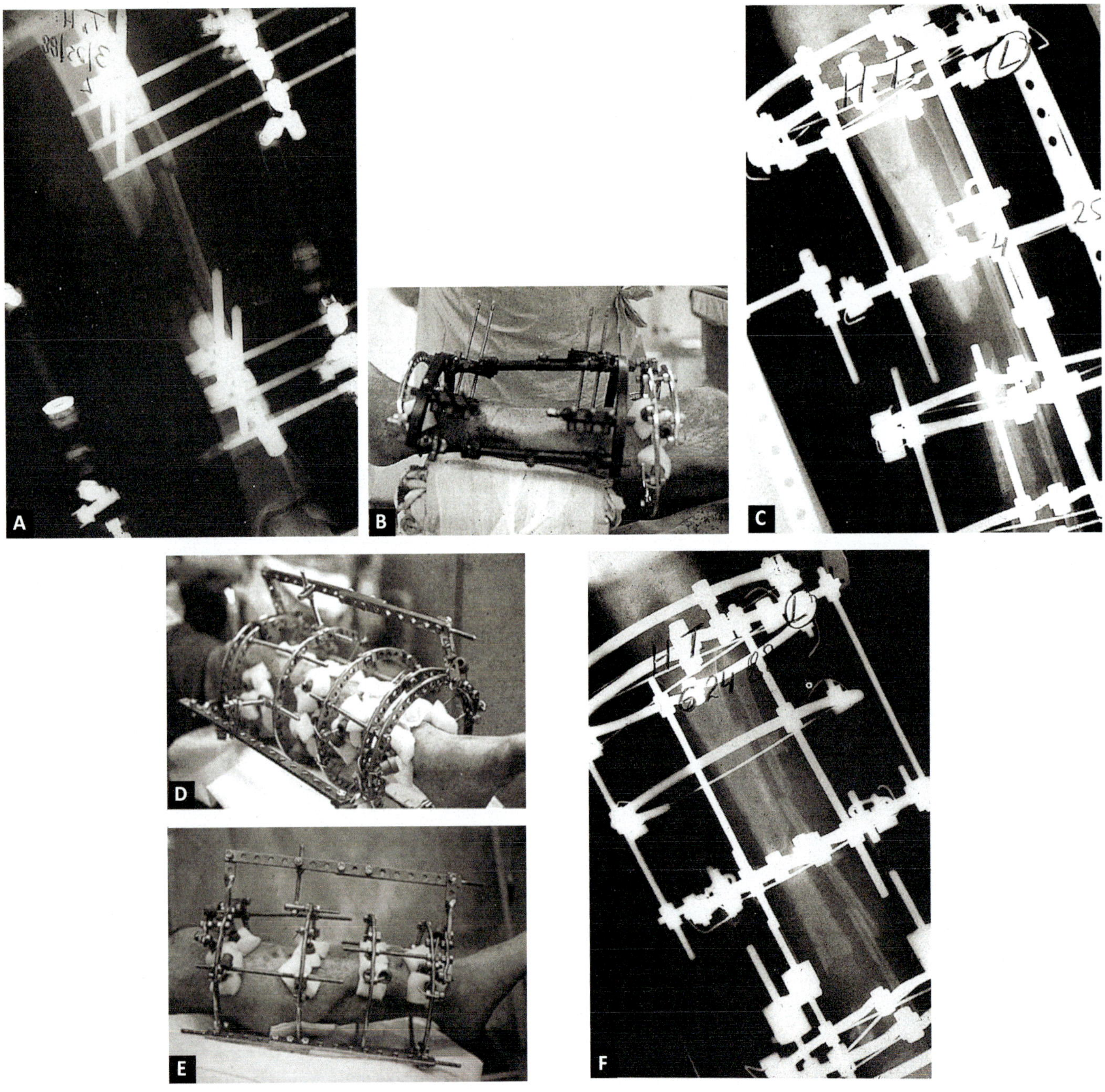

Figure 15.11: External Bone Transport for Fracture wim Bone Loss. Twenty-four-year-old man with grade C-3 left leg fracture, complicated by 6 cm of tibial bone loss, neurovascular injury, and head injury. Patient was offered below-knee amputation immediately after the injury. It was refused, and temporary fixation of the leg by bilateral frame and musculovascular flap was performed elsewhere. **A,** AP radiograph of leg before surgery. **B,** replacement of the bilateral fixator with the Ilizarov fixator. **C,** AP radiograph of leg 2 months after bifocal corticotomy and external bone transport sliding of two bone segments toward each other. Postoperative complications included development of severe swelling and moderate disturbance in blood circulation. Distraction was delayed by 2 weeks, and the proximal corticotomy healed prematurely. **D** and **E,** two views of leg 3 months after surgery. For bone segment deviation correction, the frame is reinforced by the long connecting plates, and the pulling-pushing devices are introduced. **F,** AP radiograph of leg 2 months after surgery. Bone transport of the distal fragment is accomplished, and 4-cm-long regenerate is seen

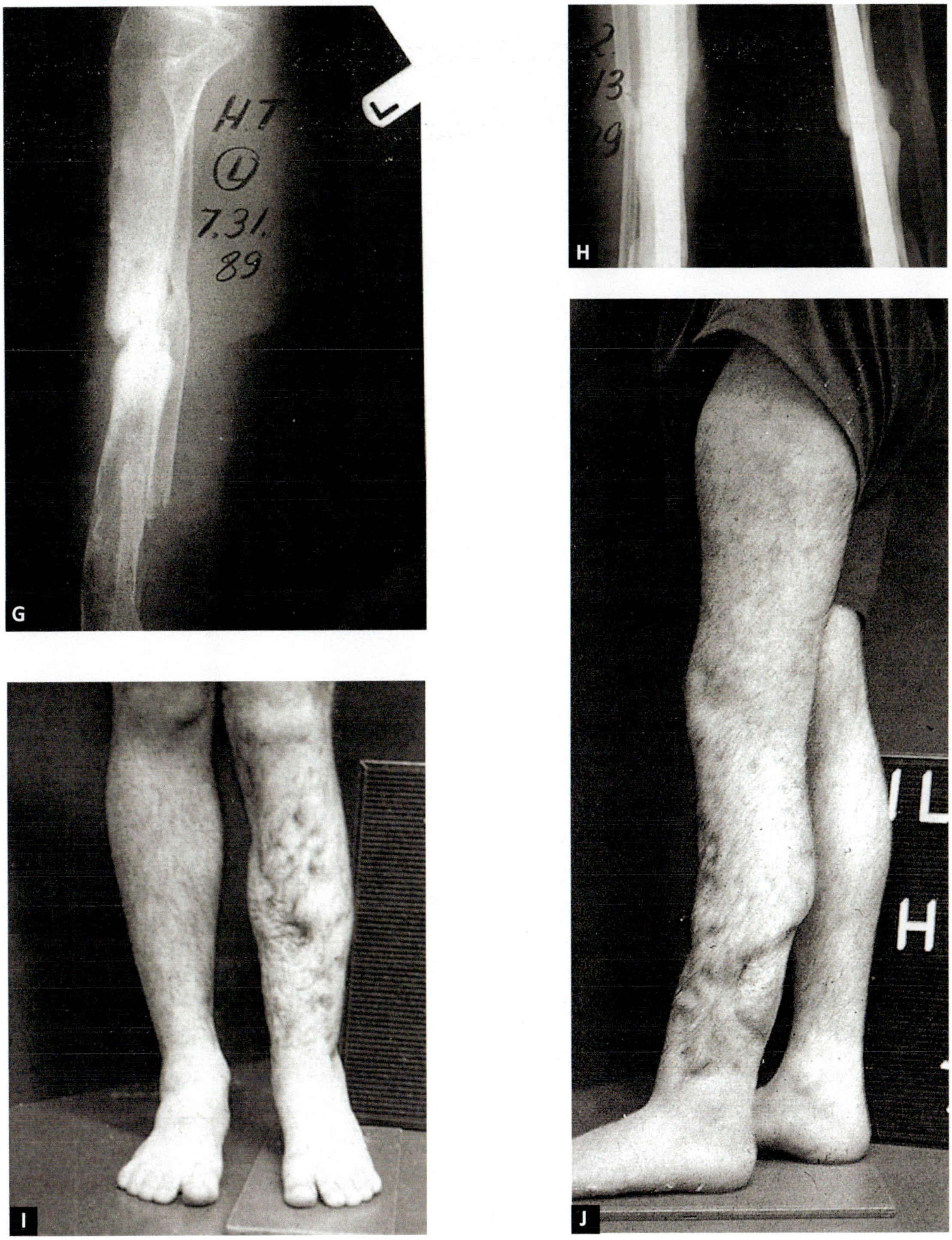

Figure 15.11 (Contd): G, lateral radiograph of leg 16 months after surgery. Proximal corticotomy site has healed, and distal transported fragment left well-calcified regenerate. The opposed bone fragments are in contact, but without sufficient signs of healing. H, radiograph of the middle segment of the leg 20 months after Ilizarov fixator application and 3½ months after osteosynthesis with an intramedullary rod. I and J, appearance of legs 2 years after surgery. Functionally and cosmetically insignificant 1-cm left leg shortness is present

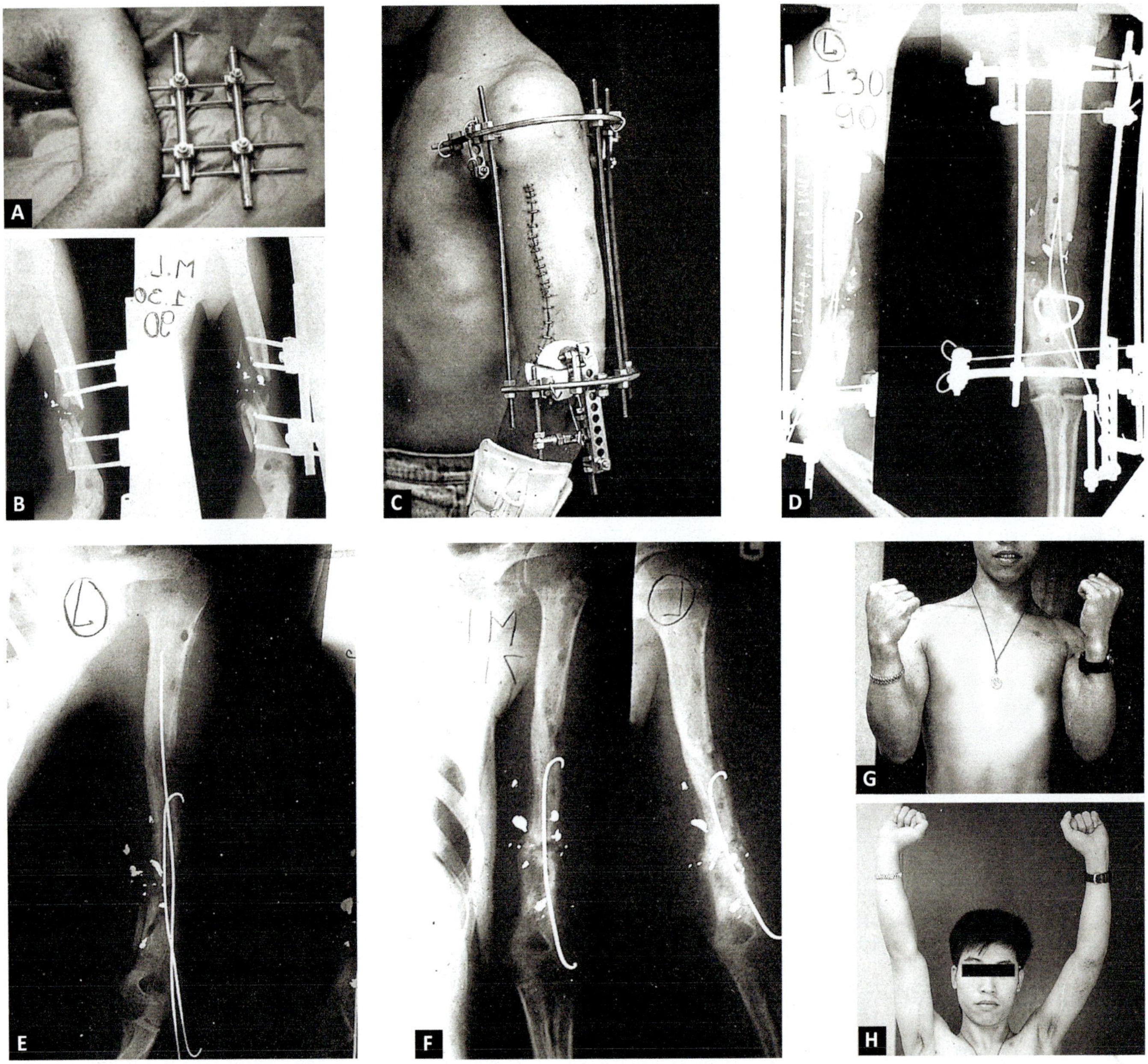

Figure 15.12: Internal Bone Transport for Fracture with Bone Loss. Eighteen-year-old man with 4 cm bone loss of the left brachius and radial nerve injury after gunshot wound. Status post-unilateral fixator and nerve revision performed elsewhere. **A,** left upper arm before surgery. **B,** AP and lateral radiographs of humerus before surgery. **C,** left arm after removal of the unilateral fixator, application of the two-ring Ilizarov fixator, proximal humerus corticotomy with introduction of intramedullary hooked wire for internal bone transport, and radial nerve revision with pulling device attached to the distal ring. **D,** lateral and AP radiographs of the arm after surgery. One of the intramedullary wires is a hooked pulling wire, another is a guidewire. The metal ring seen on AP film is a part of a forearm supporting brace, outside of the frame and the patient's body. **E,** radiograph of the humerus 4 months after surgery and removal of the fixator. Both wires were left inside temporarily. Bone transport is accomplished, calcified regenerate is seen at the site of corticotomy, and the opposed bone ends have started to heal. **F,** lateral and AP radiographs of the humerus 7 months after surgery show complete healing after the guidewire had been pulled out. The hooked wire is left in because of the technical difficulties involved in its removal. **G** and **H** appearance of the arm 2 years after surgery. Radial nerve function was fully restored

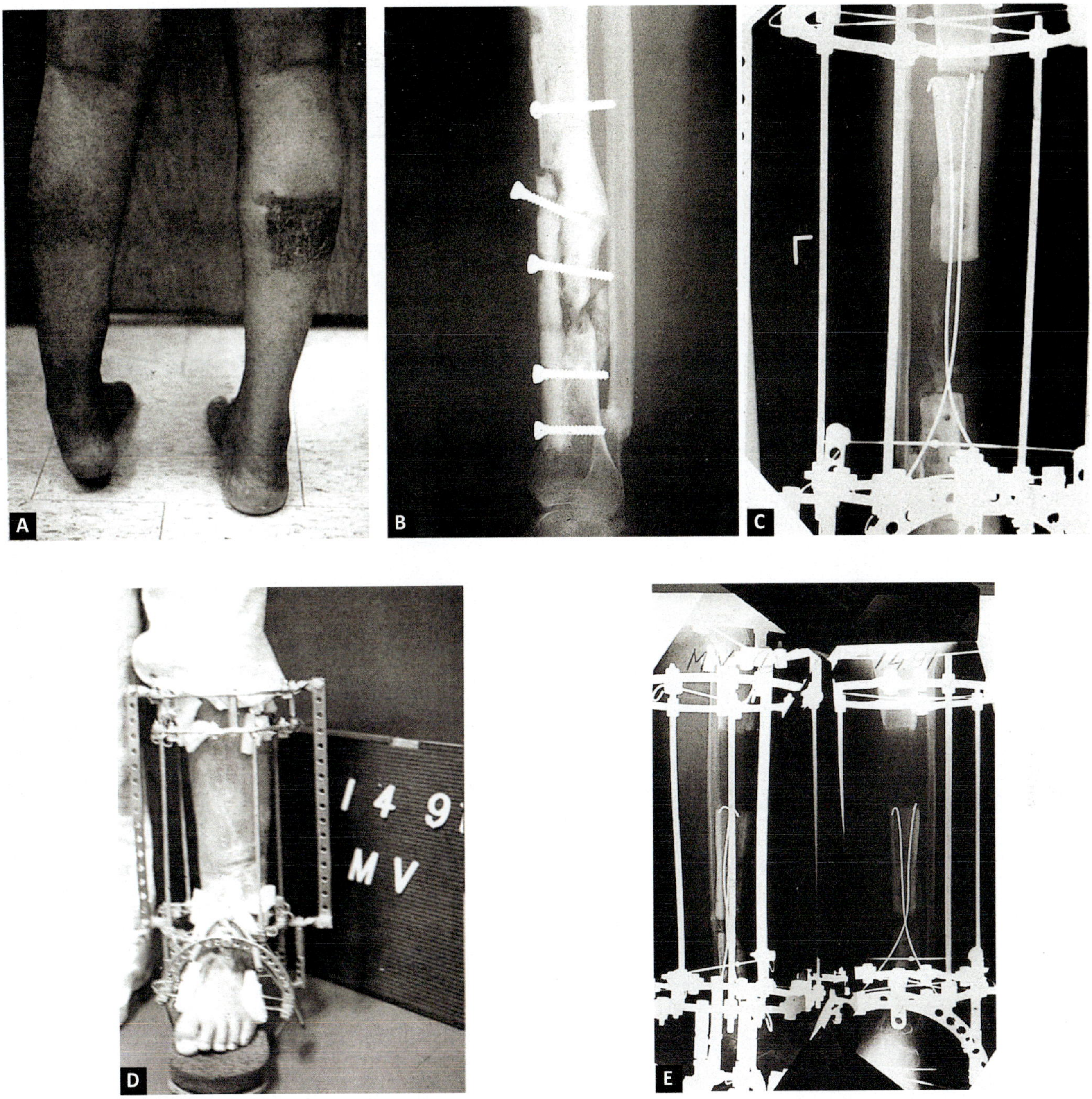

Figure 15.13: Internal Bone Transport following Resection for Osteomyelitis with Pseudocyst. Twenty-five-year-old man with nonunion and osteomyelitis with active drainage, and 3 cm shortness of the leg, with varus deformity and foot equinus. Status post-unsuccessful multiple surgeries performed elsewhere. A, legs before surgery. Note skin flap scar on the right leg. B, lateral radiograph of left leg before surgery. C, AP radiograph of leg after removal of the orthopedic screws, resection of 12 cm of the affected distal tibia, proximal corticotomy of tibia, application of the three-ring frame with the addition of a foot part, and introduction of two hooked wires for internal bone transport. Both wires have been introduced into the transported segment canal and distal tibial fragment (see Fig. 15.2C). This stabilizes the transported segment without support by the guidewire. D, leg with apparatus 6 months after surgery. E, lateral and AP radiographs of the leg 6 months after surgery. Bone transport is accomplished, but there is little regenerate behind the slided segment. Development of pseudocyst was diagnosed with radiographic and ultrasound examination

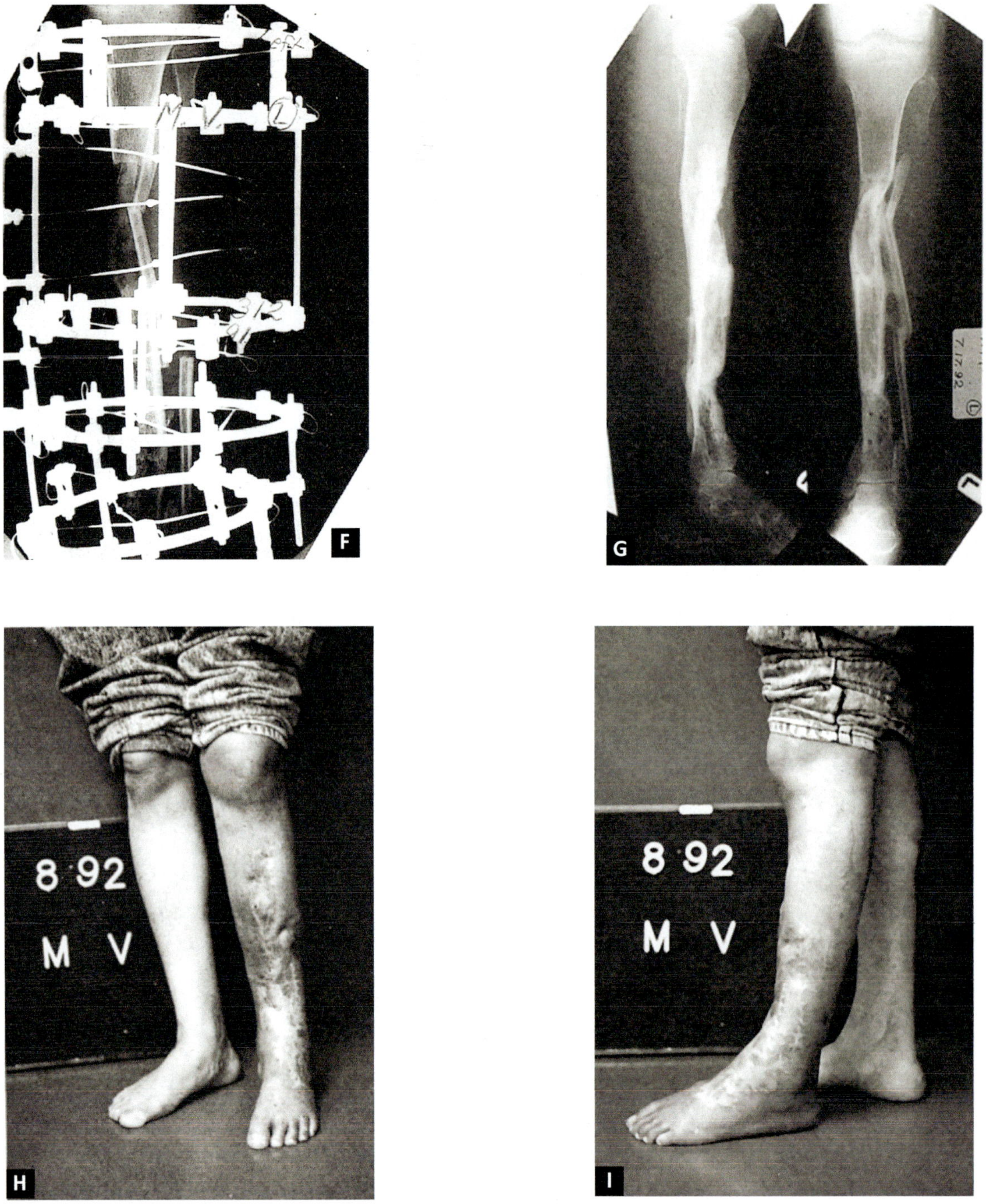

Figure 15.13 (Contd): F, AP radiograph of the leg 2 months after the second procedure, which included tibial pseudocyst debridement and autologous bone grafting, with reinforcement by the fibular segment gradually distracted to the site of pseudocyst. Because of the very short proximal fragment and the 10 cm pseudocyst, the combination of Ilizarov technique and bone grafting was used. G, lateral and AP radiographs of the leg 1 year after the second surgery. H and I, appearance of the legs 2½ years after surgery

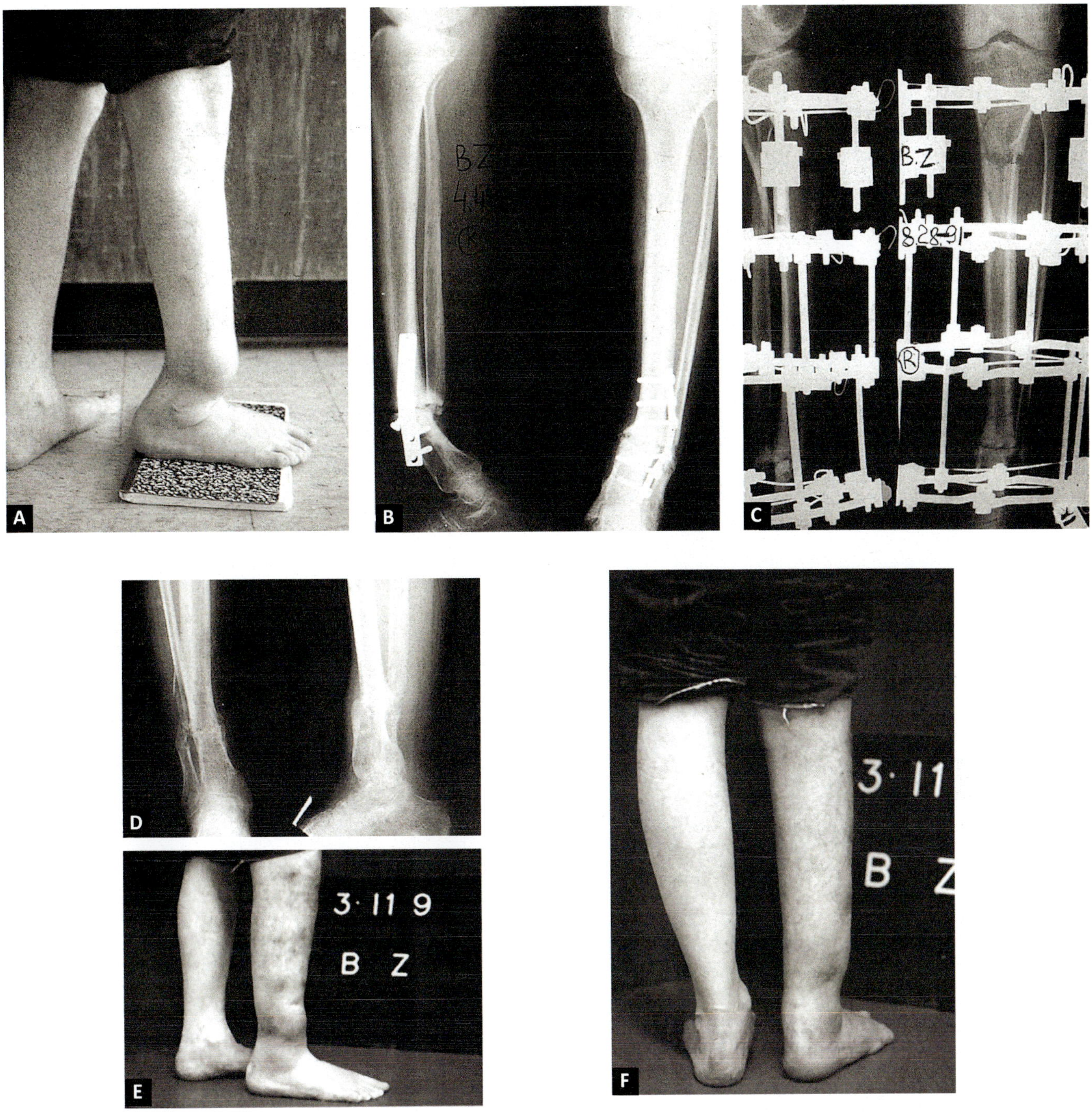

Figure 15.14: Correction of Deformity and Nonunion by Distraction-Compression. Forty-three-year-old man with right leg nonunion, 3 cm shortness, and antecurvation deformity. Status post-unsuccessful multiple surgeries. A, appearance of legs before surgery. B, lateral and AP radiographs of right leg before surgery. C, lateral and AP radiographs of the leg after surgery. Removal of the AO plate, with nonunion site resection, application of the Ilizarov four-ring apparatus, corticotomy of proximal tibia, and performance of external bone transport technique. D, AP and lateral radiographs of the leg 6½ months after surgery. There is complete healing of the nonunion site. E and F, appearance of the legs 1 year after surgery

16 Chapter

Ilizarov Fracture Management; Treatment of Foot and Hand; and Arthrodesis

The llizarov fixator may be applied for fractures produced by any loading modality, such as tension, compression, bending, shearing, torsion or combined torsion-compression, and at any level of any extremity.

Application of the Ilizarov fixator for fracture treatment requires, in some cases, a simultaneous regimen of skeletal traction. This traction aids, at least partially, in reducing angulation deformity, in achieving muscle relaxation, and in correcting shortness. The chief advantage of skeletal traction, however, is that it achieves stabilization of the limb, which enables the surgeon to approach the extremity from any direction. Such factors preclude the successful introduction of multiplanar wires.

The advantages of using the Ilizarov fixator in fracture cases are:

1. Possibility of simultaneous anatomic reduction of the displaced fragments.
2. Stable fixation provided by the wires, introduced at multiple levels and in multiple planes and orientations.
3. Early functional treatment, including joint range of motion and weight bearing, that stimulates fracture healing and shortens treatment time.
4. Possibility of correction of the secondary displacement by frame adjustment.
5. Easy approach to wounds in cases of compound fractures.

In essence, the Ilizarov circular fixator application can be considered an alternative to cast application. Frames for fracture treatment never can be assembled in advance. Fractures cannot be anticipated, and the varieties of fracture lanes and fragment displacements are too diverse to be taken into consideration prior to the particular case. In acute trauma cases, Ilizarov therefore recommends so-called progressive-concentric construction of the frame, piece-by-piece over the limb.

Biomechanic considerations for the Ilizarov fracture frame are important:

1. The sites of wire introduction must be chosen in accordance with the level and type of fracture and wounds.
2. Multiplanar positioning of many wires stabilizes fixation (Fig. 16.1).
3. For displacement reduction, the orientation of some crossing wires may be "off center" of the ring, with subsequent correction via their tensioning (Fig. 16.2).
4. Introduction of olive wires must be performed using the Ilizarov rule of thumb, that is, closer to the fracture on the convex side of the bone and farther from the fracture on the concave side (Fig. 16.3).
5. In anticipation of post-trauma swelling, the choice of rings should be at least one size larger than those normally used.
6. Displaced fragments must be corrected in order, that is, elimination of length reduction, straightening of angulation, correction of rotational deformity, and setting of the aligned fragments in a stable position, with some compression.

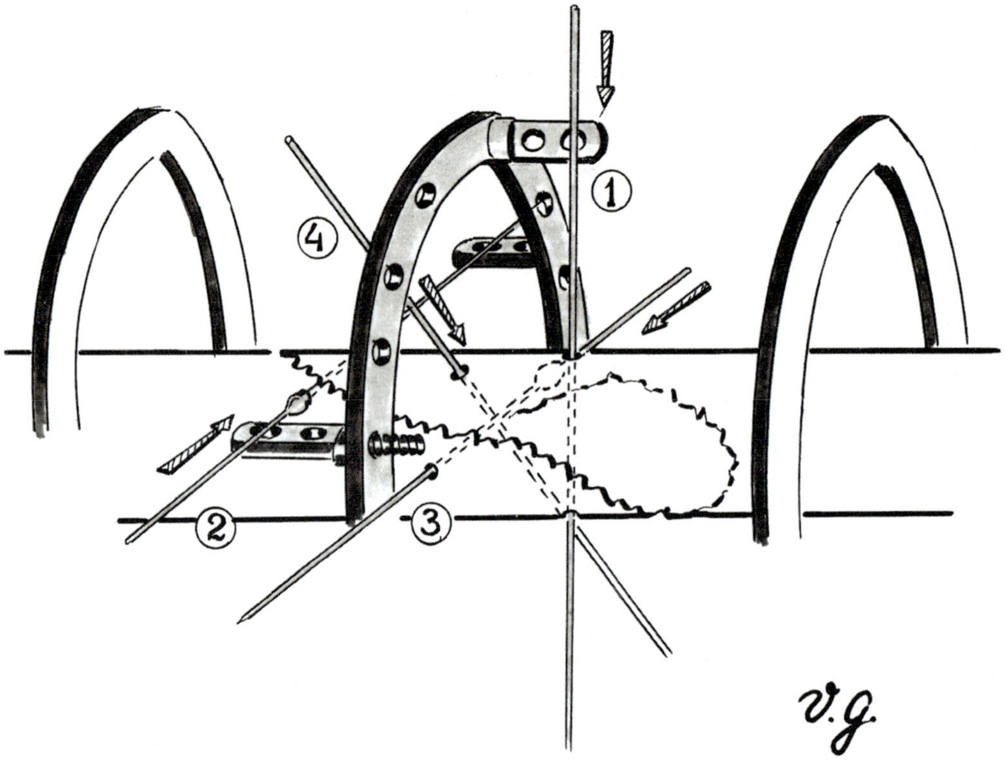

Figure 16.1: Multiplanar positioning of four wires for treatment of spiral fracture. Partial view of the frame segment applied at the level of the fracture. The wires are numbered in order of their introduction. *Arrows* indicate direction of wire introduction. The transverse wire (1) is introduced to fix and reduce the fracture. The other wires are introduced to stabilize reduction; some must be olive wires

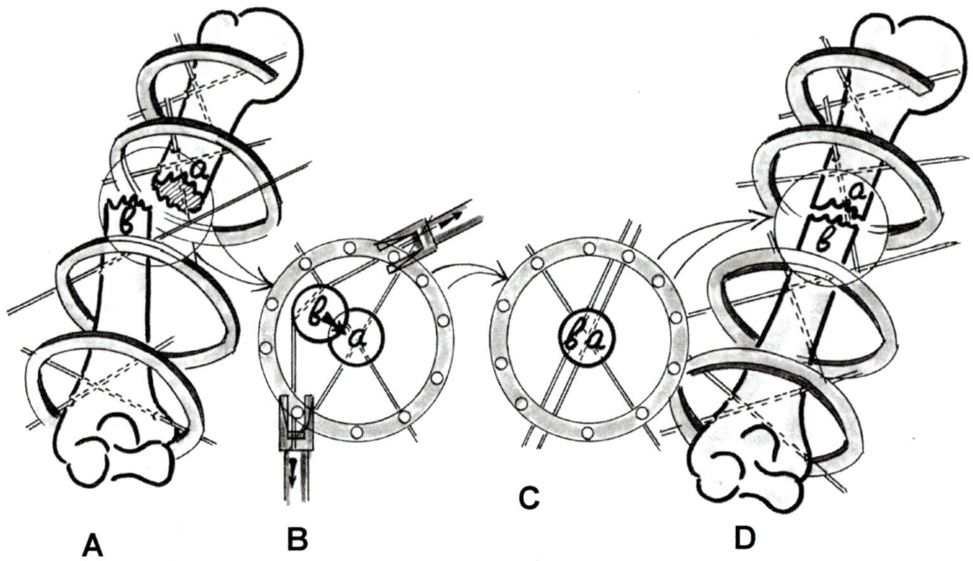

Figure 16.2: Displacement reduction via wire tensioning. Transverse displacement of fragment *b* in relation to fragment *a* is shown in different views before and after reduction. A, four-ring frame is transfixed to the bone for side displacement fracture. Proximal fragment *a* and distal end of fragment *b* are transfixed with correct centering. For the displaced end of fragment *b* the wire is oriented off-center. B, displacement at the level of the off-center wire, with tensioning at both sides. *Arrow* indicates direction of reduction. C, view after tensioning is accomplished. D, after correction of displacement, additional wires are introduced to stabilize fragment position

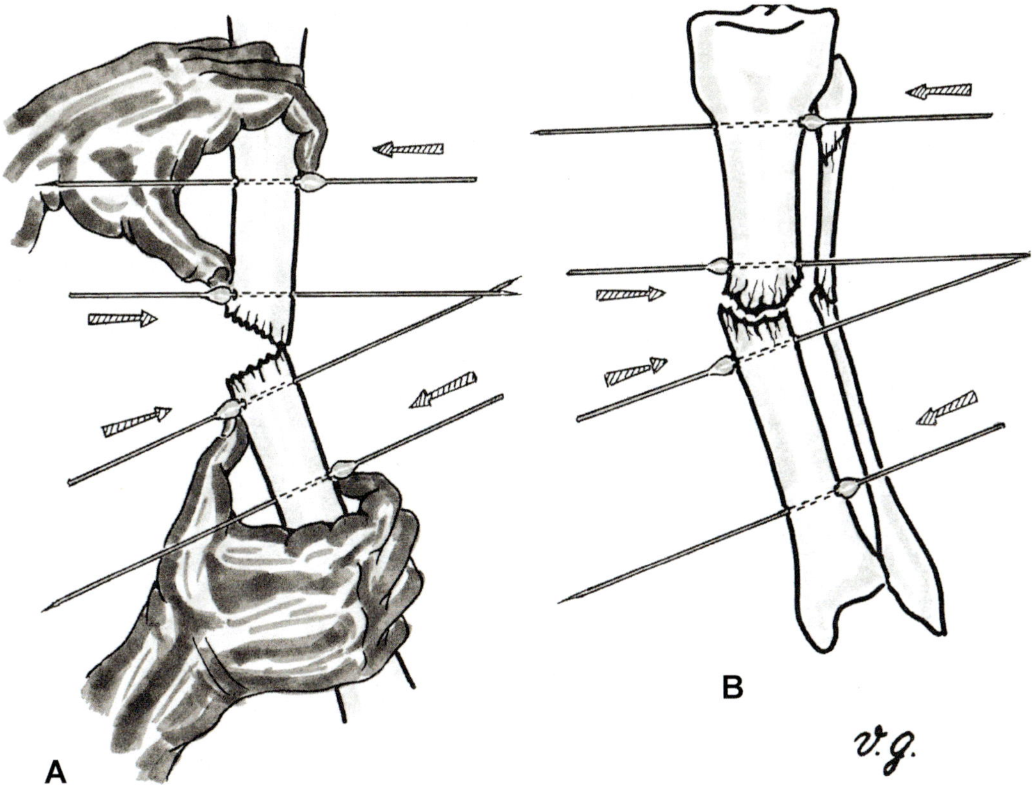

Figure 16.3: Introduction of olive wires for correction of displacement. Arrows indicate direction in which wires are introduced, which corresponds to direction of the correcting forces. A, position of physician's hands for straightening angulatory displacement of a fractured shaft. Pushing forces are applied by the thumbs to the convex side, close to the site of the fracture. Pulling forces are applied by the index fingers to the concave side, farther from the fracture site. B, fracture of the tibia with angulatory displacement. Pushing and pulling forces are applied as in A

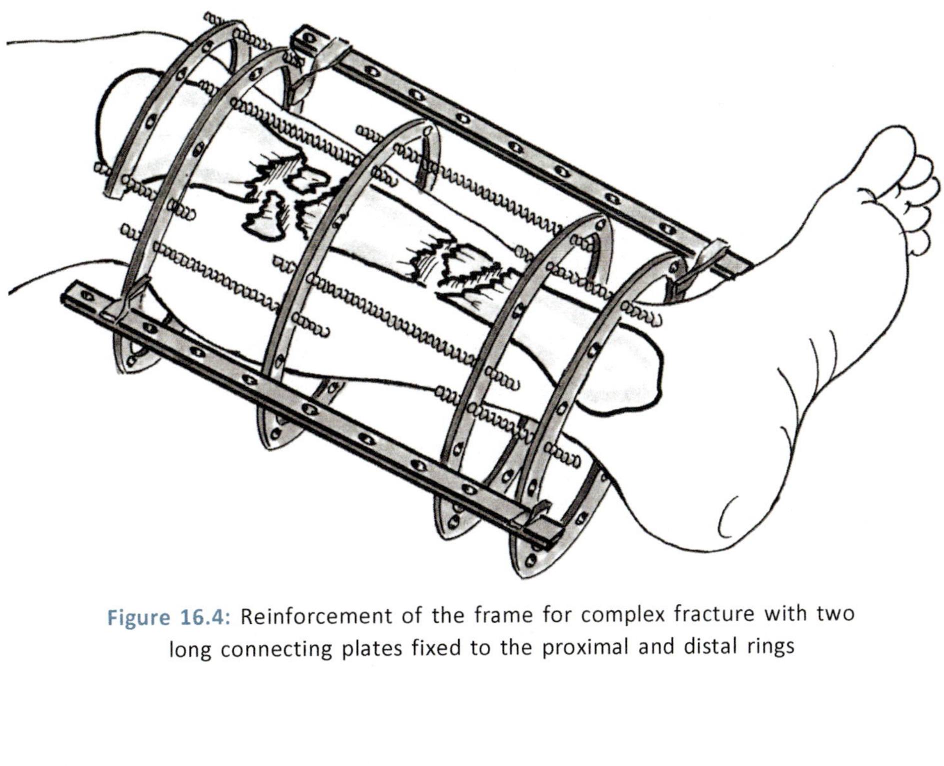

Figure 16.4: Reinforcement of the frame for complex fracture with two long connecting plates fixed to the proximal and distal rings

7. After elimination of length reduction, two or more long connection plates must be fixed to the proximal and distal rings for reinforcement of the frame and for introduction of distraction devices to correct angulation and shearing deformities (Fig. 16.4).
8. In the case of oblique and/or spiral fracture, transfixion by additional olive wires can be performed as soon as alignment of the fragments is achieved (Fig. 16.5).
9. In a case in which not all of the displaced fragments can be reduced on the operating table, additional corrective devices must be added to the frame for extended gradual reduction.

INDICATIONS FOR ILIZAROV FRACTURE TREATMENT

Indications for the Ilizarov external fixator application in traumatic fracture include the following:

I. Complex open and closed fractures of long bones:
   A. Displaced fractures of shaft (Fig. 16.6).
   B. Transverse fracture of shaft (Fig. 16.7).

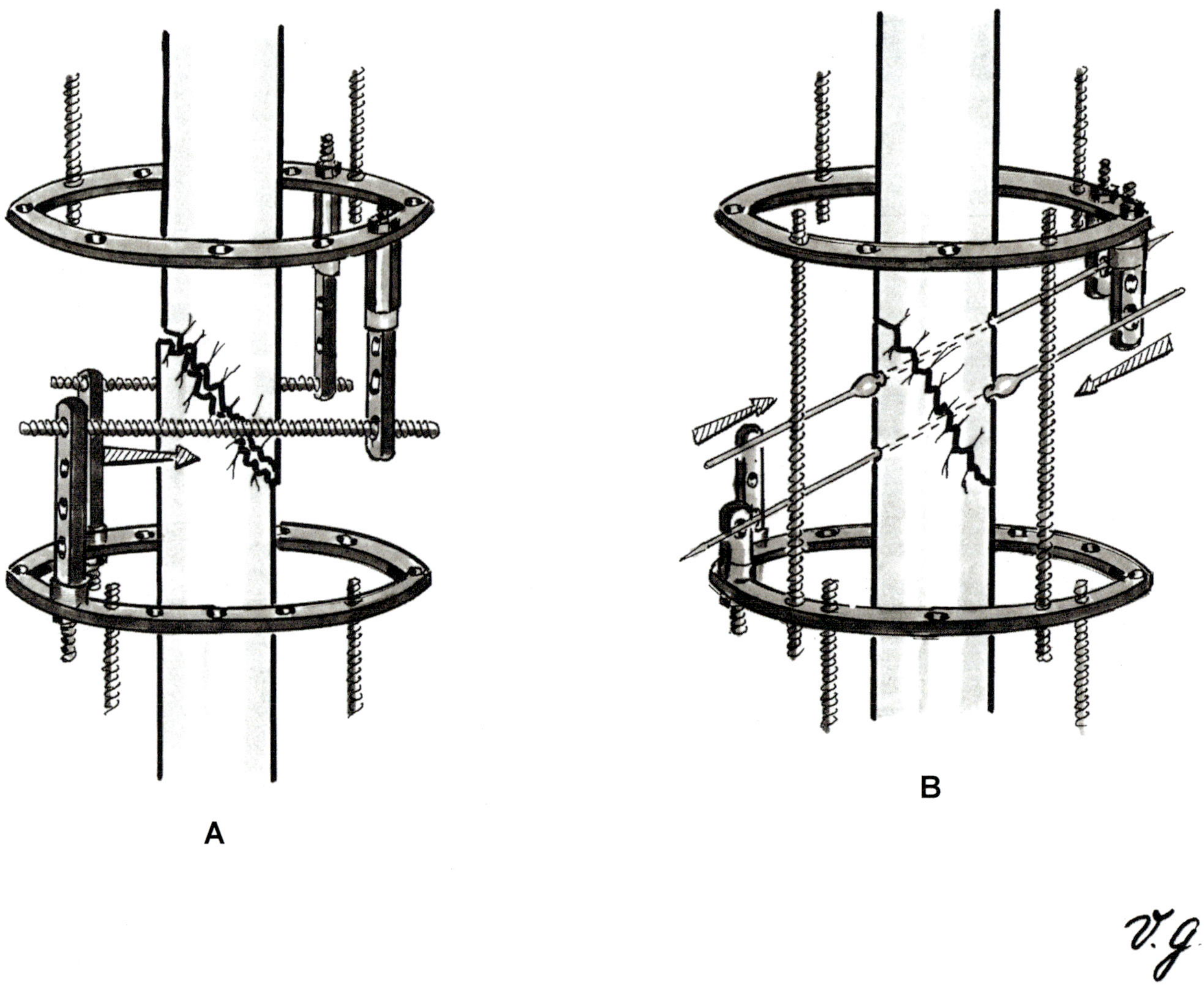

Figure 16.5: Transfixion of reduced oblique fracture by additional olive wires. Section of the frame is shown; *arrows* indicate direction of reducing and reinforcing forces. A, displaced oblique fracture is reduced by two translation devices. B, for reinforcement, two oblique wires are introduced, transfixing bone fragments in opposite directions. They are tensioned and fixed by the supports

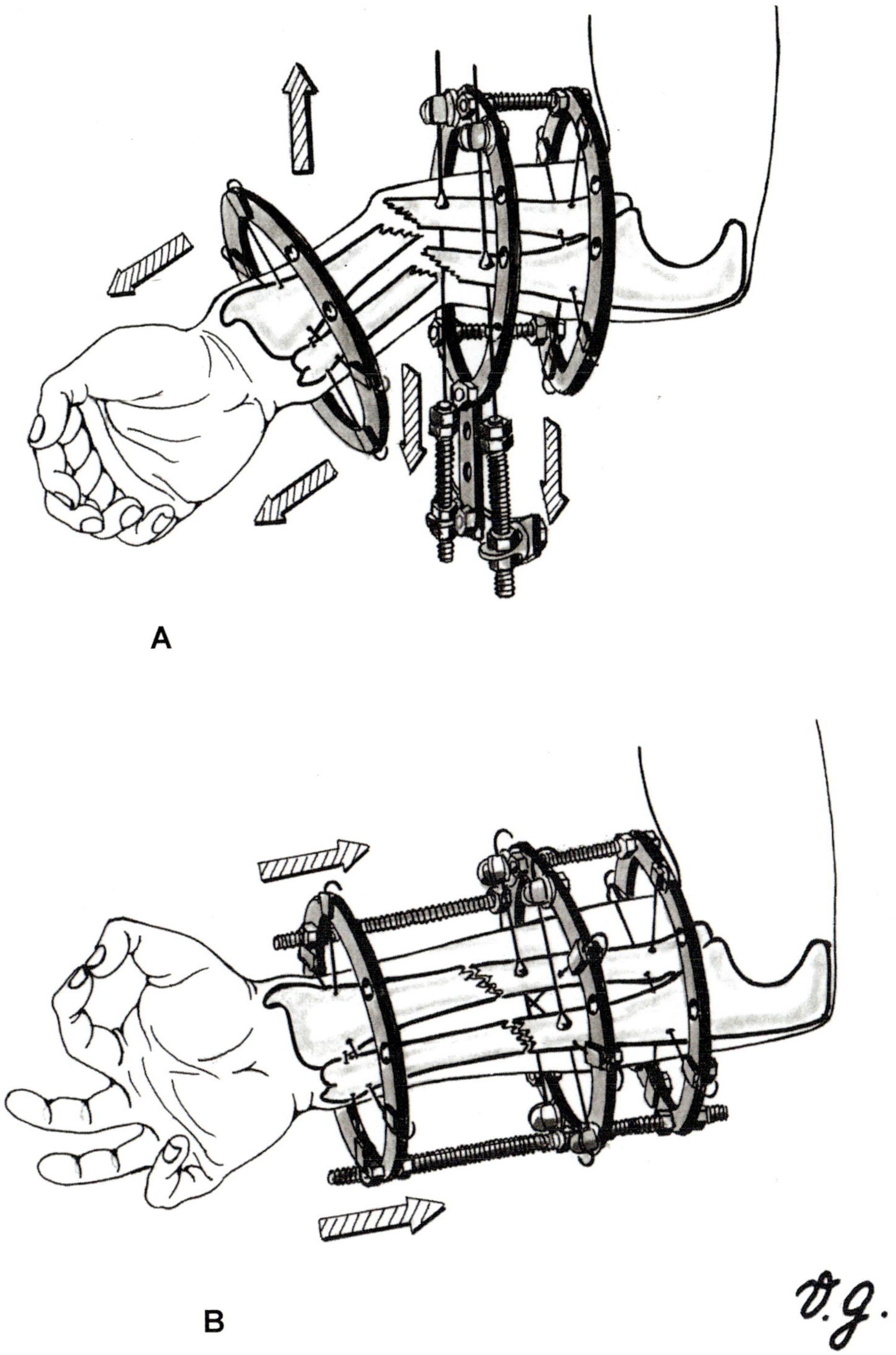

Figure 16.6: Technique of displacement reduction in a forearm fracture. *Arrows* indicate direction of reduction. A, three rings are applied to the limb. Stabilization of the proximal fragment is achieved with temporary introduction of pulling devices. B, after reduction is complete, compression of the fragments is recommended

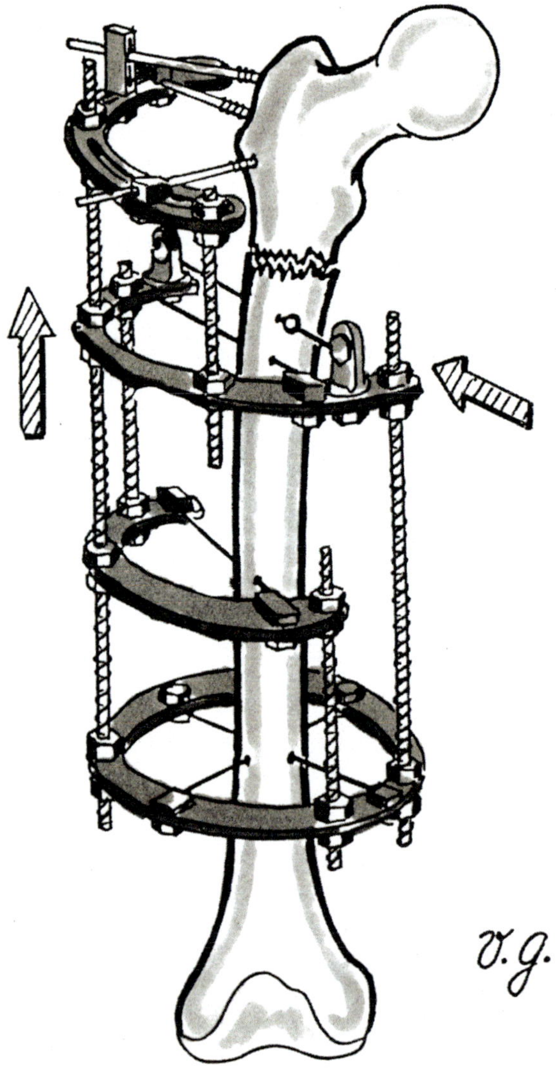

Figure 16.7: Technique of applying the Ilizarov fixator to treat transverse subtrochanter femur fracture. *Arrows* indicate direction of compression

C. Spiral fracture of shaft (see Fig. 16.1).
D. Butterfly-type fracture of shaft (Fig. 16.8).
E. Segmental fracture of shaft (see Fig. 16.4).
F. Near joint fracture (Fig. 16.9).

II. Intra-articular fractures:
A. Fracture dislocation (Fig. 16.10).
B. Condylar fracture (Fig. 16.11).

III. Comminuted fractures:
A. Unstable.
B. With bone loss (segmental defect).

IV. Compound fractures:
A. With soft tissue loss.
B. With compartmental syndrome.

V. Grade C-3 fractures.

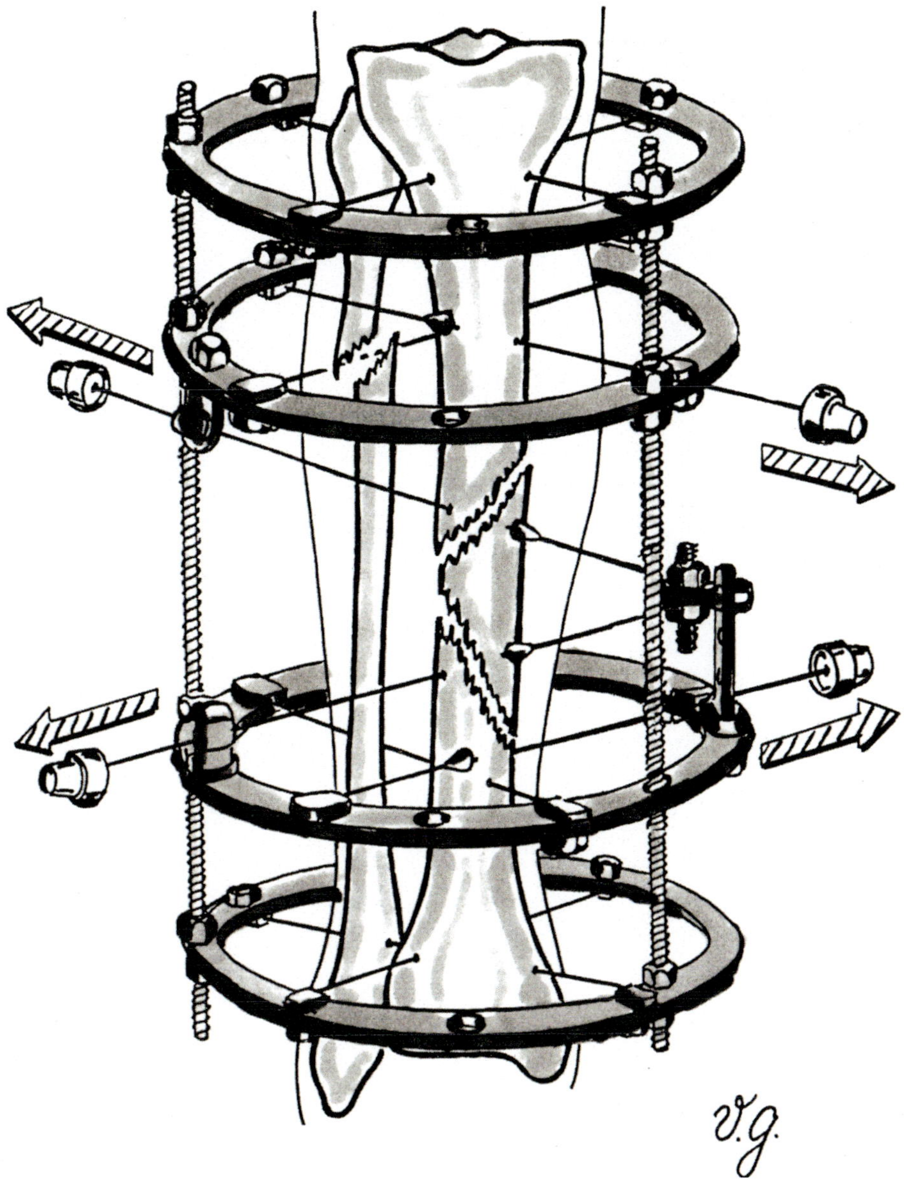

Figure 16.8: Technique of applying the Ilizarov fixator to treat butterfly-type fracture. *Arrows* indicate direction in which the olive wires pull

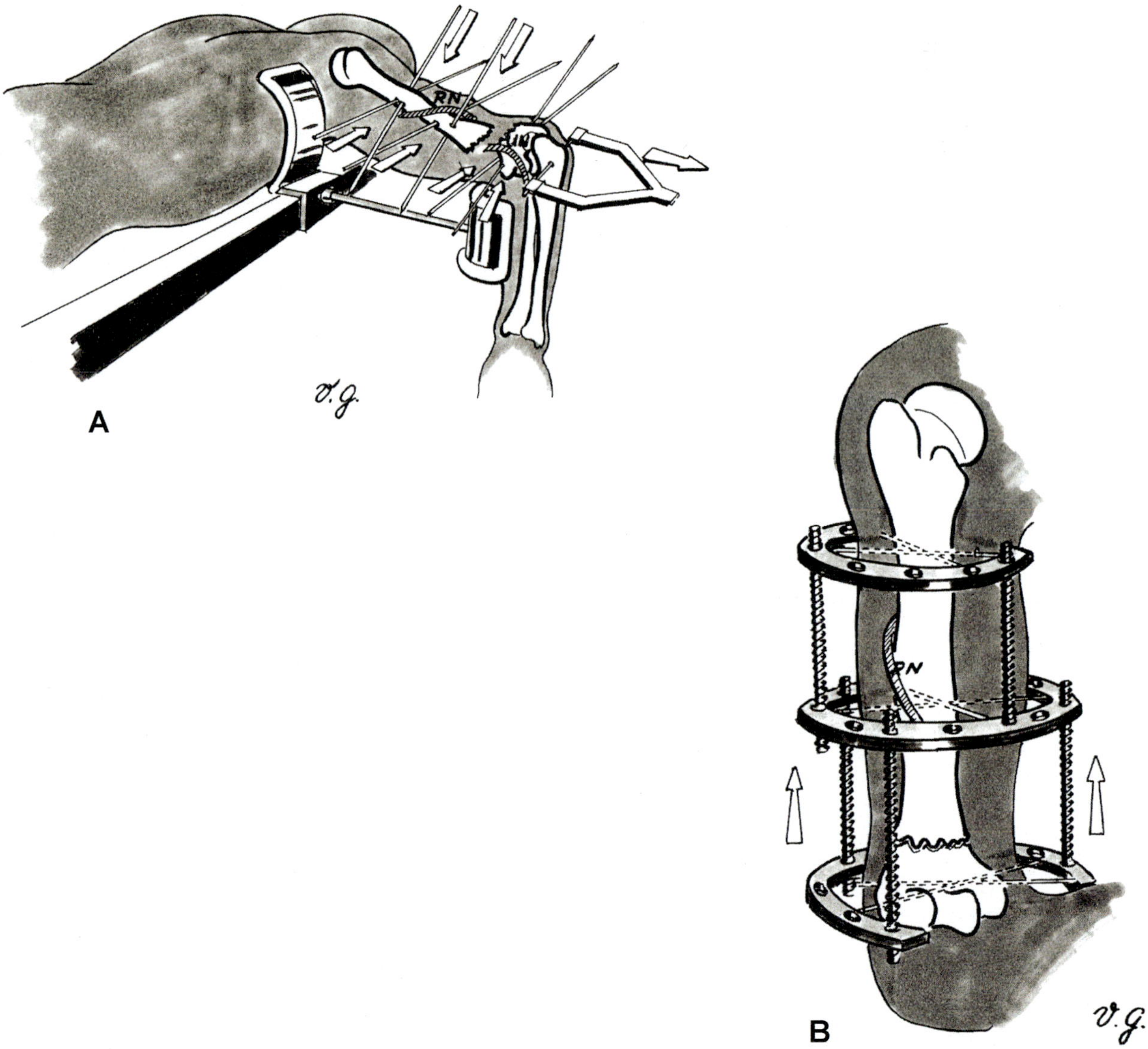

Figure 16.9: Technique of applying the Ilizarov fixator for supracondylar humerus fracture. A, wires introduction. Patient is supine on the operating table. The injured upper extremity is stabilized with skeletal traction through the olecranon and supported by the table extender. The suspended humerus position provides an excellent approach to the limb. Direction of wire introduction is shown by *arrows*. *RN* and *UN* = radial and ulnar nerves, respectively. B, frame consisting of two five-eighths rings and one full center ring Is placed on the upper arm. With careful manipulation the fracture is reduced and fixed with compression *(arrows)*

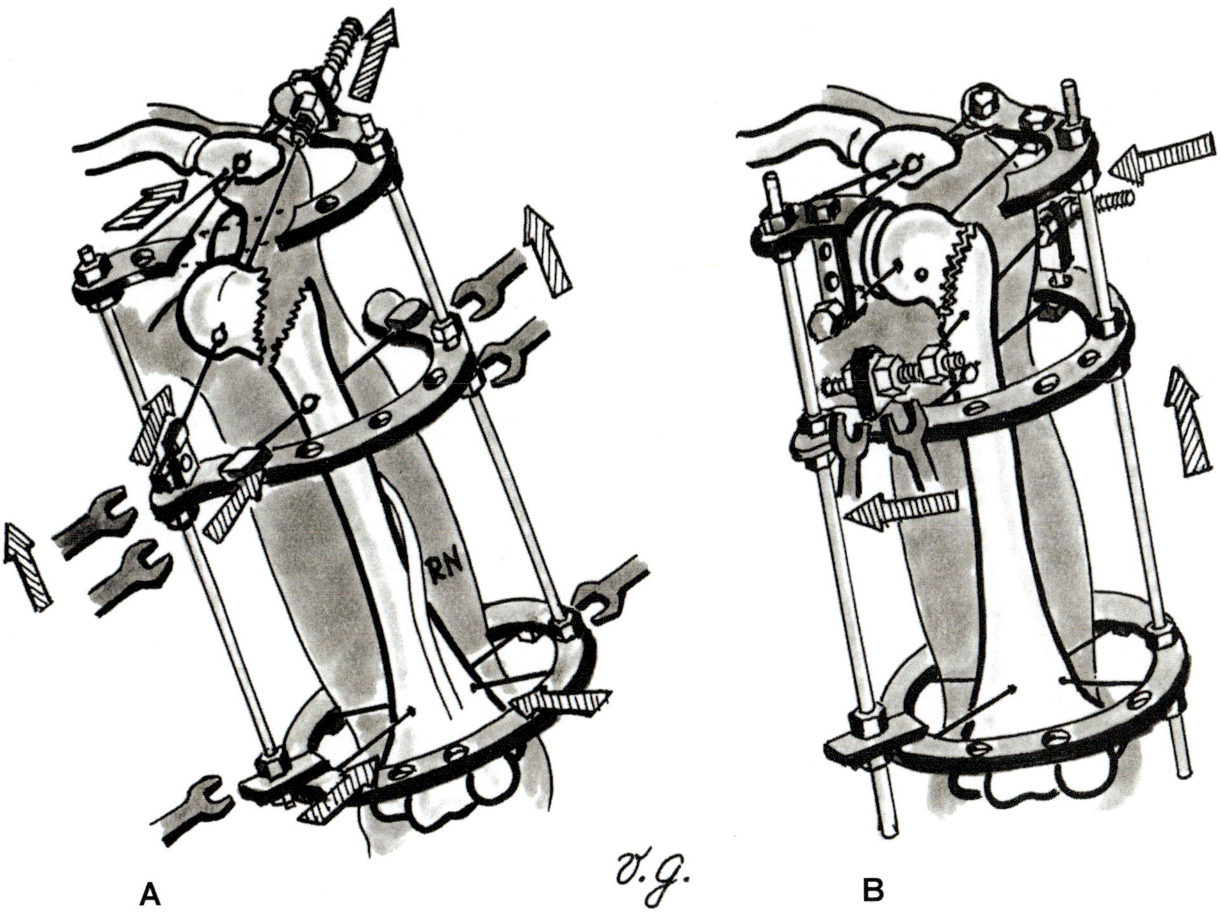

Figure 16.10: Ilizarov technique of reducing shoulder fracture and dislocation. *Arrows* indicate direction of pulling by the olive wires; *wrenches plus arrows* indicate direction of compression. The frame consists of two five-eighths rings and one distal ring. *RN* = radial nerve. An anterior section of the proximal five-eighths ring is not shown. A, olive wire is introduced through the humerus head in a direction opposite that of the dislocation. Another olive wire is introduced just below the fracture site. Both are gradually and simultaneously pulled until reduction is achieved. This maneuver must be controlled, and done under an image intensifier. B, with the head dislocation reduced the olive wire can be replaced with a standard wire. Compression of the distal fragment stabilizes the fracture reduction, which is reinforced by the introduction of additional wires

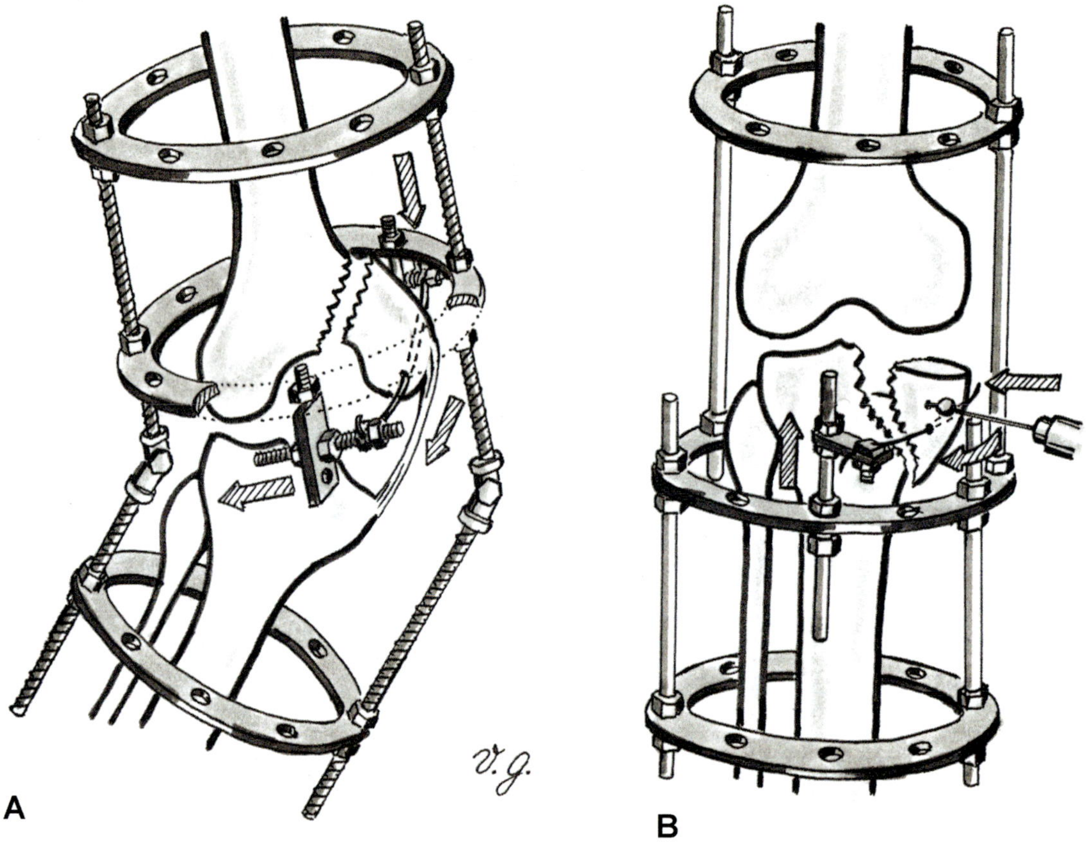

Figure 16.11: Ilizarov technique for reduction of knee condylar fractures. *Arrows* indicate pulling direction of the wire. A three-ring frame is applied (for the purpose of demonstration, an anterior section of the proximal ring is not shown). A, in a femoral medial condyle fracture two rings are placed at the femur and one ring below the knee. Fracture reduction is achieved by wire tensioning. The obliquely introduced wire is pulled to the lateral side. Both ends of the wire are pulled laterally by the distraction devices connected to the ring. The hinges at the knee gap level allow early joint motion. B, in a tibial medial condyle fracture two rings are placed at the level of the tibia and one ring at the level of the femur. After reduction is achieved the olive wire is introduced for reduction stabilization. Axial loading of the extremity is allowed several days after reduction

Professor Ilizarov developed techniques for the treatment of short bone fracture. In particular, the treatment of olecranon and clavicle fractures with displacement represents an interesting innovation because it allows motion in the nearby joints immediately after surgery (Figs 16.12 and 16.13).

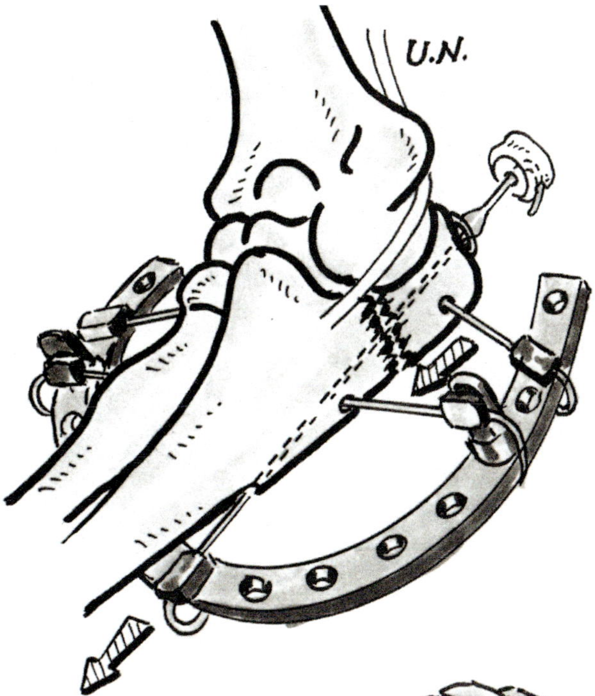

Figure 16.12: Ilizarov technique for olecranon fracture treatment. *Arrows* indicate the direction of compression. *UN* = ulnar nerve. Without incision, the first wire is introduced from the medial to lateral, distal to the fracture line and just posterior to the crista muscle supinator. This is the supporting wire, and is attached to two posts seated at the middle level of the five-eighths ring. The second wire is introduced in the same direction through the displaced olecranon, and drilled approximately 1 cm posteriorly to the ulnar nerve, carefully avoiding the nerve. This wire is slightly bent, with the concave side facing the fracture, and fixed to the ring with approximately 50 kg of tension. This reduces the displaced olecranon and creates compression at the fracture site. In addition, the olive wire is introduced through the olecranon transversely to the fracture plane. It is fixed to the tip of the ring under some tensioning. It is useful to protect the olecranon from olive wire penetration by inserting a washer before the olive stopper

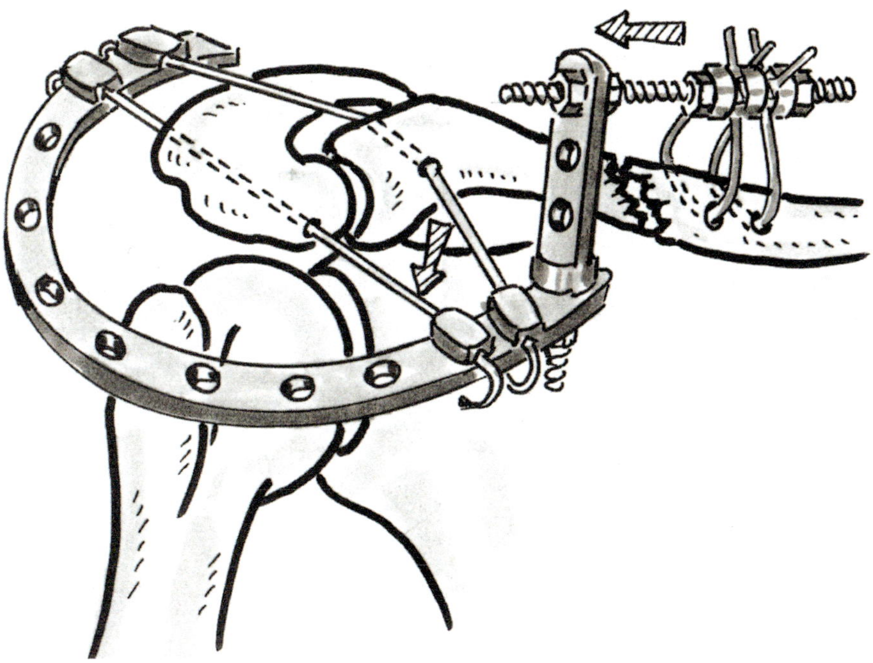

Figure 16.13: Ilizarov technique of reduction of the acromioclavicular joint and fracture of the clavicle. *Arrows* indicate direction of compression. Without incision, the first wire is introduced from posterior to anterior through the acromion. This is the supporting wire, and is transfixed to the five-eighths ring at the middle level. The second wire is introduced in the same direction through the clavicle. It is slightly bent, with the concave side facing the shoulder joint, and fixed to the ring with approximately 50 kg of tension. This reduces clavicle displacement and creates the necessary compression. For fracture reduction, two wires are introduced through the clavicle proximally to the fracture line. The direction of introduction must be from anterior to posterior, pressing back the supraspinas muscle. Both ends of these wires are bent, creating wire loops. The pulling device is attached to the anterior leg of the ring. Depending on the displacement size, a two-, three-, or four-hole post is chosen to support the device, consisting of a threaded rod with 2-mm slotted washers. The long ends of the wires are cut short. Displacement reduction is achieved by fixing the bent wires to this device, and compression of the reduced fracture by pulling the wire loops laterally

ILIZAROV TECHNIQUE FOR CORRECTING FOOT DEFORMITIES

In the 1970s and 1980s Ilizarov developed many original methods to correct various types of foot deformities. All are based on the general Ilizarov principles of distraction and compression used with the external fixator. The Ilizarov biologic law has greater importance for the foot than for any other anatomic structure. The shape-forming process acting on bone tissue depends on the magnitude of the load, the application of the frame and wires to the bone, and the adequacy of blood supply at the site of this load application.

The chief anatomic features of the foot are the arrangement and structure of closely placed small bones and their physiologic importance in the crucial weight-bearing mechanism. The anatomy of the blood vessels and nerves in the foot is also very compact. All of these factors urge the surgeon to exercise a large measure of caution and care when introducing wires through the foot.

In the foot the wire must be introduced in the correct direction on the first attempt. Multiple holes from many attempts will promote postoperative pain, weaken the bones, leave hematomas with dangerous consequences (e.g. compartment syndrome), and even delay healing. It also is important to introduce the wires slowly, to avoid any burning of the bone and soft tissues and to prevent gross injury to the blood vessels and nerves (Fig. 16.14).

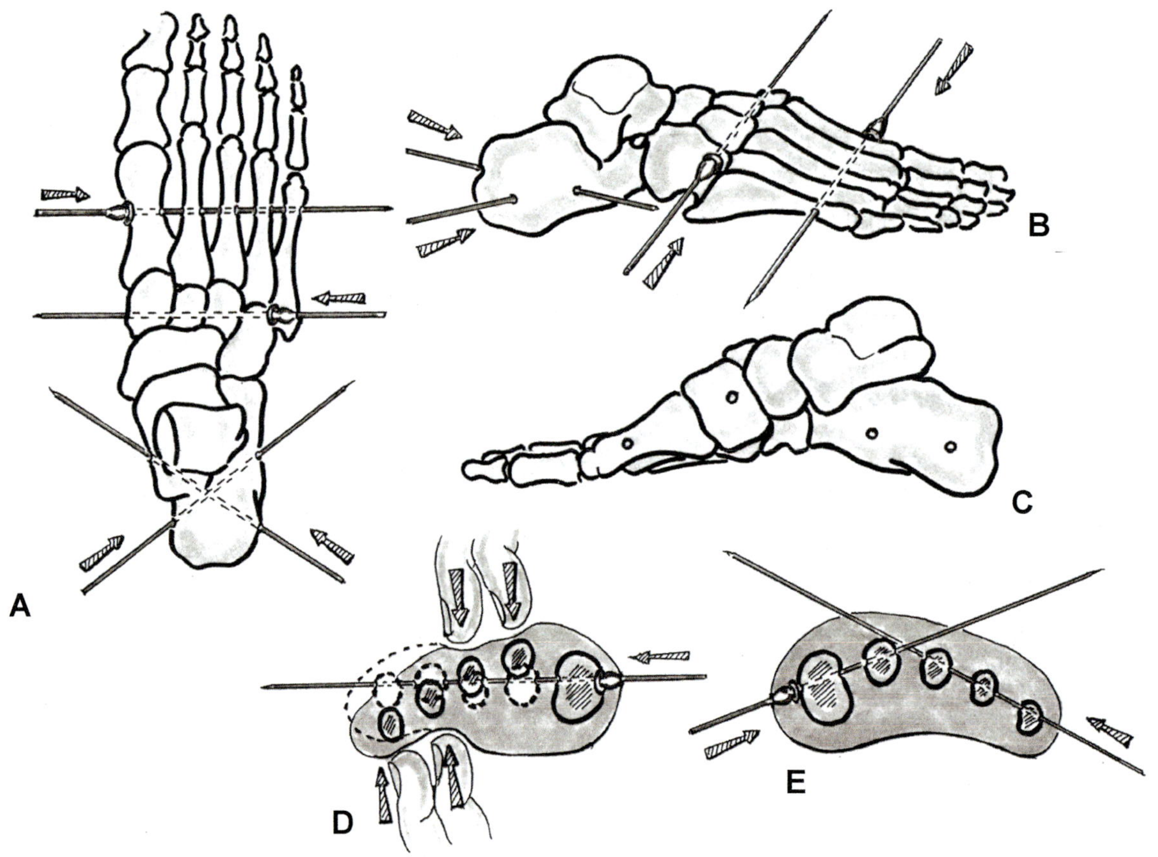

Figure 16.14: Recommended location and direction of wire introduction through the bones of the foot. A, dorsal view. B, lateral view. C, medial view. D, anterior view of metatarsal bones. The wire is introduced through all five metatarsals, which is difficult to achieve and requires slow wire introduction under control of finger pressure on each metatarsal bone head. E, in this method of wire introduction two wires transfix the five metatarsal bones. These two wires must be firmly transfixed to the frame, because if not properly tensioned they may cause intolerable pain

The frame for the foot in most of the recommended technique variations is complex, and difficult to assemble in advance. General principles of foot frame assembly include the following:

1. Most frames consist of a supporting component, a hindfoot component, and a forefoot component.
2. The supporting foot frame component is a two-ring frame (sometimes one ring with additional offset wires) attached to the tibia (Fig. 16.15). The level of its attachment depends on the size and complexity of the rest of the frame: the more complex the forefoot and hindfoot components the higher the level of the supporting component is attached.

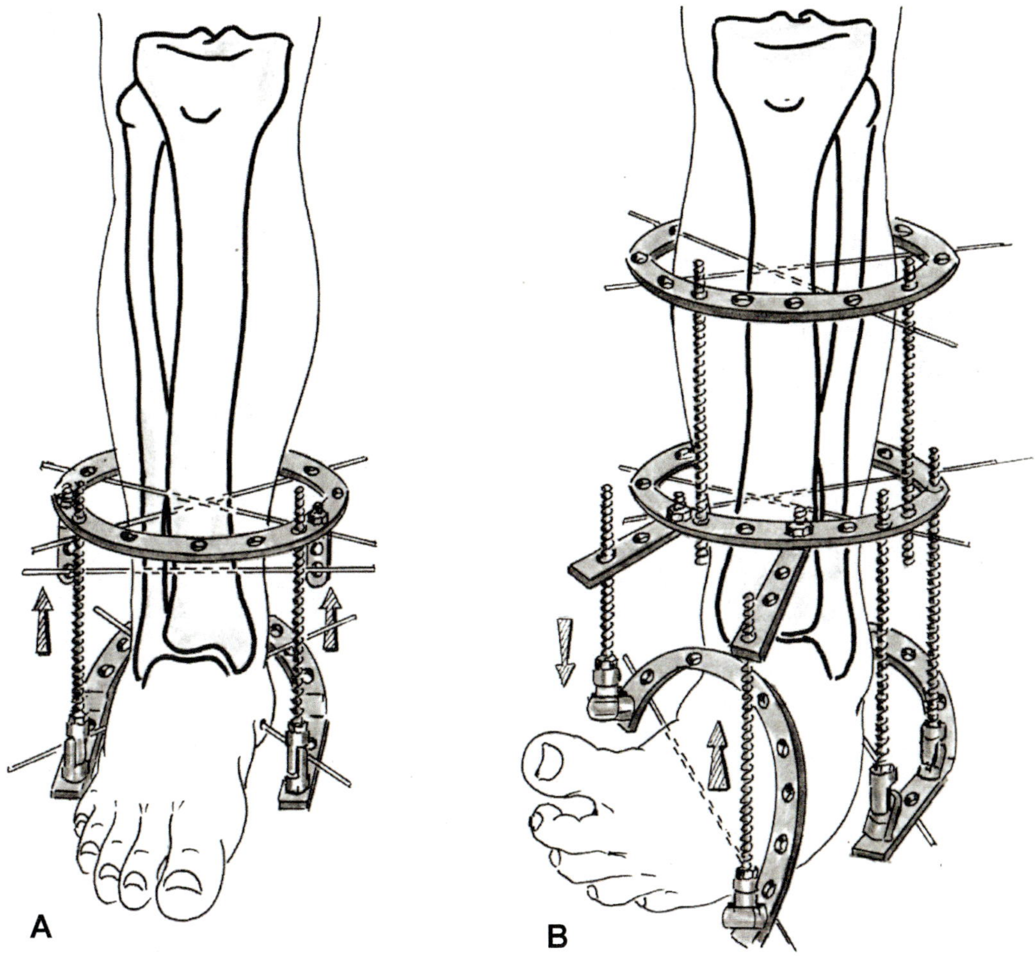

Figure 16.15: A and B, supporting component of the foot frame. The more complex the foot frame, the higher the level attachment to the tibia

3. The hindfoot component consists of a half-ring placed around the heel. In most cases both "legs" of this half-ring must be made longer by the firm attachment of connecting plates (Fig. 16.16).

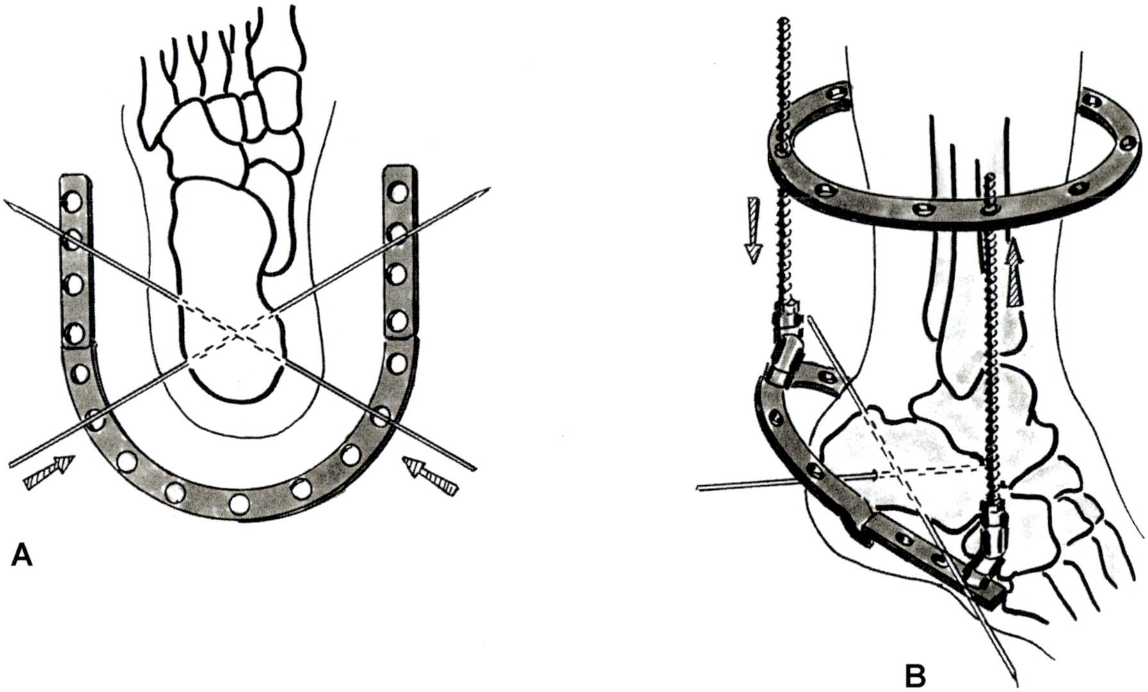

Figure 16.16: Hindfoot component of foot frame. A, plantar view. B, side view with a segment of the supporting component

4. The forefoot component consists of the half-ring placed around the dorsal surface of the forefoot. In most cases both legs of this half-ring are connected to the middle part of the connecting plates by half-hinges. This component always is connected to the supporting component (Fig. 16.17).

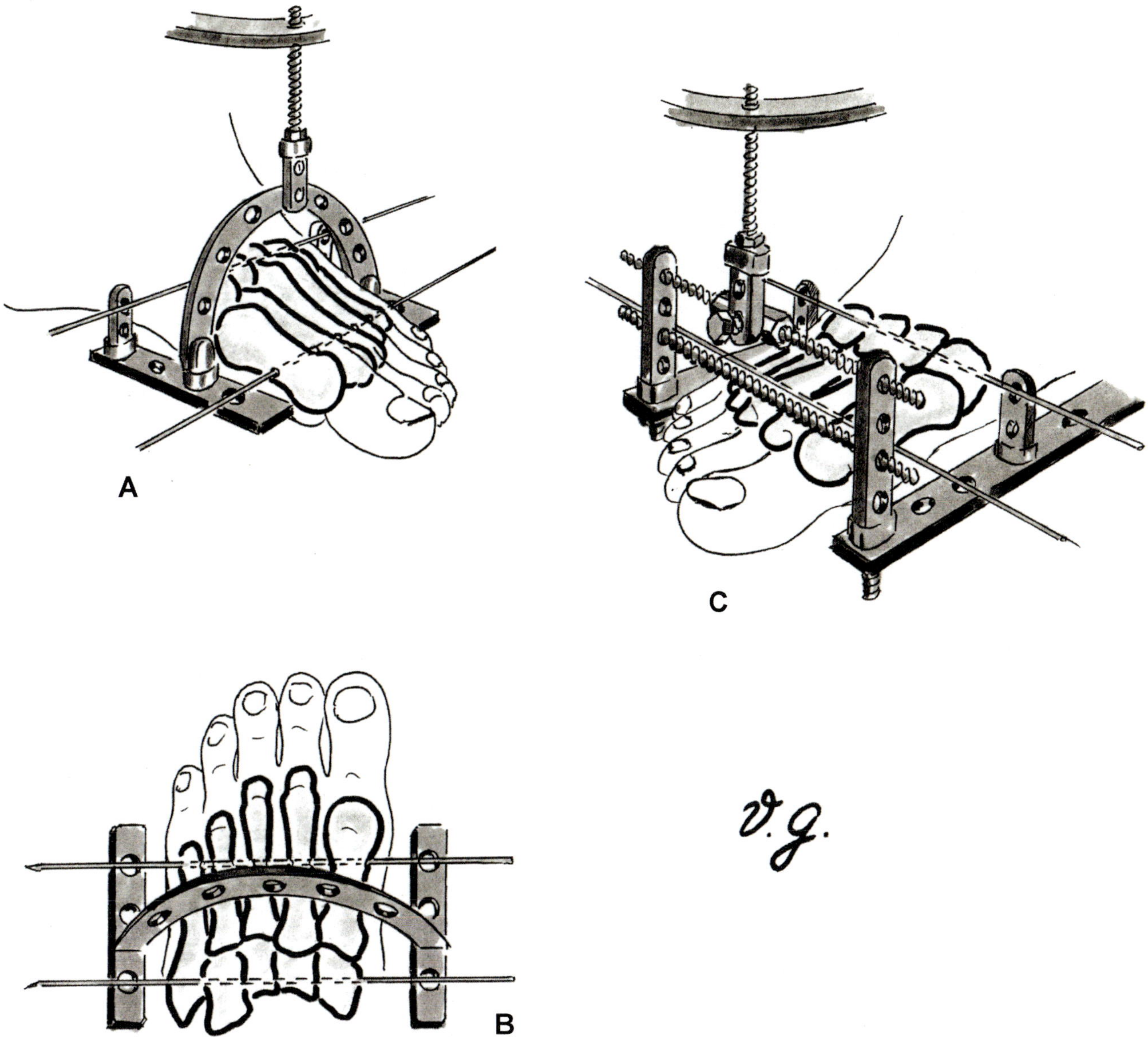

Figure 16.17: Forefoot component of foot frame. Connecting plates are attached with half-hinges. A, side view with the segment of supporting component. B, dorsal view. C, version of the forefoot component consisting of two supports with threaded rods replacing the half-ring

5. In certain cases the forefoot component consists of two long connecting plates attached to the hindfoot component and the supporting component (Fig. 16.18).

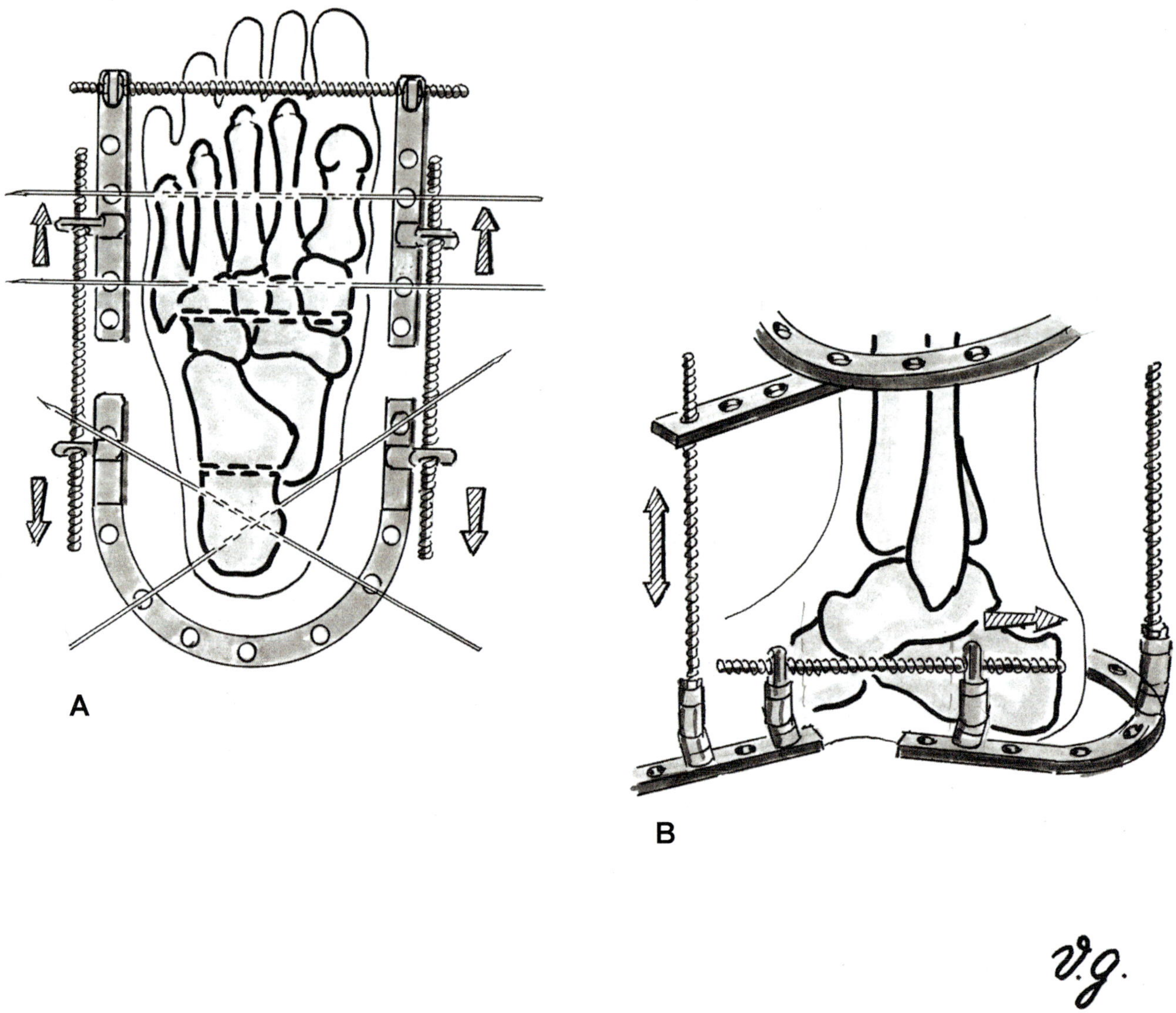

Figure 16.18: Forefoot component consisting of two long plates. *Arrows* indicate direction of distraction. A, plantar view with hindfoot component. *Interrupted lines* indicate sites of osteotomy for foot lengthening. B, side view with a segment of the supporting component, showing their connection. Hinges are introduced to the connecting threaded rods to position the forefoot component in proper angulation in relation to the hindfoot

6. The forefoot and hindfoot components may or may not be connected to each other, depending on the goal of treatment.
7. Connection between the forefoot and hindfoot component should be flexible in most cases (Fig. 16.19).
8. In the foot frame assembly the need to introduce and use hinges is more common than in any other type of frame. In certain cases such hinges must have two axes (see Fig. 16.17) for simultaneous correction of two different types of deformities.

Bearing in mind these main principles, many different types of foot deformities can be corrected with the Ilizarov technique and apparatus (Figs 16.20 to 16.22; see also Fig. 14.14).

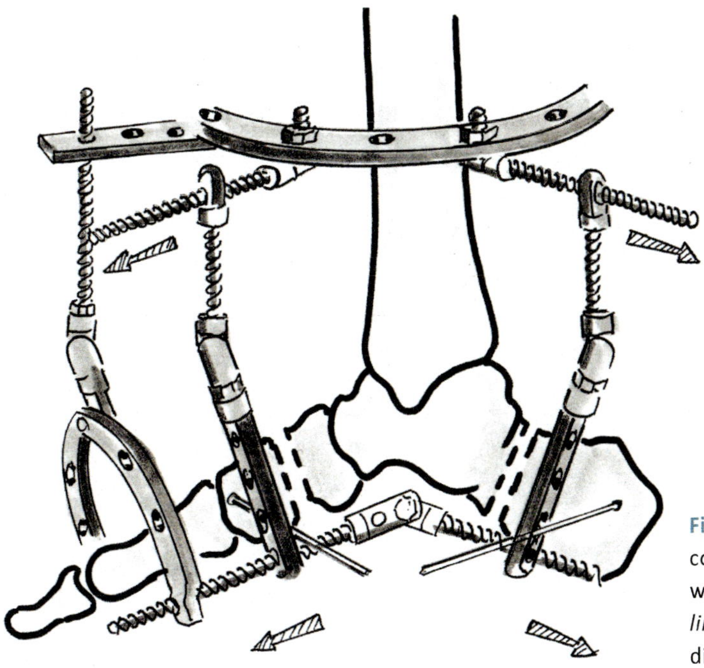

Figure 16.19: Connection between the forefoot and hindfoot components for the purpose of foot lengthening. Side view with a segment of the supporting component. *Interrupted lines* indicate osteotomy sites; *arrows* indicate direction of distraction

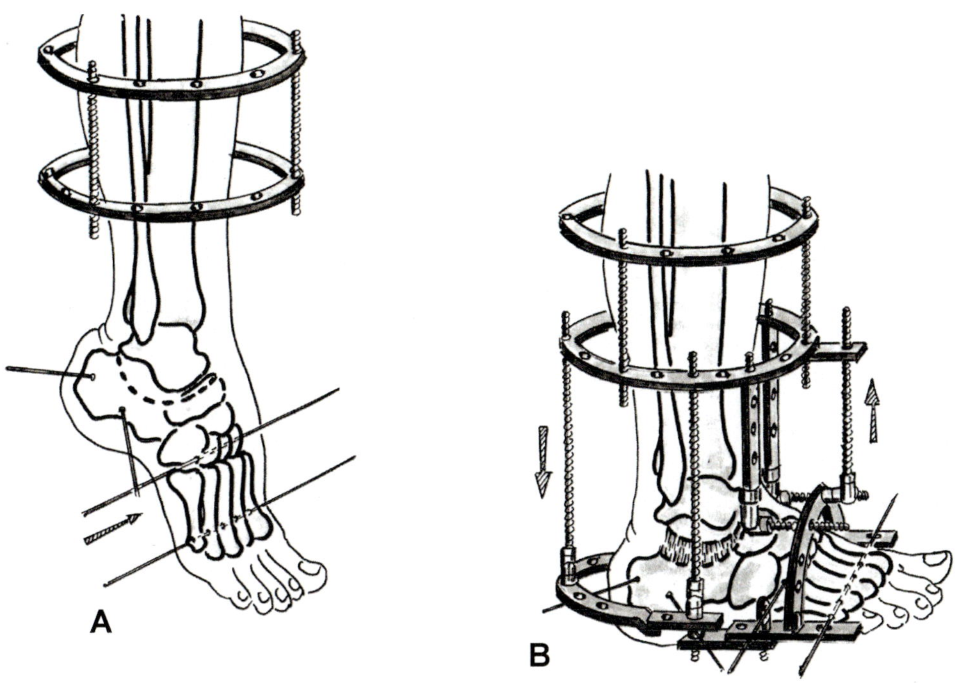

A

B

Figure 16.20: Ilizarov technique for equinus correction with U-shaped foot osteotomy *(interrupted line)*. **A,** foot in equinus position with two supporting rings on leg. Wires are introduced in preparation for application of the foot component of the frame. **B,** foot component of the frame is applied and gradual equinus correction completed. *Arrows* indicate direction of corrective forces of the pulling-pushing mechanisms

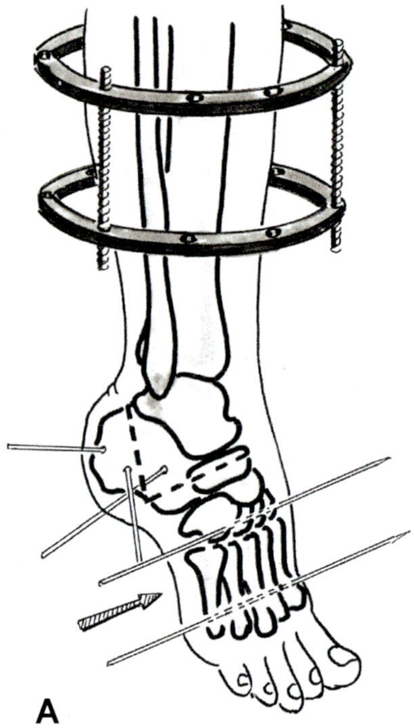

Figure 16.21: Ilizarov technique for equinus correction with V-shaped osteotomy *(interrupted line)* **A,** foot in equinus position with two supporting rings on leg, Wires are introduced in preparation for application of the foot component of the frame. **B,** foot component of the frame is applied and gradual equinus correction completed. *Arrows* indicate direction of corrective forces of the pulling-pushing mechanism

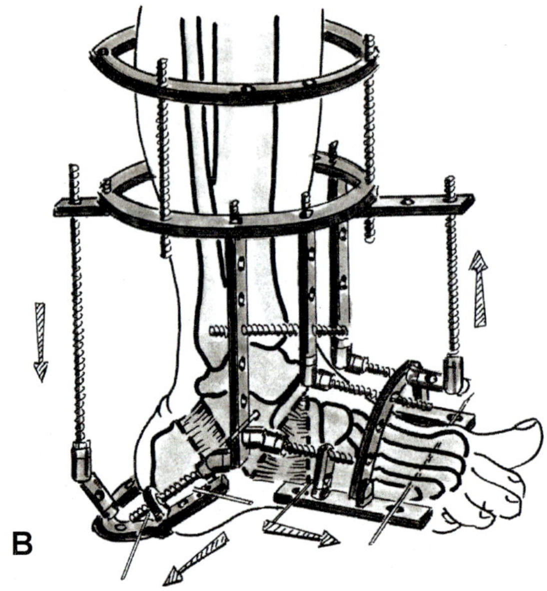

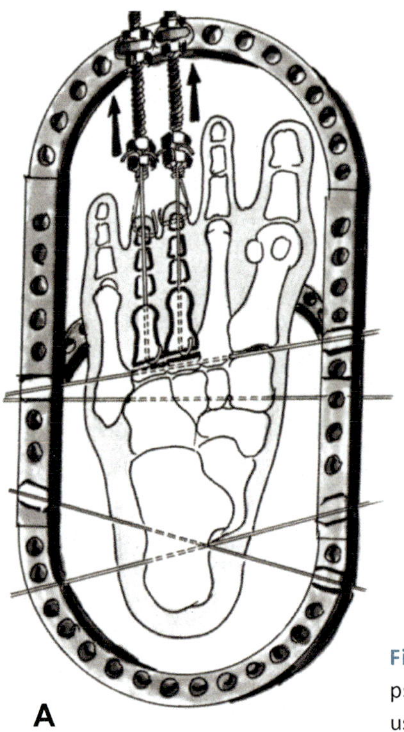

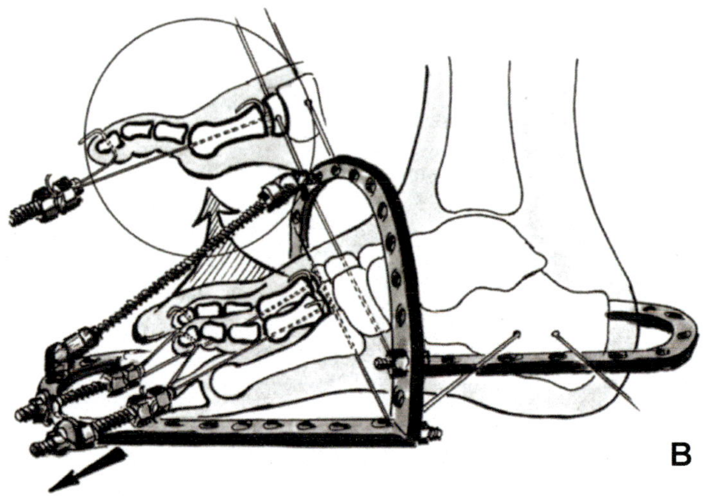

Figure 16.22: Technique of metatarsal bone distraction for lengthening toes. In type 1 pseudohypoparathyroidism, the metatarsal bones can appear symmetrically shortened, usually the second and third or the third and fourth metatarsals. This cosmetic defect can evoke much unhappiness in the patient. Based on the Ilizarov principles, the technique of metatarsal bone lengthening was developed by Vladimir Golyakhovsky. **A,** plantar view. To simultaneously lengthen the metatarsal bone and the corresponding toe, the two pulling hooked wires are attached to the same pulling device. **B,** side view. The frame for this treatment is not necessarily stabilized by the supporting frame

ILIZAROV TECHNIQUE FOR CORRECTIVE HAND PROCEDURES

For correction of hand deformities, Ilizarov has designed a miniapparatus, one-fourth the size of the original fixator. Corticotomies of metacarpal and phalangeal bones are performed through a 4-mm incision, and the osteotome for this procedure is of a correspondingly small size. Such procedures, however, must be performed by surgeons specially trained in the principles of plastic surgery and microsurgery. The frames for Ilizarov technique lengthening of the hand and for the treatment of syndactyly are shown in Figures 16.23 and 16.24.

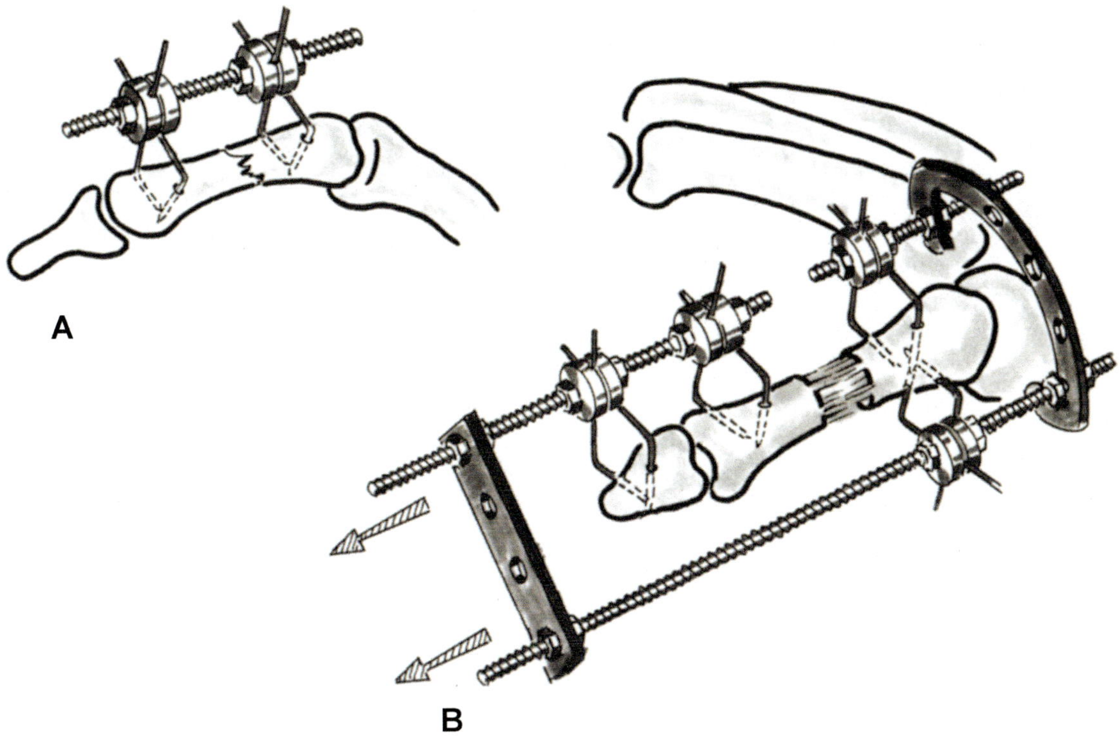

Figure 16.23: Basic assembly of the Ilizarov fixator for hand treatment. A, for finger fracture and lengthening. B, for metacarpal bone fracture and lengthening. *Arrows* indicate direction of distraction

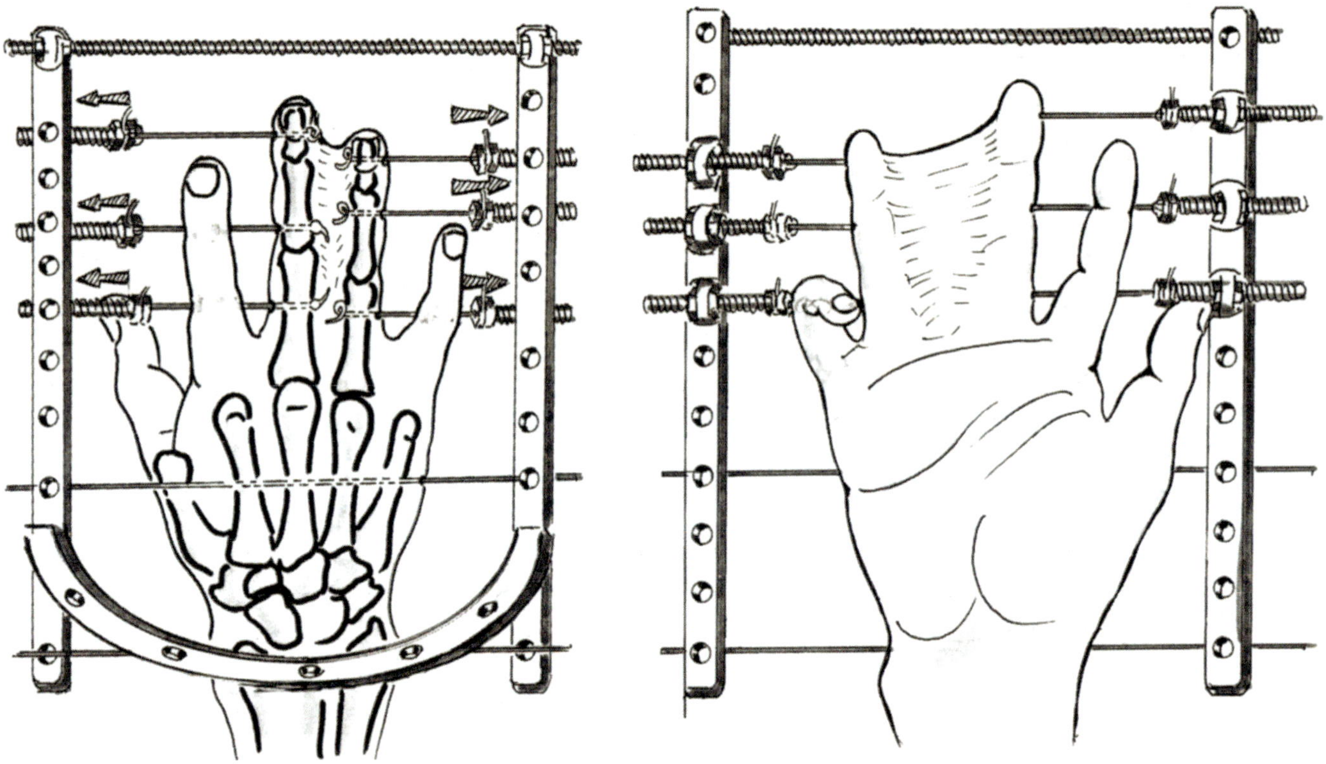

A B

Figure 16.24: Ilizarov technique for treatment of syndactyly. **A,** dorsal view. *Arrows* indicate direction of skin stretching. **B,** anterior view after skin is stretched

ILIZAROV TECHNIQUE FOR COMPRESSIVE ARTHRODESIS

Along with resection of deformed joint surfaces, it is necessary to achieve fusion by stabilizing and compressing the bone fragments. Both of these procedures may be accomplished relatively easily with the Ilizarov fixator. In certain cases compression-distraction can be performed simultaneously, allowing the surgeon to lengthen the resected joint and to compensate for limb shortness (Figs 16.25 and 16.26).

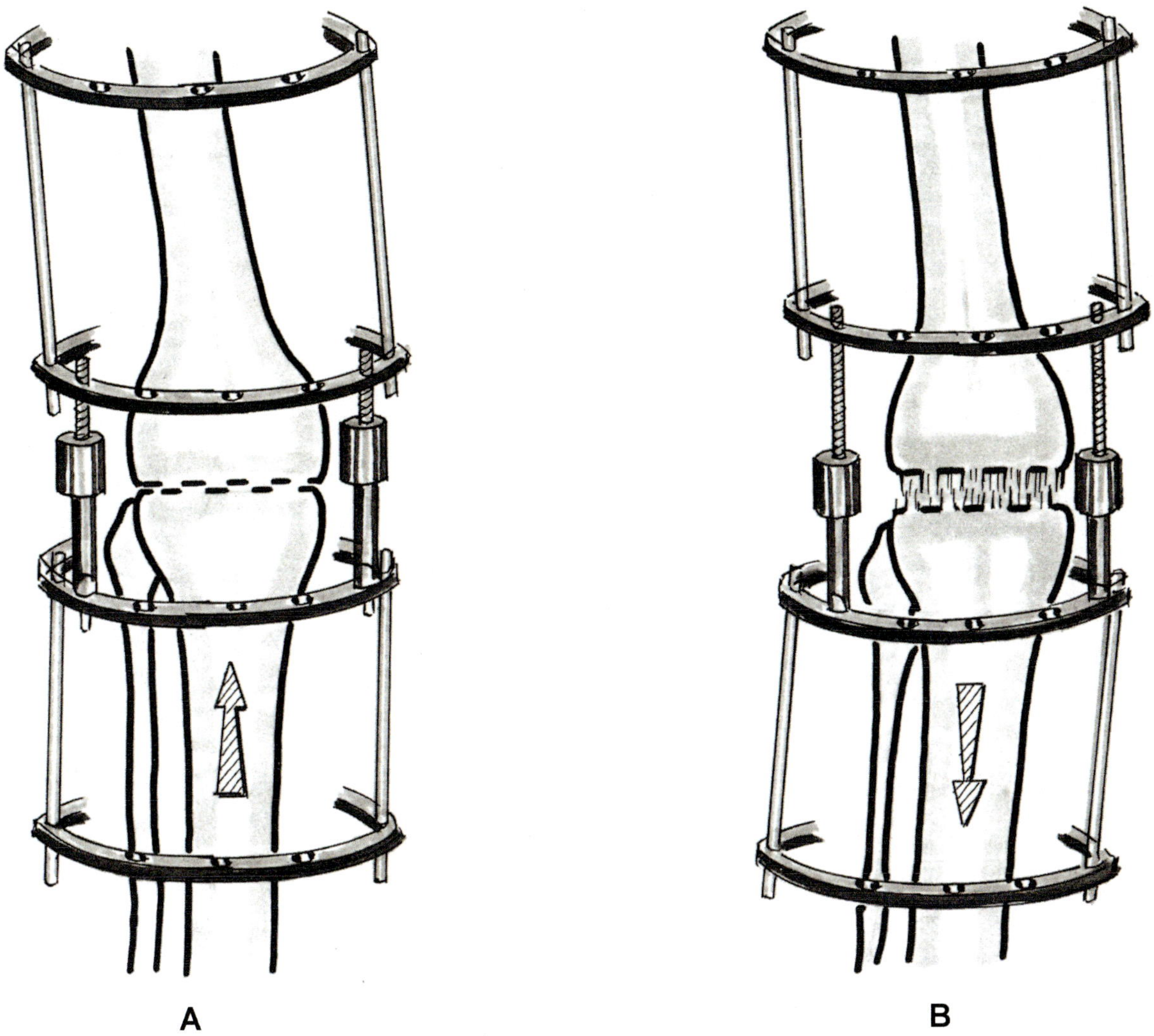

Figure 16.25: Ilizarov compression-distraction technique for knee arthrodesis. *Arrows* indicate direction of compression-distraction. A, compression after resection is continued for 2 weeks at a low rate, 0.25 to 0.50 mm/day. B, after 2 weeks of compression and a 1-week waiting period, distraction is begun at a rate of 0.25 mm twice a day

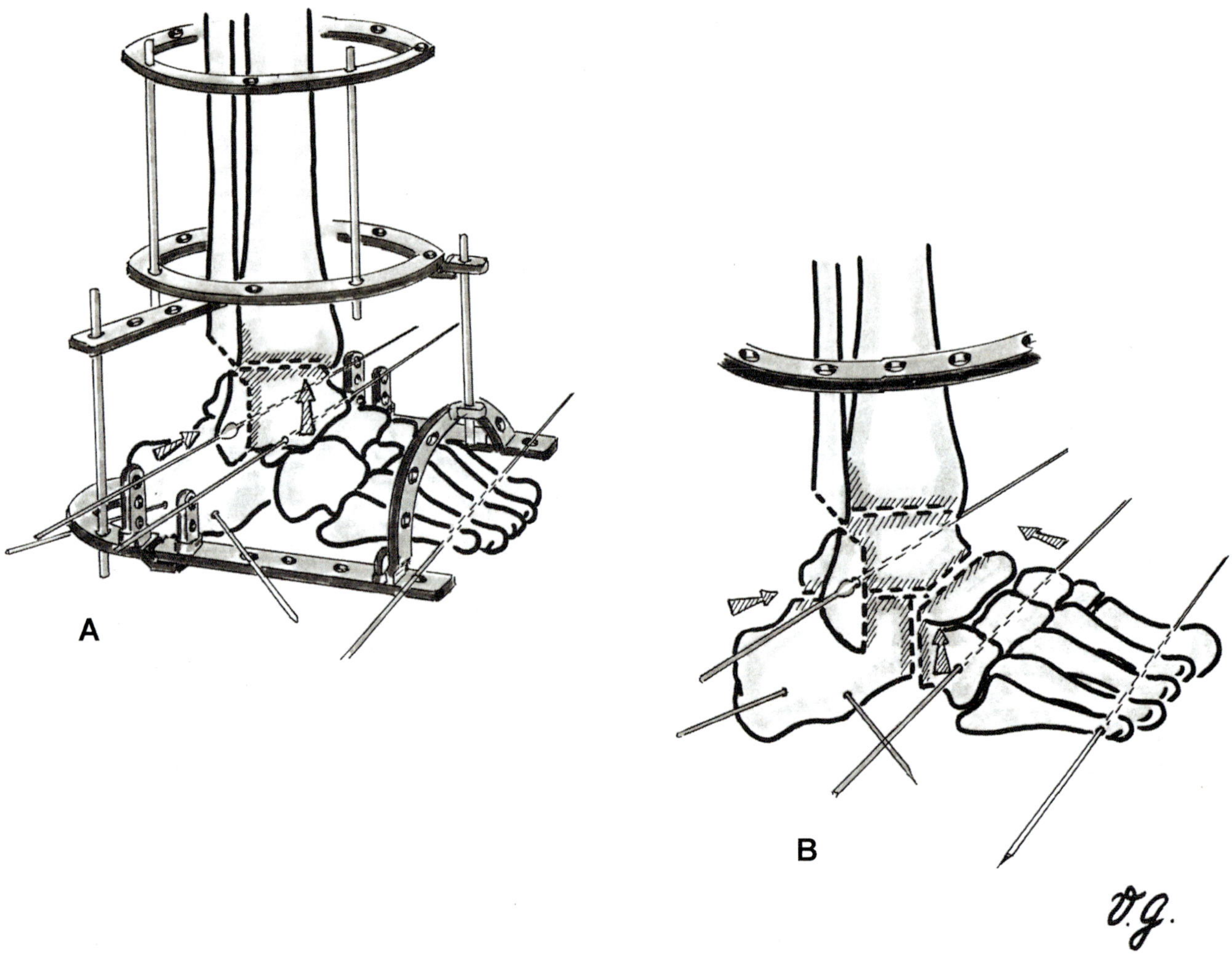

Figure 16.26: Ilizarov compression technique for ankle arthrodesis. *Arrows* indicate direction of compression; shaded areas indicate resected joint surfaces. **A,** Using the foot frame with a leg support component, compression of the shifted lateral malleolus and tibiotalar joint is undertaken. **B,** with additional resection of the talonavicular, subtalar, and talocuboid joints the triple arthrodesis can be performed

ILIZAROV TECHNIQUE FOR STUMP LENGTHENING

Lengthening of a short tibial stump was the first case of distraction Ilizarov performed, in the early 1960s. Application of the fixator for short stump lengthening is indicated for both the upper and lower extremities. The advantage of this technique is that lengthening of the bone promotes local vascular neogenesis and improves the condition of the stump skin and soft tissues (Fig. 16.27).

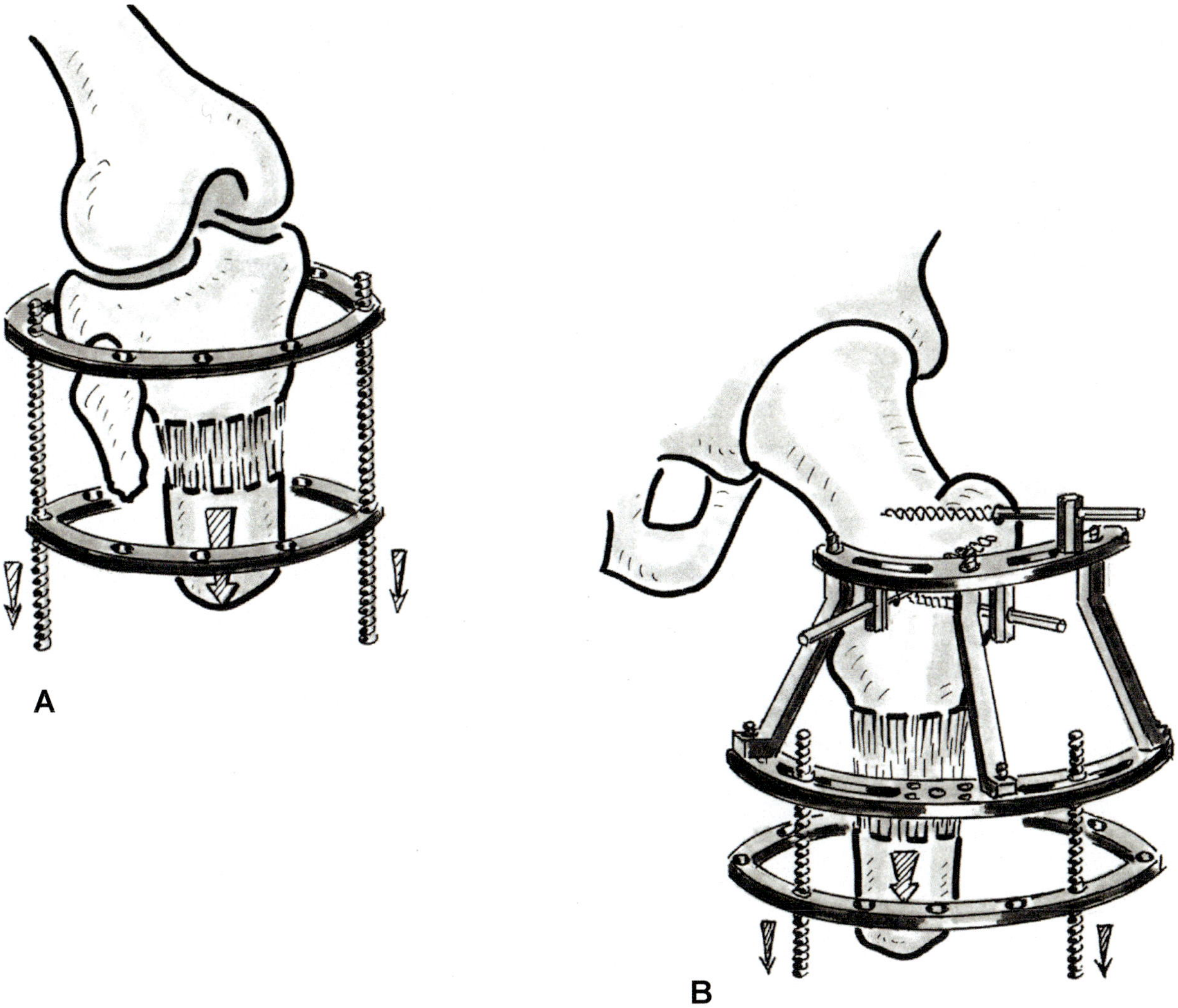

Figure 16.27: Ilizarov technique for short stump lengthening. *Arrows* indicate direction of distraction. A, short tibia stump lengthening. B, short femur stump lengthening

CASE ILLUSTRATIONS

Figures 16.28 to 16.30 illustrate cases in which the Ilizarov apparatus was used in the treatment of foot and knee fractures, arthrodesis, and for femoral stump lengthening.

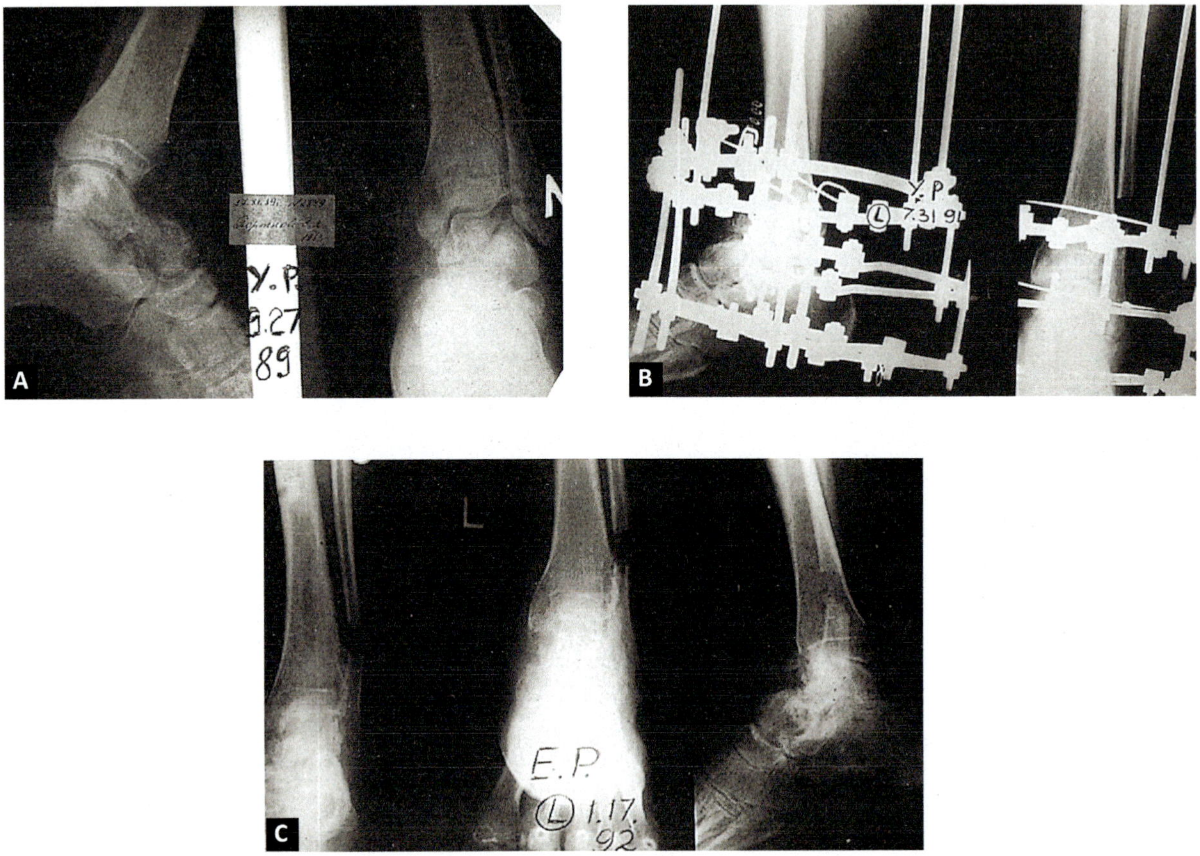

Figure 16.28: Ankle Arthrodesis. Twenty-seven-year-old man with valgus deformity, restricted range of motion, and pain in the left ankle. Patient had a history of fracture-dislocation of the left foot. Two years earlier, conservative treatment (closed reduction and plaster cast application) had been tried. **A,** lateral and AP radiographs of left ankle before surgery. **B,** radiographs after ankle resection and application of the Ilizarov fixator for compression arthrodesis. **C,** radiographs 1 year after surgery show complete ankle fusion

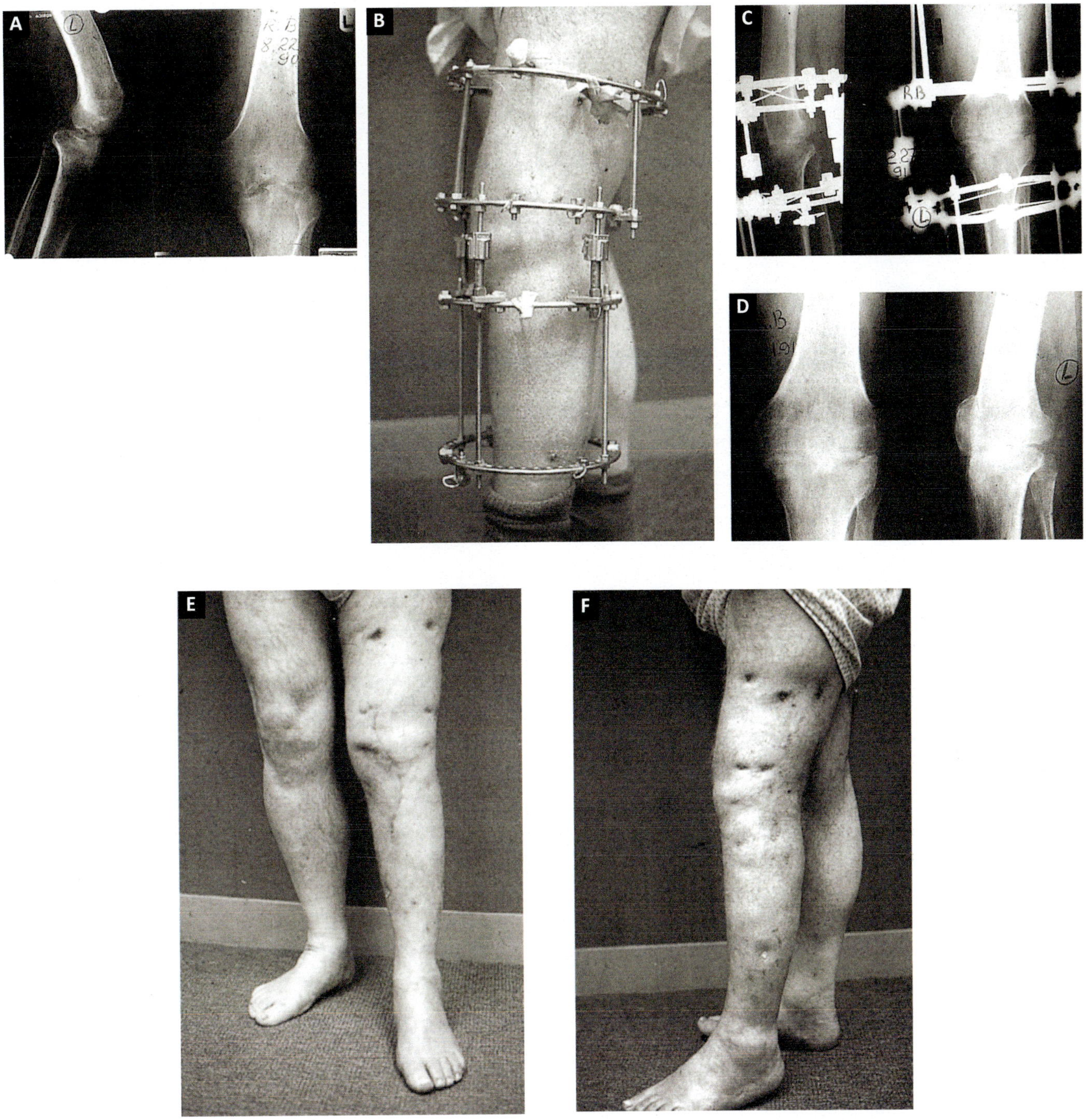

Figure 16.29: Knee Arthrodesis. Fifty-eight-year-old man with history of tuberculosis in the left knee; severe arthritis developed. A, lateral and AP radiographs of left knee before surgery. B, leg after left knee resection and application of the Ilizarov fixator and compression arthrodesis. For the purpose of stability, the femoral and leg components of the apparatus are large, and include two-rings connected by four graduated telescopic rods. C, lateral and AP radiographs of left knee 5 months after surgery show complete knee fusion. D, radiographs after removal of the fixator 6 months after surgery. E and F, appearance of left leg 1 year after surgery

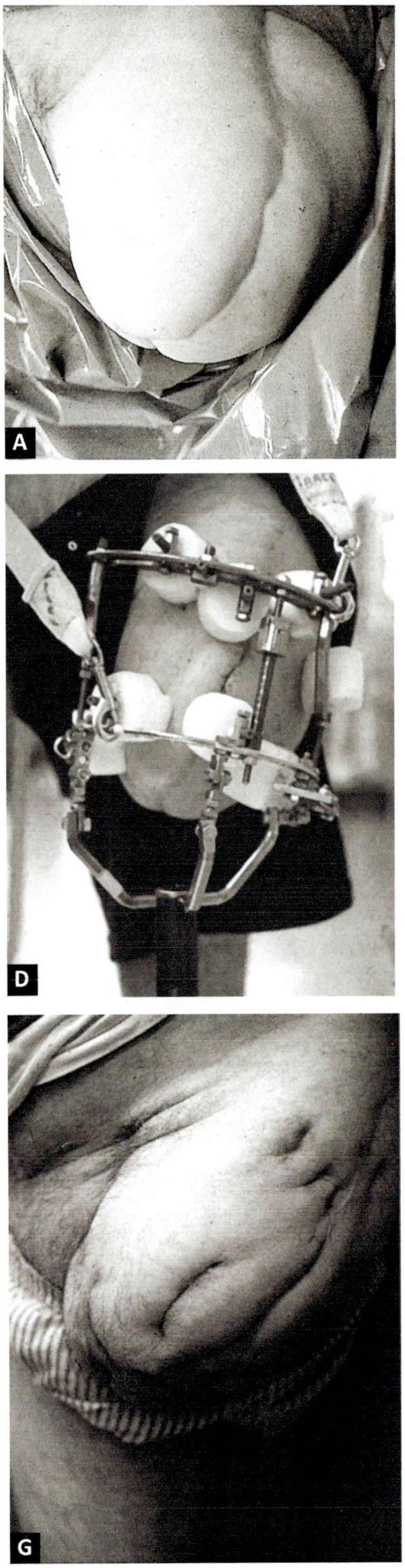

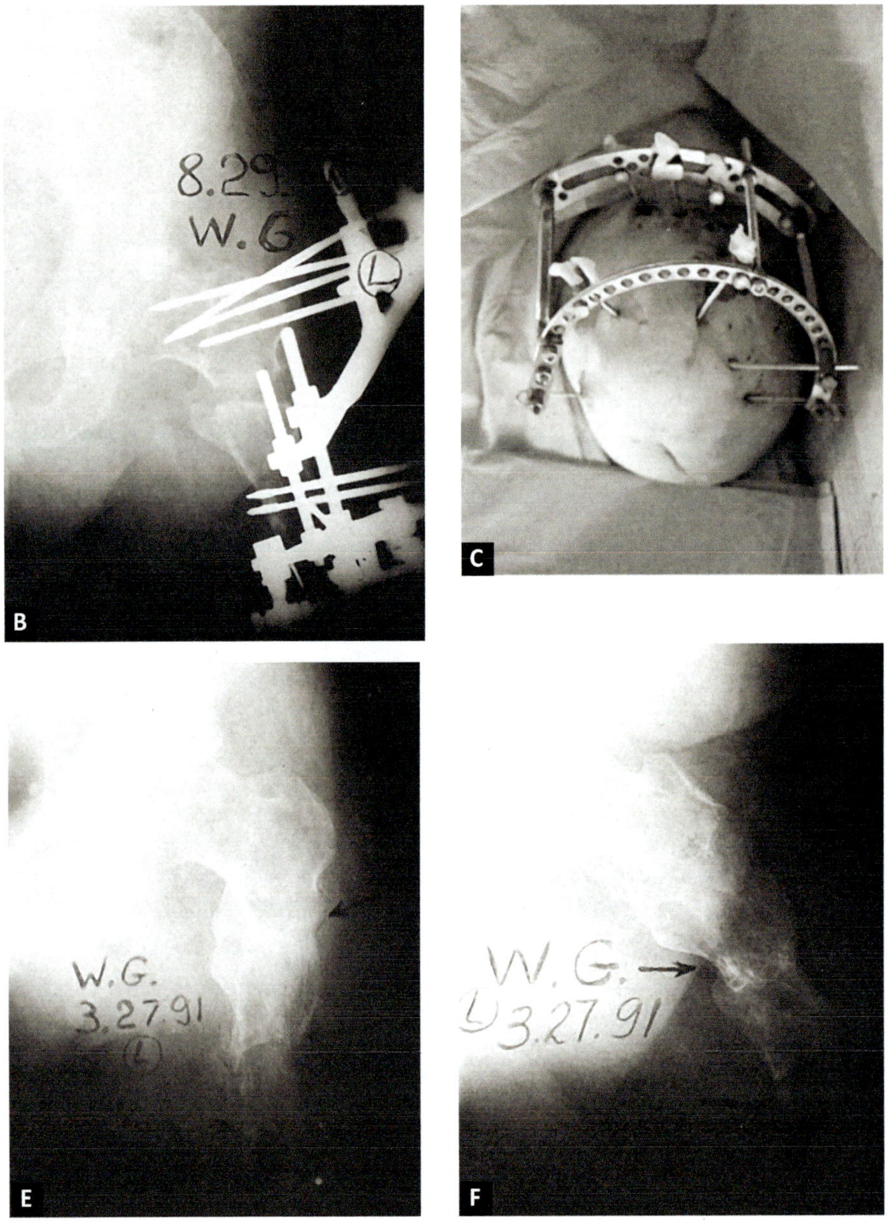

Figure 16.30: Short Femur Stump Lengthening. Sixty-seven-year-old man with a short left femur stump after amputation 10 years earlier because of severe chronic vascular disease. Patient complained that the stump was too short to fit a prosthesis. **A,** appearance of stump before surgery. **B,** radiograph of stump after subtrochanteric corticotomy and application of the fixator. **C,** stump after surgery with frame applied. **D,** stump with fixator and supporting frame for axial loading 2 months after surgery. **E,** AP radiograph of stump 7 months after surgery. **F,** lateral radiograph of stump 7 months after surgery. **G,** appearance of stump 1 year after surgery

17

Chapter

Fixator Removal and Complications of Ilizarov Technique

Treatment with the Ilizarov technique consists of five stages:

1. Fixator application and a following latency period of 4 to 7 days.
2. Period of distraction/compression of 1 to 4 or 5 months (depending on the case).
3. Period of immobility and fixation of the bone position. This usually takes twice as long as distraction-compression.
4. Discontinuation of distraction-compression and frame dynamization 15 to 20 days prior to fixator removal.
5. Period of immobilization with a cast or brace. This is not compulsory, and depends on the case.

CRITERIA FOR FIXATOR REMOVAL

Before treatment the patient must be informed of the duration of the Ilizarov therapeutic course. During the initial period in the hospital the patient is trained in pin care and distraction-compression. If the patient is a child the parents are trained to do this.

During distraction-compression the patient is seen by the physician in the clinic or office weekly at first, then monthly. The appearance of early radiodense regenerate should be observed in this period. On radiographs the first new bone shadow can be seen as early as 3 to 4 weeks after distraction is begun. Taking into account that radiographic appearance is always 10 to 14 days behind real tissue development, the physician can coordinate the rate and rhythm of distraction at this stage. After further distraction the defined columns of new bone oriented in the direction of distraction appear in 6 to 8 weeks. At this stage the quality of new bone can be evaluated radiographically. If the regenerate maintains a constant diameter, normal development is taking place. Rapid regenerate development, seen mostly in young patients and in patients with achondroplasia or Ollier disease, can lead to premature regenerate ossification.

Tomographic evaluation of regenerate quality is recommended at least once before the end of the distraction-compression period. The best way to evaluate regenerate development is to verify it on computed tomographic (CT) scan. If normal it appears fully cylindrical and in the same cross-section with the corticotomized bone ends. Because metallic materials interfere with the CT image, they have to be replaced temporarily with nonmetal connectors at the time of the procedure.

It also is possible to evaluate the regenerate sonographically. This method has some advantages, in particular, lower cost.

To achieve regenerate calcification complete immobility is necessary. This is the third period of fixation. The patient's physical activity, on the other hand, is increased with physical therapy and axial loading. Toward the end of this period the radiographic appearance of the regenerate is verified.

With satisfactory appearance of the regenerate calcification and its complete recanalization, the formation of cortex is seen. At this stage the cessation of distraction-compression is accomplished by loosening the nuts at the sides of the connecting rod attachments (Fig. 17.1). This dynamizes the immobilized bone fragments and the regenerate between them. The patient continues to apply axial loading to the bone for 15 to 20 days more before the apparatus is removed. It should be emphasized that the criteria for removal of the Ilizarov apparatus are positive results of evaluation of the regenerate at the final stage of its development and clinical and radiographic evaluation during all periods of treatment. The choice of the type of cast or brace and its duration on the extremity depends on the particular case.

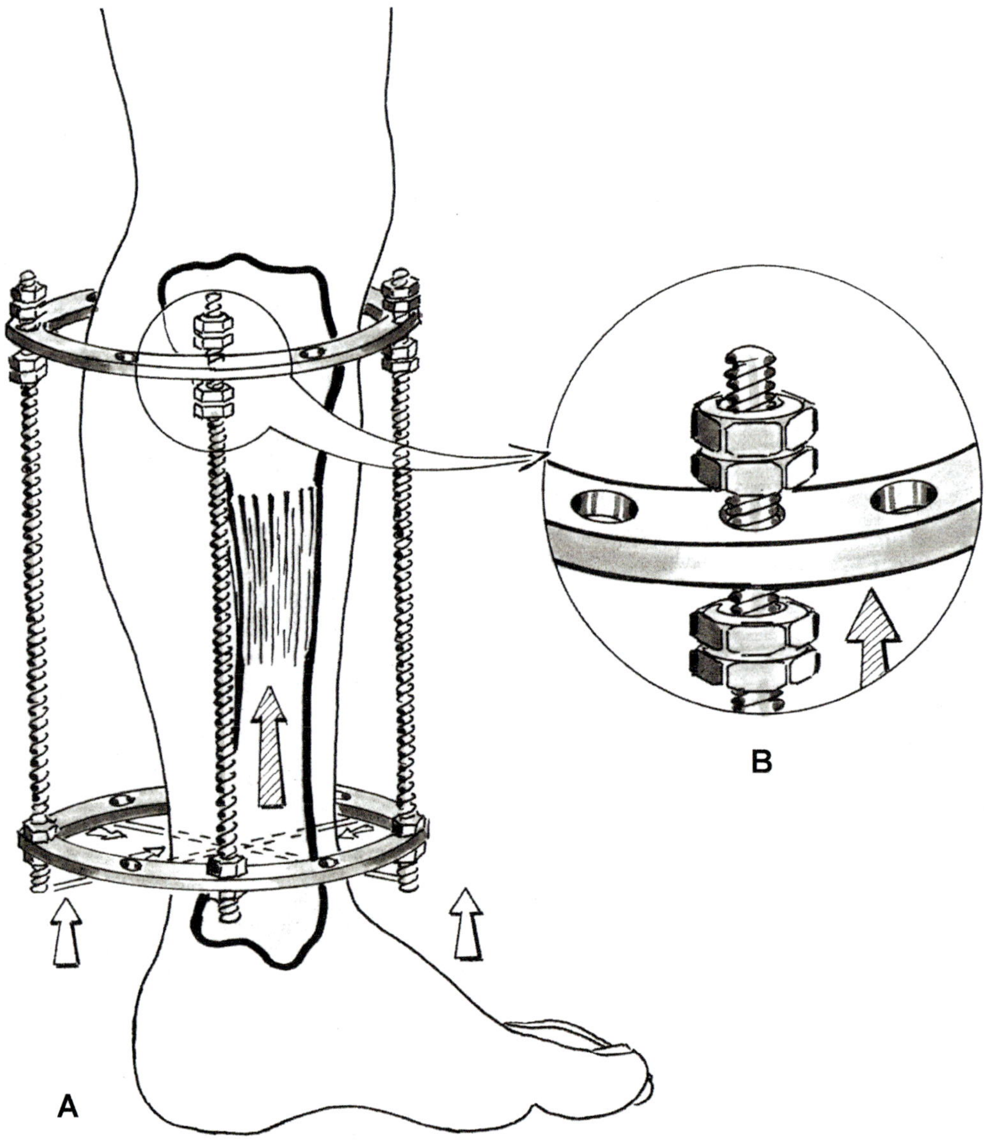

Figure 17.1: Dynamization of the fixator at completion of Ilizarov treatment. A two-ring frame with loose nuts on the proximal ring is shown. A, distraction forces are released by loosening the nuts. *Arrows* indicate direction of frame dynamization. Full weight-bearing is now directed onto the regenerate. At the same time, the rings with transfixed wires prevent axial displacement. B, enlarged view of the technique of loosening the nuts. Each nut above and below the ring wall is locked by the second nut, leaving 4 to 5 mm of space between the nut and the ring surface

TECHNIQUE OF ILIZAROV FIXATOR REMOVAL

This procedure may be performed while the patient is under general anesthesia in the operating room or with local anesthesia in the clinic or surgeon's office. The decision depends on several factors:

1. Size and complexity of the frame (large and complex frames must be removed in the operating room).
2. Presence or absence of complete regenerate development or bone healing. If there is any doubt about regenerate or healing quality, the fixator must be removed in the operating room.
3. Presence or absence of infection. When there is infection, the fixator must be removed in the operating room, with subsequent debridement.
4. Presence of half-pins in the frame dictates fixator removal in the operating room.
5. Evaluation of the patient's psychologic condition. The patient's ability to withstand some pain is necessary. In children and psychologically fragile patients the fixator must be removed in the operating room.

The following is a list of the four most important factors in the Ilizarov fixator removal technique.

1. The tension of all wires must be released before they are cut. Because the wires are under tension of more than 100 kg, cutting them produces extreme pain, which the patient can feel even under sedation and superficial anesthesia. Moreover, when the wire is cut while still under tension microinjury and even stress fracture in the regenerate may be provoked.
2. All olive wires (or the other wires with stoppers) must be removed by extraction toward the stopper. Sometimes this requires the application of considerable strength. There also may be a blood vessel near the stopper, which will cause some bleeding to occur. This requires that the surgeon apply pressure with the finger for several minutes.
3. Extraction of the wires with large pliers must be done strictly in the direction of the wire position and orientation in the bone.
4. Removal of the half-pins requires careful turning of the T-shaped hand drill because of their tendency to break in the bone. Because these pins are under tension for a long time, metal fatigue and microfailure can develop, causing the pins to break when turned.

After the wires are cut near the rings and the half-pins are screwed out, the rings must be separated by removing the connectors and taken off one by one. Clinical evaluation of the regenerate must be done at this time. Careful checking with both hands determines strong or weak healing.

Radiographic evaluation of healing in the operating room with anteroposterior and lateral films absolutely is necessary. Only after such evaluation can the decision to apply or not apply a cast be made. In certain cases, with regenerate bone of questionable strength, the two wires above and below the regenerate must be left in and incorporated into the cast (Fig. 17.2). This helps prevent collapse of the regenerate until it is mature enough to withstand axial loading.

After fixator removal the patient must be seen by the surgeon in 1 to 2 months and a new radiographic control evaluation of the regenerate performed. The full calcification of regenerate bone can be expected 6 months to 1 year after fixator removal. This depends largely on the functional loading of the healed bone.

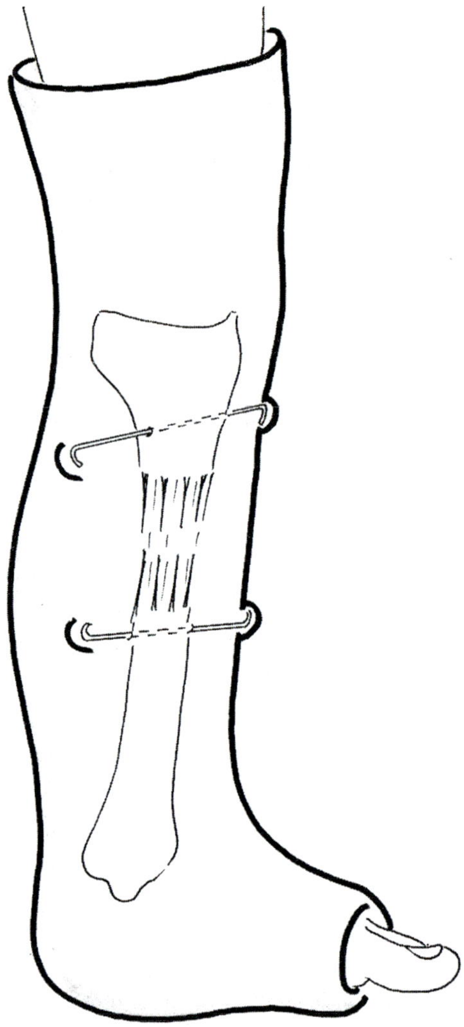

Figure 17.2: Technique of incorporating the wires into the cast after Ilizarov fixator removal. Ends of the wire must be bent and embedded in the cast wall

COMPLICATIONS

Many complications may arise during the long course of treatment with the Ilizarov technique. **Most, however, are preventable or correctable and will not interfere with successful results of treatment.**

Complications of the Ilizarov technique can be classified as: (1) general, due to the method; (2) specific, related to technique; and (3) inflammatory (Table 17.1).

Complications due to method or technique are related to application of the apparatus and may become apparent soon after the procedure is performed; however, some may not develop until after the patient has been discharged from the hospital. Thus it is important to see the patient in the office or clinic soon after discharge. For the first 3 to 4 weeks after discharge the patient should be seen at least once a week, so that any early complications can be corrected as soon as possible.

Correction of some complications may necessitate that the patient be readmitted to the hospital because procedures must be performed that may require general anesthesia. Two common complications due to distraction are posterior subluxation of the tibia (Fig. 17.3) and foot equinus (Fig. 17.4).

Table 17.1: Complications of Ilizarov technique

Complication	*Likely cause*
General complications, related to method	
1. Immediate	
a. Neurologic compromise	Wire transfixion
b. Vessel penetration	Wire transfixion
c. Comminuted fracture of osteotomized bone	Corticotomy, at moment of osteotome twist
d. Displacement of osteotomized fragment	Corticotomy, at moment of cracking of posterior cortex
2. Delayed	
a. Pain	Neurologic reaction to wire impingement and/or distraction
b. Compartment syndrome	Hematoma from vessel penetration by wire and/or comminuted fracture at corticotomy site
c. Muscle contracture	Imbalance of flexor-extensor muscle strength; inadequate physical activity
d. Neurologic compromise	Secondary to distraction
e. Local edema	Lymphostasis and/or hematoma secondary to distraction
f. Hypertension	Increased blood circulation secondary to tissue regeneration
g. Joint subluxation (Figs 17.3 and 17.4)	Imbalance of muscle tension secondary to distraction
Specific complications, related to technique	
1. Early complications	
a. Local skin tightness	Negligent wire orientation
b. Local edema with compromise of circulation	Deflection of ring(s) due to improper wire positioning
c. Premature healing at corticotomy/osteotomy site	Incomplete corticotomy/osteotomy (of fibula; delay in start of distraction; failure to create an initial gap at osteotomy site; failure to fix osteotomized fibula to both ends of tibia)
d. Local pain with motion	Wire penetration of muscle or tendon at site of active motion
2. Delayed complications	
a. Break in wire(s)	Initial tension too strong
b. Axial deviation of distracted fragment	Unstable frame and/or improper use of olive wires
c. Joint stiffness	Imperfect frame assembly and/or inadequate physical therapy
d. Partial development of regenerate (not across full diameter of bone)	Compromise of bone marrow and/or periosteal blood supply
e. Delayed development of regenerate	Improper rate and rhythm of distraction; inadequate physical therapy
3. Late iatrogenic complications	
a. Development of pseudoarthrosis	Improper use of compression-distraction forces; insufficient evaluation of all components of treatment
b. Angulation of regenerate	Premature removal of apparatus and/or inadequate casting/bracing
c. Fracture of regenerate	Failure to secure proper conditions for prevention of fracture
d. Psychologic incompatibility	Failure to evaluate patient's ability to tolerate pain, duration of treatment, care of apparatus; inadequate support services
Inflammatory complications	
1. These complications can arise at any time in the course of treatment, and include pin tract infection, phlebitis, osteomyelitis	Inadequate care of treatment site, history of previous infection

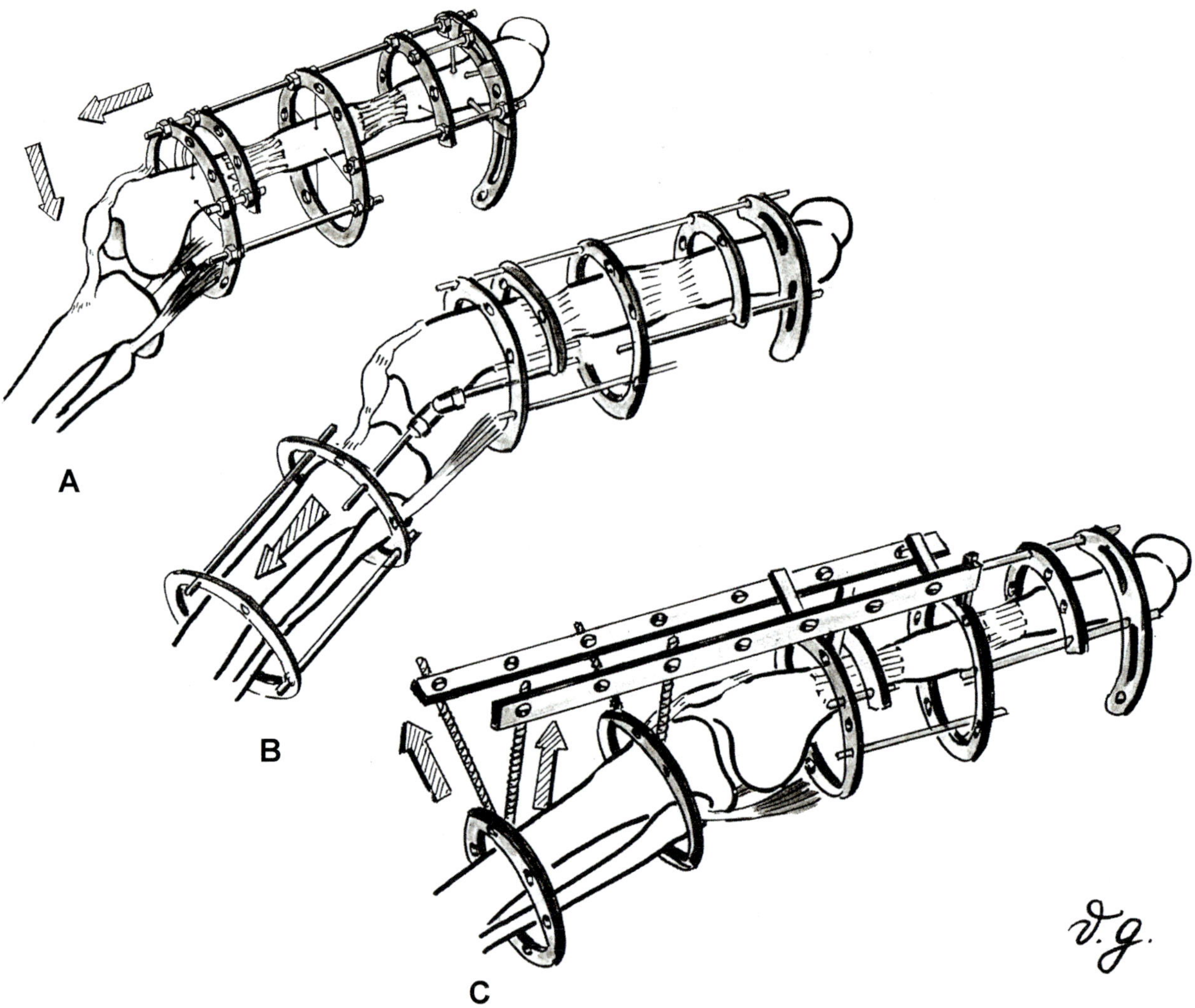

Figure 17.3: Posterior subluxation of the tibia resulting from femoral lengthening, and its correction. *Arrows* indicate direction of pulling-distraction. A, with a bifocal corticotomy and significant bone lengthening, the hamstring muscles are unable to accommodate, and their tendons become overtensioned. This may lead to gradual posterior tibial subluxation. B, two-ring frame is applied to the leg, and distraction at the knee level is produced. C, with the knee distracted, the corrective pulling device is adjusted to both frames, and subluxation is corrected

The possibility of complications must be explained fully to the patient before treatment is begun. This is especially important because the patients (or their parents or other relative) actively participate in the process of treatment. They take care of the skin, change dressings near the pins, and perform daily distraction by turning the nuts or graduated rod cylinders of the apparatus. In the course of doing this, patients can cause or prevent some complications.

One of the remarkable features of the Ilizarov technique is that correction of some kind almost always can prove efficacious. Even inflammatory complications, which develop toward the end of treatment, can be corrected with adjustment of the apparatus and additional procedures. Development of hypoplastic regenerate or pseudoarthrosis may necessitate other plasty procedures (e.g. bone grafting, plate placing, intramedullary rod introduction).

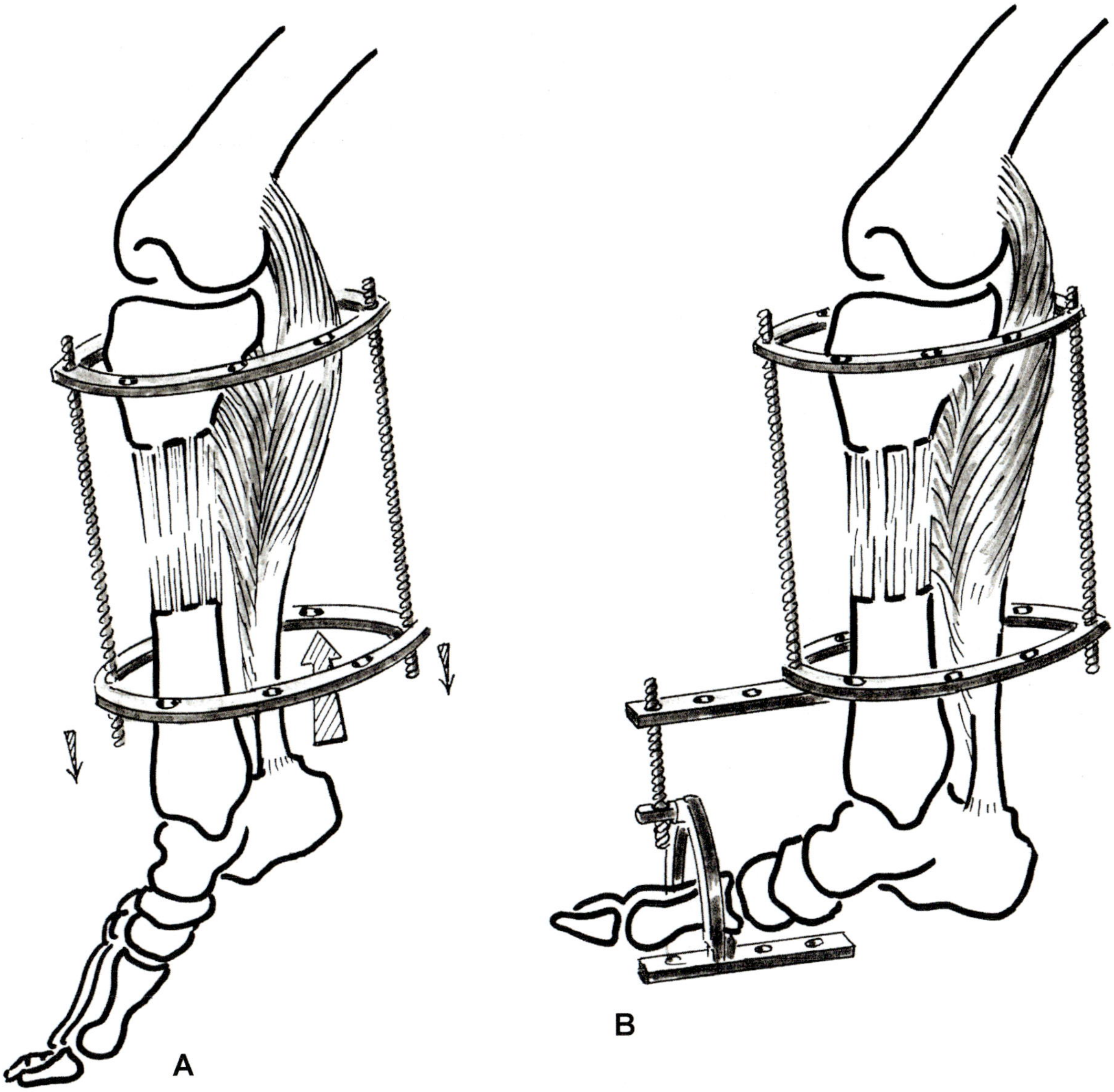

Figure 17.4: Foot equinus, and technique for its correction. *Arrows* indicate direction of pulling-distraction. A, with tibial lengthening greater than 4 cm, the posterior leg muscles became overtensioned, leading to gradual development of equinus. B, foot frame is adjusted, and gradual correction of equinus is effected

Successful correction of difficult skeletal problems by the Ilizarov technique does not depend necessarily on the number and severity of complications. Quick recognition and full immediate correction of these complications can assure the desired results of treatment.

PART FOUR

The New Development of the Method

18 Chapter

The New Modifications of the Ilizarov Technique

The apparent simplicity and clarity of the Ilizarov technique provoked many orthopedic surgeons around the World to offer their own modifications, as it always happened to the great inventions. Some of the new modifications are based on advanced technology of new materials for fixator parts, there are introductions of aluminum rings, and carbon rings, and titanium rods.

Because the whole frame, and the rings in particular, have to bear tremendous load up to 300 kg or more for a long period of time, the best material to sustain it remain stainless steel. Some modifications consist of small technical innovations. All these modifications are governed by the principles discovered and technique developed by Dr. Ilizarov.

The most essential innovation of the Ilizarov treatment is an addition of the computer programming to the calculation of bone deformity correction. The computer assisting control helps the doctors and the patients to produce precalculated bone reduction, correction, compression and lengthening. Several special software programs including Internet based programs are available.

At the present time several modifications are in use in different countries, which produce essentially the same kind of treatment as it is done by the original Ilizarov frame.

The most popular of the Ilizarov modifications is so called "Taylor Spatial Frame" (TSF), produced by Smith and Nephew Co, Memphis, TN, USA.[1] In 1996, Dr. Taylor unveiled his three dimensional "Spatial Frame". This frame shares a number of components and features of the Ilizarov frame. The biomechanics of TSF is based on the use of the Stewart platform (1965) hexapod (six "legs") principles of the French engineer Moniot, who described it in 1986 in a patent claim. The TSF circular external fixator consists of two aluminum rings connected by six telescopic linkage rods called "struts". The full rings and partial rings are of several diameters and have a flat surface with multiple holes. The shape of the rings are different from the Ilizarov's rings by six outer protuberances, and each of them has three additional holes (Fig. 18.1). Two rings are connected to each other by six telescopic struts. Each strut has the virtual hinges at the both ends. These hinges are the universal joints free to rotate, and any combination of six struts length can be a valid for a treatment frame. Each strut has the + or – signs and an arrow showing direction for finger turning (Fig. 18.2).

The Ilizarov system utilizes hinge and translation mechanisms specifically oriented for a given clinical case. By the Dr. Taylor suggestion, with the introduction of the

[1]The Smith and Nephew Co. advertises the Taylor's frame as "the revolutionary yet simple solution for trauma and deformity correction".

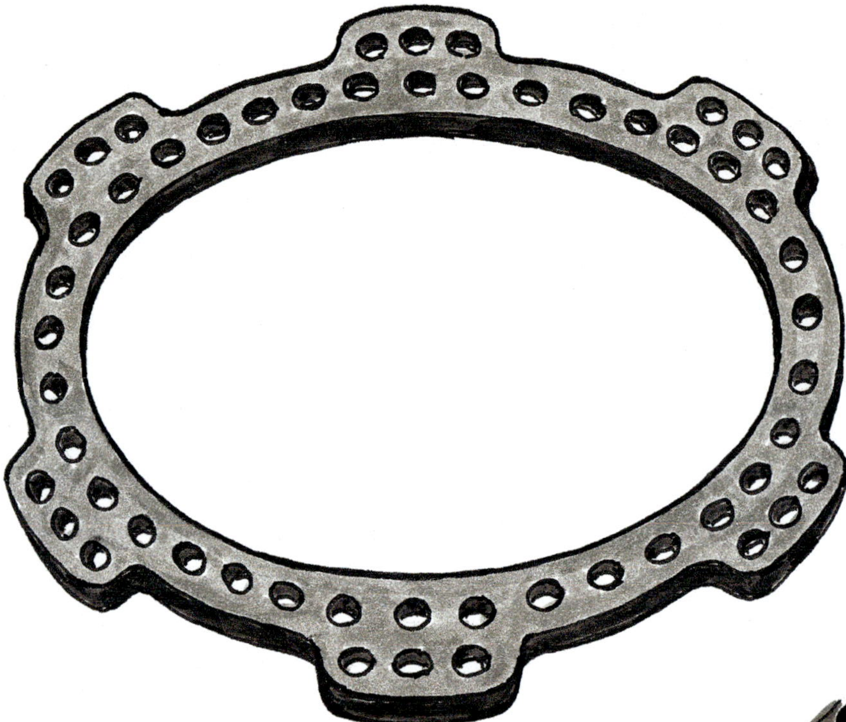

Figure 18.1: The Taylor system full ring. It is made of aluminum and is different from the Ilizarov's ring by the six protruding outside ledges, with three holes each, for the connection with the struts

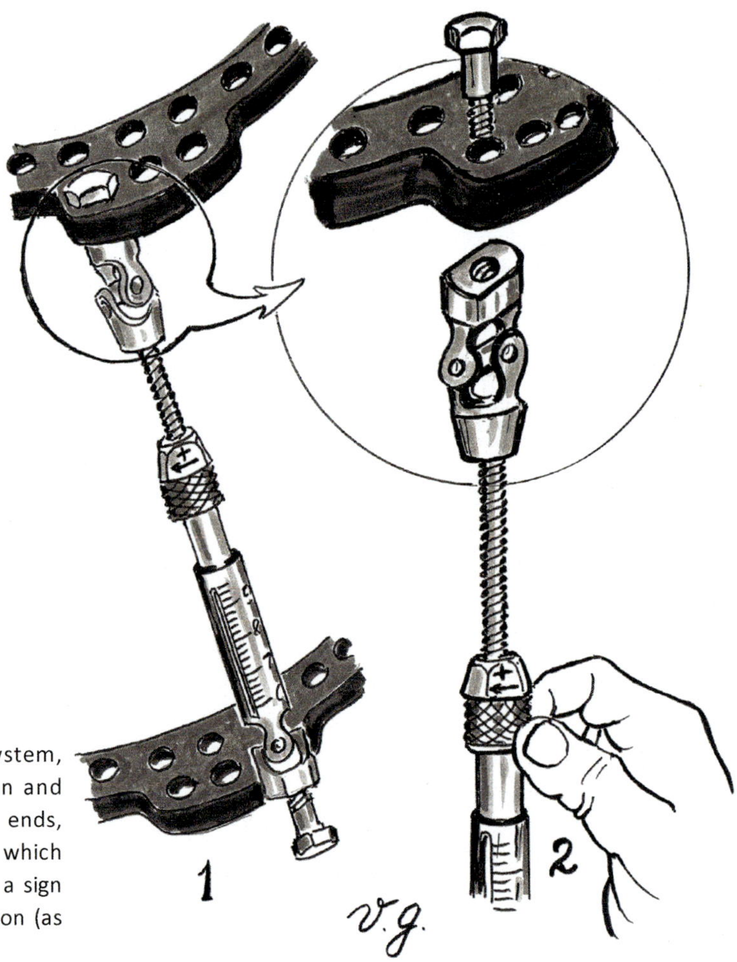

Figure 18.2: Two connecting struts of the Taylor system, struts length is valid for the ring position angulation and inclination. (1) The strut with two hinges at the both ends, connected to one ring. (2) Enlarged view of the hinge which is a virtual universal joint free to rotate, each strut has a sign + or – with an arrow indicator of the movement direction (as shown)

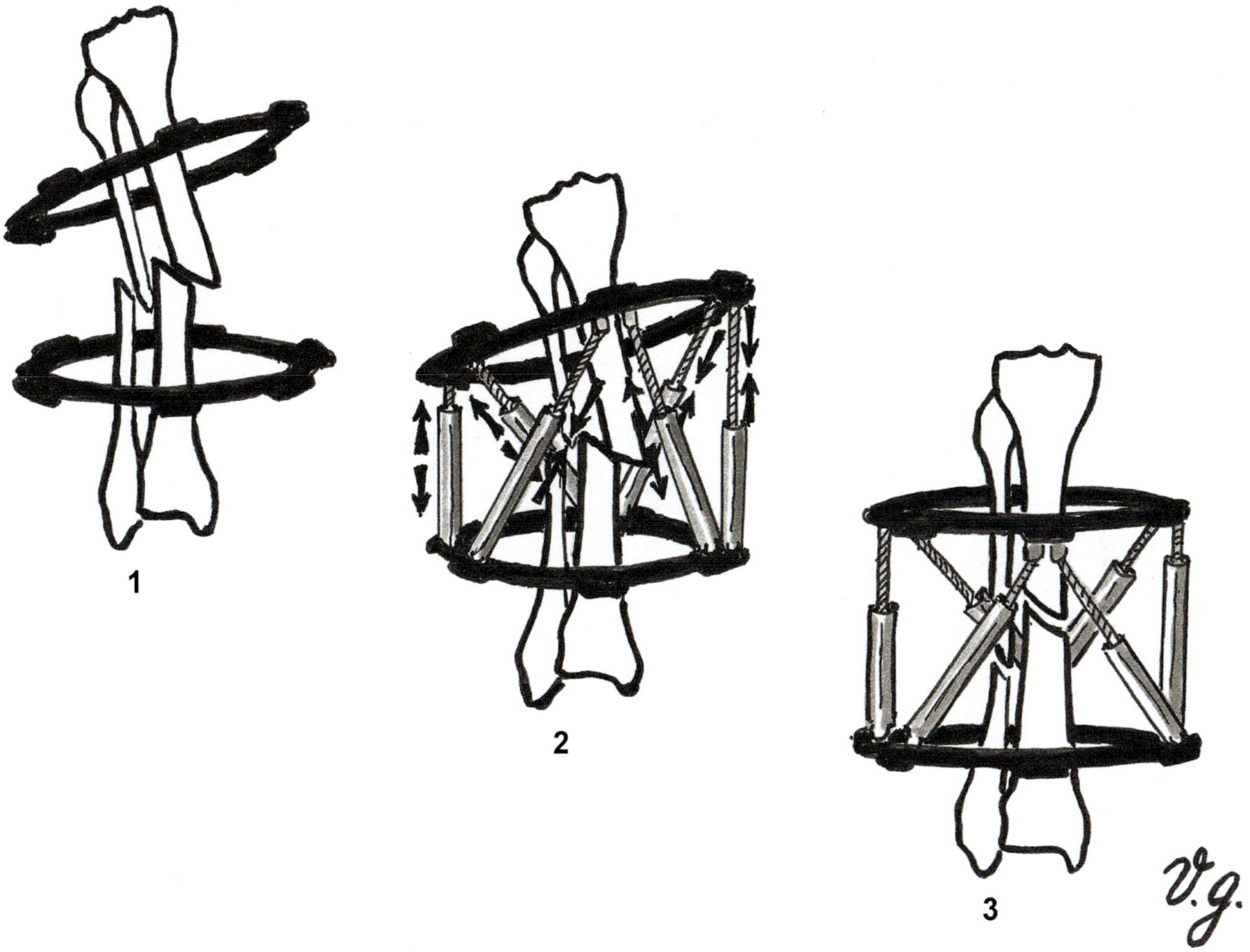

Figure 18.3: Schematic representation of the Rings First Method of Deformity Correction of an acute tibia-fibular fracture. (1) Two rings are mounted orthogonaly to each bone fragment; as distinguished from the Ilizarov method, only one ring is transfixed to one fragment. Note that proximal and distal rings are positioned perpendicular to the long fragment's axis, as recommended by Ilizarov. (2) Six struts are attached between rings in the Spatial Frame configuration. Note that the struts are shorter at the outer side of a limb; the arrows near each strut indicate the direction for returning them to their neutral length to produce a necessary correction. Neutral strut length is determined by measuring the distance from a ring to the interior end for each fragment. The neutral strut length can be determined with the software. (3) The struts are returned to their neutral length. Note that rings inclination is changed, and with this position the bone fragments are reduced. At this stage there is a need for the compression for the fracture healing

virtual free hinges the correction of deformity can be achieved just by adjusting length of struts in any type of deformity (Fig. 18.3).

Two rings are fixed to the bone fragments by the half pins and K-wires exactly on a manner of the Ilizarov ring connection[2] (Fig. 18.4). Bone fragments attached to the rings can be moved through simultaneously.

Six deformity parameters needed to fully define a clinical deformity correction of variety of displacements (anteroposterior, varus/valgus, lengthen/shorten).

[2]Unlike Ilizarov principles Dr. Taylor suggest constant use of the half-pins.

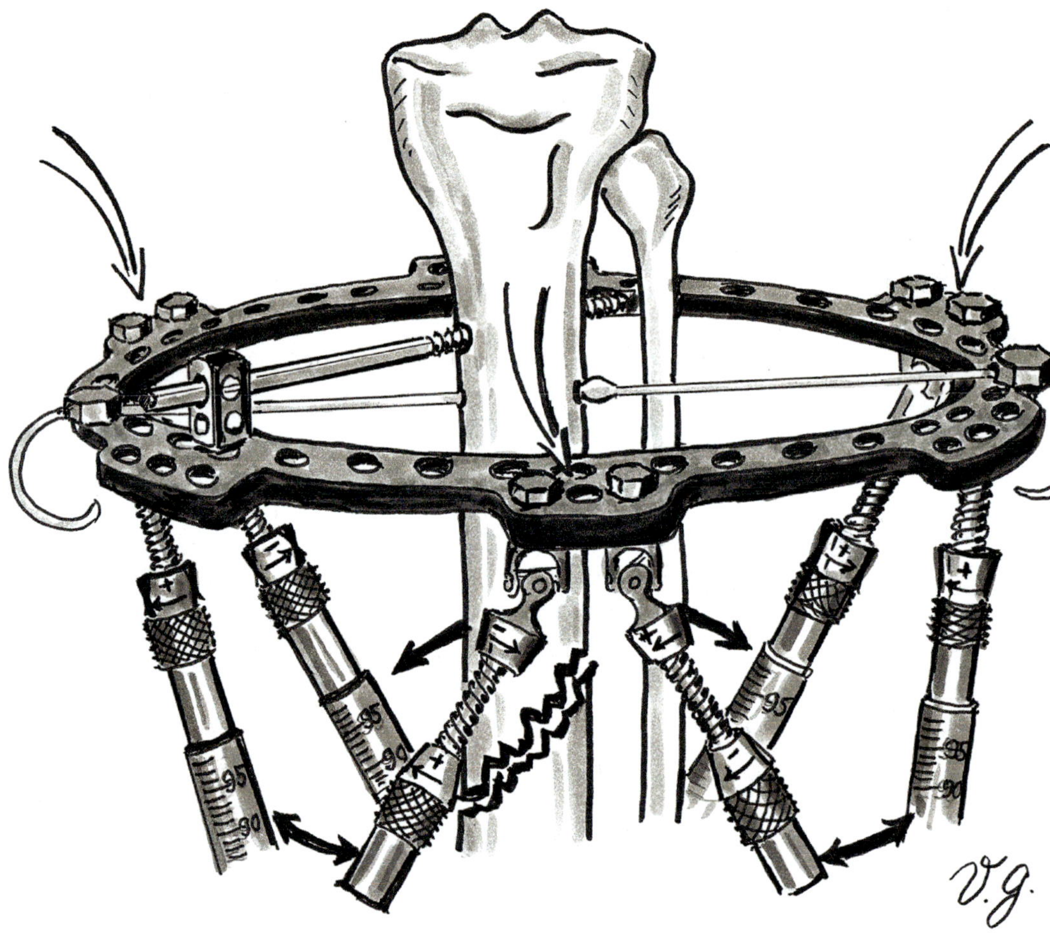

Figure 18.4: The representation of a Taylor Spatial Frame fixation to the fractured tibia. Partial view, the proximal part of frame with a supporting ring is shown. The ring transfixed to the bone by a half-pin and K-wire with a stopper. The half-pin provides for stiffness but at the same time deprives of the elasticity which generates more rapid callus formation and maturation. The white arrows point to the three protruding outside ledges of the ring to which the universal hinges are attached, the black arrows point to the pairs of the six struts which support the frame stability. Because the hinges are the virtual universal joint free to rotate the stability may not always be firm enough

Attached to the bone, the rings allow to correct bone deformity in variety of fractures, nonunions, and malunions. This is done by altering the length of the six struts. The relationship between the rings can be varied in three dimension space. According to Dr. Taylor the advantage of this innovation is that, unlike the Ilizarov frame, there is no need to modify his frame as the adjustments to the struts are made. Regardless of the complexity of the fracture or chronic bone deformity the same two rings of TSF fixator can be used.

Reduction of the acute fractures is produced manually or by the conventional Ilizarov technique and the struts are locked in position. In conjunction with a hand-held computer, analyzing the starting and ending position of the rings, is checked. This provides information about the necessary adjustments of the rings. Using this computer information a doctor can change the relative position of the rings and reduce the fragments displacement in all six axes by adjusting the length of the struts.

For the treatment of nonunions, malunions, and for lengthening and shortening a bone, the TSF could be assembled prior to mounting exactly mimic existing deformities. This is done as it is recommended with the Ilizarov method. The two rings and connected telescopic struts are adjusted to a position matching the skeletal deformity, and then fixed to the bone as it also done with the Ilizarov technique.

One particular innovation of TSF is that the skeletal deformity can be corrected in conjunction with a computer software program. The TSF is a true computer-assisted product, driven by the powerful operative planning software. In other words, the computer gives suggestion how to correct deformity after the "Spatial Frame" application, and a doctor just follows this suggestion and translates it to a patient.

Based on anterior-posterior and lateral X-ray films, physician measures the six deformity parameters and the four mounting parameters. These parameters are input to a Total-Residual Deformity Correction Program (TDCP). They enter into specialized software along with parameters of ring size and initial strut lengths. The Internet-based software that goes with this system creates a specific day-by-day "prescription" for strut length changes and correction of deformity. The returns of 6 struts length adjust the frame to exactly mirror the deformity and it will be fully corrected when the struts moved to their specified length in neutral position. The patient is given exact printed instruction for the daily schedule of correction corresponding to software program. This instruction shows in details what direction and with which rhythm and speed the patient has to move the struts.

Usually it is given to the patient as a printed list with the indications for turning particular strut by the following parameters: medial translation, lateral translation, anterior translation, posterior translation, varus translation, valgus translation, apex anterior, apex posterior, internal rotation, external rotation and the parameters of lengthening for each particular strut.

Under periodical control of a doctor and in conjunction with this program, the distraction or compression is produced by the patient himself in a manner it is done with the original Ilizarov frame.

The undesirable effect of universal joints is that they have some tuft and not always produce sufficient stability. Because of this the two rings of TSF frame do not always stable enough. This is especially evident with a complex deformity of a big limb. To support stable position in some cases the frame needs a placement of additional struts or has to be used in combination with the original Ilizarov frame (Fig. 18.5).

The Canadian research group of doctors[3] proposed a technique to apply the inverse kinematics of the Taylor Spatial Frame to calculate the initial position of the frame and fixation pins, the strut length, and the daily schedule of correction. The group claims that by using TSF it improved accuracy of the method by giving a surgeon greater flexibility in frame placement. It is done by removing the need to measure the 13 frame parameters preoperatively and by calculating the correction based on 3D coordinates. The group recommends to do this on the basis of CT data rather than by the measurement from radiographs. This and many other deviations of the Taylor recommendation prove variability of original Ilizarov method.

Another modification of Ilizarov circular fixator in the market is a device named "Smart Correction". It is a hexapod based frame essentially similar to TSF but with carbon fiber rings and with the titanium struts which makes the frame MRI compatible. The rings have variable strut's holes. As the TSF it is used in connection with software which produces direction to the strut length changes in order to correct the bone deformity.

The same year of 1996, at which the TSF was developed in America, the German company "LITOS" has developed the "Ilizarov Hexapod System". According to the detriments, this system can be applied with Ilizarov and other fixator systems, it

[3]From the School of Computing, Queen's University, Kingston, Ontario, Canada.

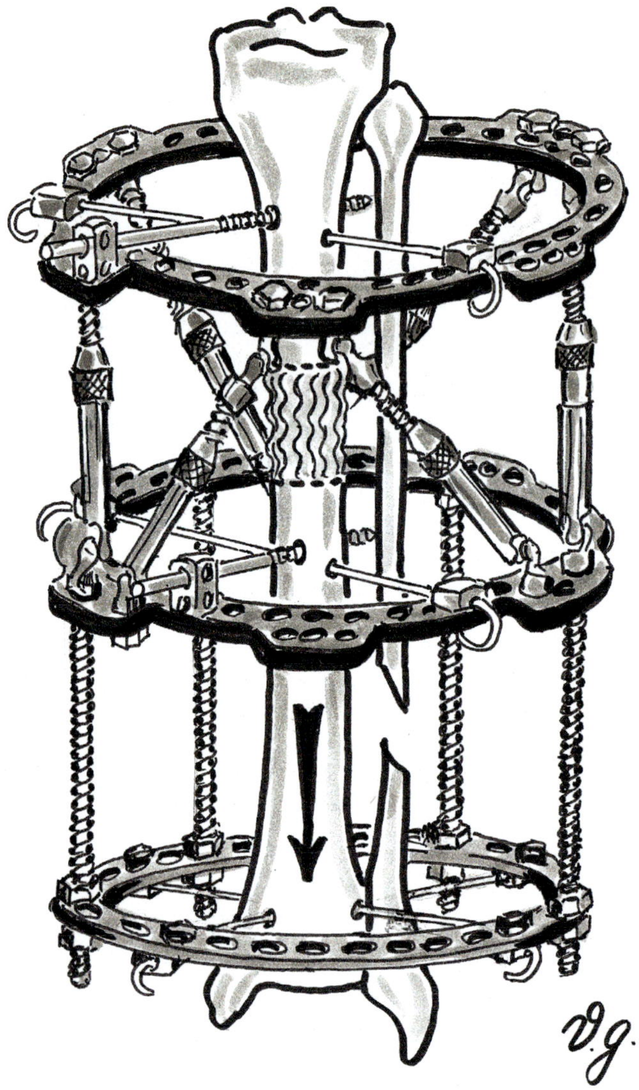

Figure 18.5: Schematic representation of a combination of the Taylor-Ilizarov frame. The bone lengthening is done by the Taylor Spatial Frame with six struts. The arrow shows a direction of distraction for lengthening, the wavy vertical lines show new bone formation at the site of corticotomy, which is marked by the interrupted line. This drawing shows that two Taylor rings with the virtual hinges free to rotate may not provide enough stability for such a long treatment needed for lengthening and that way are supported by the addition of the Ilizarov ring distally

provides a universal and precise 3-demensional bone movement; the path of reduction/correction can be easily modified.

It is based completely on the original Ilizarov frame and designed in such a way that can be combined with other parts. The fixation of the rings is provided by the tensioned K-wires.

The main difference is that the rings are connected by six special distractors of different length (105 to 235 mm). At the both ends of a distractor there are spherical hinges. These hinges are attached to the Ilizarov ring by a special Y-Adapter (Fig. 18.6), and provide free motion of the distractor as it is with the universal joints of the Taylor struts.

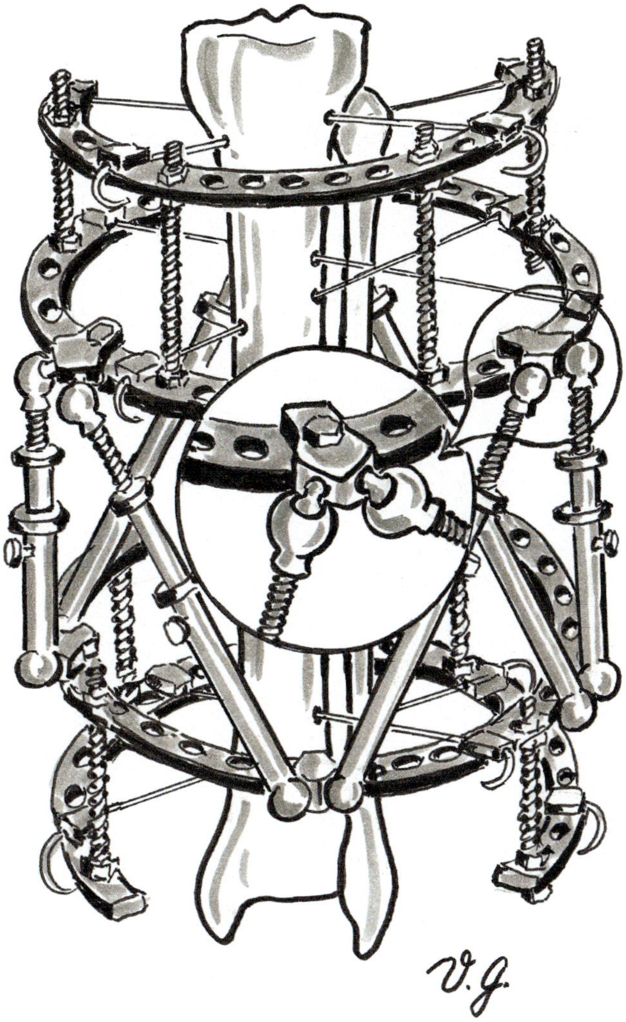

Figure 18.6: The Ilizarov Hexapod System of a German company "Litos" mounted on the tibia. This is an essentially four-ring Ilizarov frame utilizing the rings fixation by the K-wires. The rings are connected by the Ilizarov rods. Just the two main rings providing correction, reduction, compression and distraction of the bone fragments are connected to each other by the six distractors with the spherical hinges at the both ends. These hinges are attached to the rings. An enlarged section shows the part of ring with the attached Y-shaped adapter and spherical hinges. This type of connection provides free rotation of distractors. Stability of the frame is secured by the combined support of four rings

As a new development the Litos/hexapod Co. produce the technology of two more systems – "Poli Hes" and "Easy hex". Software provides adjustment parameters for both systems.

The "Poli hex" system is compatible with other fixator systems and is based on combination of a standard unilateral fixator with the Ilizarov frame which is directed by the hexapod distractors. This is a very complicated system of bone deformity correction, which could surprise the late Dr. Ilizarov. It requires three stages surgery:

1. At first the application of a unilateral fixator with a fixation by half-pins is done; no correction of deformity is performed at this stage.
2. Then the application of Ilizarov frame follows as an addition to the unilateral frame; with the combination

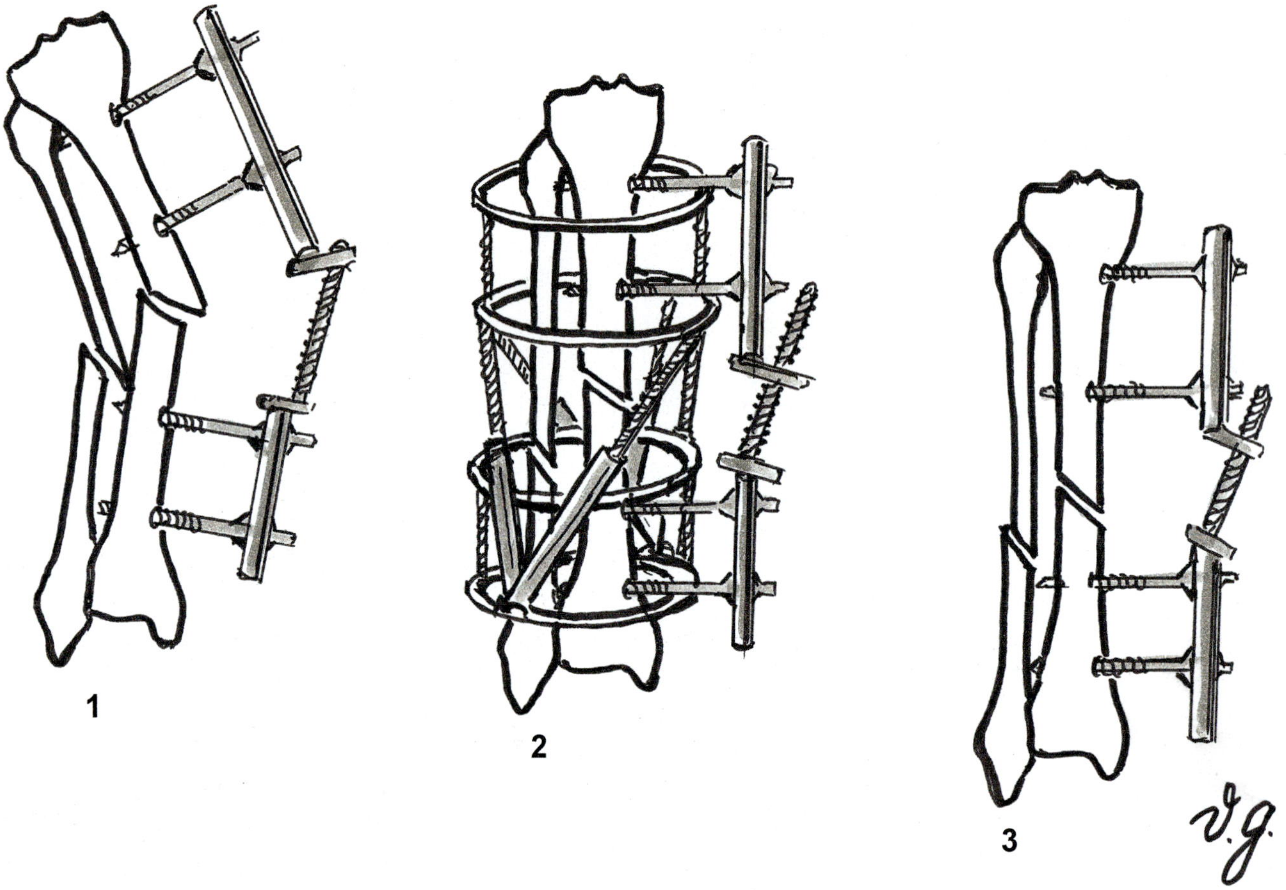

Figure 18.7: Schematic representation of the three stage reduction and treatment of tibia-fibular fracture by the "Poli hex" system. (1) The application of a unilateral fixator before the correction of angular deformity. (2) Additional application of the four ring Ilizarov frame with gradual reduction by the distractors with spherical hinges. The unilateral fixator is locked in the achieved position. (3) The Ilizarov frame is removed and the treatment continues with the unilateral fixator

of two frames attached to the bone the gradual correction of deformity is performed by the Ilizarov.

3. After deformity reduction the Ilizarov is dismantled but the unilateral fixator is remounted for continuation of treatment until the complete bone healing (Fig. 18.7).

The "Easy hex" system is used primarily for rapid bone displacement reduction. The frame consists of two open tubular rings with holders for the Schanz screws. The hexapod distractors are attached directly to the tubular rings. This provides stable, quick and easy assembly and successful reduction by the fixation with half-pins (Fig. 18.8)

The computer assisting control allows continuous reduction with the bone fragments movement along a path and available with both systems for determining the adjustment parts of the hexapod robot.

One more modification of the Ilizarov frame is so called "TRUE/LOK" system – the lightweight metal/plastic flexible ring fixator, developed at Texas Scottish Rite Hospital for Children (USA). It is designed as a preassembled functional block. It has some insignificant innovations like telescopic Linear and Angular Distractors if compared to the original Ilizarov frame, and is used for reduction of fractures, correction of deformities, and bone lengthening. The "True/Lok"

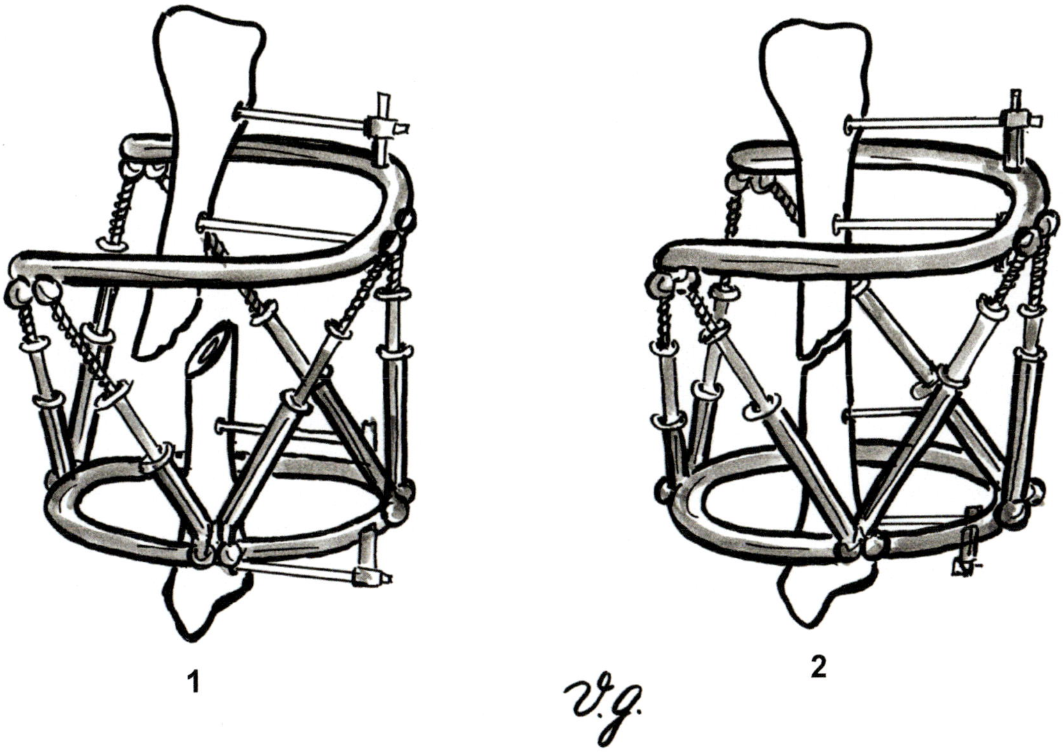

Figure 18.8: Schematic representation of the rapid reduction of tibia displacement by the "Easy hex" system. (1) The special frame consisting of one open and one full tubular rings is attached to the fragments by the four Schanz screws. This provides stability of the fragments. (2) The six hexapod distractors are attached to the tubular rings by the spherical hinges with subsequent reduction of the fragments

system is also successfully used for the foot and ankle deformities corrections.

Based on the manual hexapod fixator an "intelligent" system of robotic movement has been developed in the Institute for Micro System Technology in Hamburg, Germany. It is a bone mounted robot system for fracture control. A motorized external fixator was accomplished by implementation of motors, gears and position sensors. It mounted microcontroller system allows for autonomous adjustment of the fixator according to the planned six degree of freedom movements of the fracture fragments. According to the inventors and doctors, the "intelligent" external fixator optimizes bone healing and increases patient safety and comfort by increasing precision and frequency of the bone movements and preventing maloperation by computer-aided planning and autonomous movements.

One has to remember that in 1978 Dr. Ilizarov also developed an electromechanical autodistractor, programmed to produce a 1 mm revolution per day. The batteries for the motor were provided on the patients's belt. The device was a nonstop motor connected to the telescopic rod. Four autodistractors were attached to four telescopic rods. The device worked well but at that time there were no microbatteries and no computer programming. The autodistractor made the fixator frame heavier and more expensive, and didn't become popular.

THE CONCLUSION

The Ilizarov technique of bone fractures and deformities treatment by a circular fixator with multiplanar transfixation is a truly great innovation in the orthopedic surgery which revolutionized the fracture, bone deformities, nonunion and other bone pathology treatment. In this book we showed how to assemble and apply the Ilizarov circular fixator. The book is different from others on this subject by the detailed drawings and explanations. We presented general principles of the technique for the treatment of different types of bone fractures and deformities, and illustrated them with our clinical cases. We also found necessary to present to the reader a short biography of Dr. Ilizarov.

Working in isolation in a small Siberian Town of Russia, in 1950-70s, under very poor and primitive conditions, he was able to develop a new type of the external fixator. Working with this fixator he discovered the new biological law of tissue growth and developed the Tension Stress Concept for its control. In fact, he was the first to develop a doctrine of tissue generation under the influence of bone distraction. This way Dr. Ilizarov opened the new chapter in the whole discipline of orthopedic surgery.

The techniques developed by him were the first methods of minimal invasive surgery for the bone treatment. They now became popular around the world and thousands of orthopedic surgeons successfully use them in their practice. These techniques have almost unlimited potentialities for a great advances and improvements. There are several new modifications of the Ilizarov fixator which are included in this last chapter of the book. These modifications reflect further development of the Ilizarov achievements, based on new interpretations of his principles.

It is difficult to imagine how the Ilizarov external fixator will look in 20 or 30 years but one can foresee that any further developments and improvements will be based on the Dr. Ilizarov great discoveries.

Selected Bibliography

1. Bianchi Maiocci A, Aronson J (Eds). Operative Principles of Ilizarov Fracture Treatment, Non-union Osteomyelitis, Lengthening, Deformity Correction. Baltimore, Williams and Wilkins, 1991.
2. Cattaneo R. Ilizarov from Kurgan ti Lecco and to the world. European Orthopaedic Bulletin of EFFORT, 1997;Issue 6:10-1.
3. Edelman M, Bialik V, Katzman A. Correction of deformities in children using the Taylor. Orthop B 2006;15(6): 387-95.
4. Edelman M, Bialik A, Katzman A. The use of the Taylor spatial frame in adolescent Blount's disease: is fibular osteotomy necessary? J Child Orthop 2008;@(3):199-204.
5. Fauro C, Merloz P. Transfixation. Atlas of Anatomical Sections for the External Fixation of Limbs. New York, Springer-Verlag, 1989.
6. Feldman DS, Shin S, Madan S, Koval KJ. Correction of tibial malunion and nonunion with six-axis analysis deformity correction using the Taylor Spatial Frame. J of Prthop Trauma 2003;17:549-54.
7. Frankel VH, Gold S, Golyakhovsky V. The Ilizarov technique. Bulletin of the Hospital for Joint Diseases Orthopaedic Institute 1988; 48:17.
8. Golyakhovsky V, Gavriel A Ilizarov. "The magician from Kurgan"; Bulletin of the Hospital for Joint Diseases Orthopaedic Institute 1988;48:12.
9. Golyakhovsky V, Gavriel A Ilizarov. "The magician from Kurgan", 1988; Bulletin (Hospital for Joint Diseases), 1997;56:54.
10. Golyakhovsky V, Frankel VH. Ilizarov bone transport in large bone loss and severe osteamyelitis. Bulletin of the Hospital for Joint Dieases Orthopaedic Institute, 1991;51(1):63-73.
11. Green SA. Complications of External Skeletal Fixation. Springfield, Ill, Charles C. Thomas, 1981.
12. Green SA (Ed). Basic Ilizarov techniques. Tech Orthop 1990;5:4.
13. Green S. Taylor Spatial Frame Disorients Ilizarovians. Distraction, The Newsletter of ASAMI – North America, 1997;5(1).
14. Ilizarov GA. Transosseous Osteossynthesis; Theoretical and Clinical Aspects of the Regeneration and Growth of Tissues; New York, Springer-Verlag, 1991.
15. Ilizarov GA. The tension-stress effect on the genesis and growth of tissues; 1: The influence of stability of fixation and soft-tissue preservation. Clin Orthop 1989;238:249-80.
16. Ilizarov GA. The tension-stress effect on the genesis and growth of tissues; II: The influence of rate and frequency of distraction. Clin Orthop 1990;239:263-84.
17. Lehman W (Ed). Operating Room Guide of Cross Sectional Anatomy of Extremities and Pelvis. New York, 1989.
18. Lyun DP, Borschneck, Ellis RE. Computer-assisted correction of bone deformities using a 6-DOF parallel spatial mechanism. In: Niessen W, Viergever M (Eds): Medical Images, Computing and Computer Assisted Intrevention (MICCAI), Springer-Verlag, (Berlin), 2001;232-340.
19. Paley D. Current techniques of limb lengthening. J Pediatr Orthop 1988;8:73-92.
20. Paley D. Principles of Deformity Treatment; Germany, Springer-Verlag, 2002.
21. Stewart D. A platform with six degrees of freedom; Proceedings of the Institute for Mechanical Engineers, 1965;180:371-86.
22. Taylor JC. Correction of general deformity with Taylor spatial fixator. J Carles Tylor, http/www. Jcharlestaylor.com/spat/00spat/.html. Accessed April 2008.
23. Taylor JC, Paley D. Six axis deformity analysis and correction; Springer-Verlag, New York, 2002.
24. Wendland R, Wackenhut F, Seide R, Muller J. Bone mounted hexapod robot for outpatient distraction osteogenesis. In Pringer Berlin Heidelberg, IFMBE Proceedings, 2009;22:1679-82.
25. Wuckich DK, Belczyk RJ. An introduction to the Taylor spatial frame for foot and ankle; Techniques in Orthopaedics, 2006;16(1): 2-9.

Index